CASEBOOK of
Neuropsychiatry

CASEBOOK of
Neuropsychiatry

Edited by

Trevor A. Hurwitz, M.B.Ch.B., M.R.C.P. (U.K.), F.R.C.P.C.

Warren T. Lee, M.D., Ph.D.

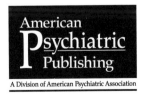

American
Psychiatric
Publishing

A Division of American Psychiatric Association

Washington, DC
London, England

If you would like to buy between 25 and 99 copies of this or any other American Psychiatric Publishing title, you are eligible for a 20% discount; please contact Customer Service at appi@psych.org or 800-368-5777. If you wish to buy 100 or more copies of the same title, please e-mail us at bulksales@psych.org for a price quote.

Copyright © 2013 American Psychiatric Association
ALL RIGHTS RESERVED

Manufactured in the United States of America on acid-free paper
17   16   15   14   13   5   4   3   2   1
First Edition

American Psychiatric Publishing
A Division of American Psychiatric Association
1000 Wilson Boulevard
Arlington, VA 22209-3901
www.appi.org

Library of Congress Cataloging-in-Publication Data
Casebook of neuropsychiatry / edited by Trevor A. Hurwitz, Warren T. Lee. — 1st ed.
    p. ; cm.
    Includes bibliographical references and index.
    ISBN 978-1-58562-431-7 (pbk. : alk. paper)
I. Hurwitz, Trevor A., 1950– II. Lee, Warren T., 1963– III. American Psychiatric Association.
[DNLM: 1. Mental Disorders—Case Reports. 2. Neurobehavioral Manifestations—Case Reports. 3. Neuropsychiatry—methods—Case Reports. WM 40]
RC346
616.8—dc23

2013005969

British Library Cataloguing in Publication Data
A CIP record is available from the British Library.

CONTENTS

Trevor A. Hurwitz, M.B.Ch.B., M.R.C.P. (U.K.), F.R.C.P.C.
Warren T. Lee, M.D., Ph.D.

Andrew K. Howard, M.D., F.R.C.P.C.

Paul Dagg, M.D., F.R.C.P.C.
Jennifer Klages, Ph.D., R.Psych.

Marie-Claire Baril, M.D., F.R.C.P.C.
Sandra J. Mish, Ph.D., R.Psych.

Jennifer Klages, Ph.D., R.Psych.
Paul Dagg, M.D., F.R.C.P.C.

Andrew K. Howard, M.D., F.R.C.P.C.

CONTRIBUTORS

Silke Appel-Cresswell, M.D.
Pacific Parkinson's Research Centre, Assistant Professor, Department of Medicine, Division of Neurology, University of British Columbia, Vancouver, British Columbia, Canada

Marie-Claire Baril, M.D., F.R.C.P.C.
British Columbia Neuropsychiatry Program; Clinical Assistant Professor, Department of Psychiatry, University of British Columbia, Vancouver, British Columbia, Canada; Psychiatrist, Interior Health Authority, Kamloops, British Columbia, Canada

Leon Berzen, M.B.B.Ch., F.F.Psych. (S.A.), F.R.C.P.C.
British Columbia Neuropsychiatry Program; Clinical Assistant Professor, Department of Psychiatry, University of British Columbia, UBC Hospital, Vancouver, British Columbia, Canada

Catherine Chiles, M.D., D.F.A.P.A., F.A.P.M.
Associate Professor of Psychiatry, Yale University School of Medicine, VA Connecticut Healthcare System, West Haven, Connecticut

Paul Dagg, M.D., F.R.C.P.C.
British Columbia Neuropsychiatry Program; Clinical Associate Professor, Department of Psychiatry, University of British Columbia, Vancouver, British Columbia, Canada; Medical Director, Tertiary Mental Health, Interior Health Authority, Kamloops, British Columbia, Canada

Marius Dimov, M.D., F.R.C.P.C.
British Columbia Neuropsychiatry Program; Clinical Instructor, Department of Psychiatry, University of British Columbia, UBC Hospital, Vancouver, British Columbia, Canada

Anthony Feinstein, M.B.B.Ch., M.Phil., Ph.D., F.R.C.P.C.
Professor, Department of Psychiatry, University of Toronto; Director, Neuropsychiatry Program, Sunnybrook Health Sciences Centre, Toronto, Ontario, Canada

Omar Ghaffar, M.Sc., M.D., F.R.C.P.C.
Sunnybrook Health Sciences Centre, Toronto, Ontario; Ontario Shores Centre for Mental Health Sciences, Whitby, Ontario; Department of Psychiatry, University of Toronto, Toronto, Ontario, Canada

Andrew K. Howard, M.D., F.R.C.P.C.
British Columbia Neuropsychiatry Program; Clinical Assistant Professor, Department of Psychiatry, University of British Columbia, Vancouver, British Columbia, Canada

Trevor A. Hurwitz, M.B.Ch.B., M.R.C.P. (U.K.), F.R.C.P.C.
Medical Director, British Columbia Neuropsychiatry Program; Clinical Professor, Department of Psychiatry, University of British Columbia, Vancouver, British Columbia, Canada

Magdalena Ilcewicz-Klimek, M.D., F.R.C.P.C.
British Columbia Neuropsychiatry Program; Clinical Instructor, Department of Psychiatry, University of British Columbia, UBC Hospital, Vancouver, British Columbia, Canada

Jennifer Klages, Ph.D., R.Psych.
Neuropsychologist, British Columbia Neuropsychiatry Program, Tertiary Mental Health, Interior Health Authority, Kamloops, British Columbia, Canada

Brenda Kosaka, Ph.D., R.Psych.
Neuropsychologist, British Columbia Neuropsychiatry Program; Clinical Assistant Professor, Department of Psychiatry, University of British Columbia, Vancouver, British Columbia, Canada

Warren T. Lee, M.D., Ph.D.
Associate Professor, Department of Psychiatry and Behavioral Science, Duke University Medical School, Durham, North Carolina

Aaron Mackie, M.D., F.R.C.P.C.
Clinical Lecturer, Faculty of Medicine, University of Calgary, Calgary, Alberta, Canada

Scott McCullagh, M.D., F.R.C.P.C.
Assistant Professor, Department of Psychiatry, Neuropsychiatry Program, Sunnybrook Health Sciences Centre, University of Toronto, Toronto, Ontario, Canada

Sandra J. Mish, Ph.D., R.Psych.
Neuropsychologist, British Columbia Neuropsychiatry Program, Tertiary Mental Health, Interior Health Authority, Kamloops, British Columbia, Canada

William J. Panenka, M.Sc., M.D., F.R.C.P.C.
British Columbia Neuropsychiatry Program, UBC Neuropsychiatry and Clinical Investigator Fellow, University of British Columbia, UBC Hospital, Vancouver, British Columbia, Canada

Robert M. Rohrbaugh, M.D.
Professor and Deputy Chair for Education and Career Development; Director of Medical Studies and Residency Program Director, Department of Psychiatry; Director, Office of International Medical Student Education, Yale University School of Medicine, New Haven, Connecticut

Anton Scamvougeras, M.B.Ch.B., F.R.C.P.C.
British Columbia Neuropsychiatry Program; Clinical Associate Professor, Department of Psychiatry, University of British Columbia, UBC Hospital, Vancouver, British Columbia, Canada

David Sherman, M.Sc., M.D.
Department of Psychiatry, University of British Columbia, Vancouver, British Columbia, Canada

Vinod H. Srihari, M.D.
Associate Professor, Department of Psychiatry, Yale University School of Medicine, New Haven, Connecticut

Robert Stowe, M.D., F.R.C.P.C.
British Columbia Neuropsychiatry Program; Clinical Associate Professor
of Psychiatry and Neurology (Medicine), University of British Columbia,
UBC Hospital, Vancouver, British Columbia, Canada

Joseph Tham, M.D., F.R.C.P.C.
British Columbia Neuropsychiatry Program; Clinical Assistant Professor,
Department of Psychiatry, University of British Columbia, Vancouver,
British Columbia, Canada

Pieter Joost van Wattum, M.D., M.A., D.F.A.A.C.A.P.
Associate Clinical Professor of Child Psychiatry and Psychiatry, Yale University
School of Medicine; Medical Director, Clifford Beers Guidance
Clinic, New Haven, Connecticut

Eugene Wang, M.D., F.R.C.P.C.
Clinical Assistant Professor, Department of Psychiatry, Forensic Psychiatry
Program, University of British Columbia, Forensic Psychiatric Hospital,
Port Coquitlam, British Columbia, Canada

Disclosure of Competing Interests

The following contributors to this book have indicated a financial interest in or other affiliation with a commercial supporter, a manufacturer of a commercial product, a provider of a commercial service, a nongovernmental organization, and/or a government agency, as listed below:

Silke Appel-Cresswell, M.D.—The author has received speaker fees from Teva and the Dystonia Medical Research Foundation Canada and travel support from Merz, Novartis, and Teva; has served as a consultant for Novartis, Merz, and Actelion; and received research support from Novartis and Allergan. She has received research grant support from the Pacific Parkinson's Research Institute, the Pacific Alzheimer Research Foundation, the National Parkinson Foundation, and the Parkinson Society British Columbia.

Paul Dagg, M.D., F.R.C.P.C.—The author has been paid to give talks or attend meetings of consultants by the following companies: Bristol Myers Squibb, Eli Lilly, Janssen, Lundbeck, and Pfizer.

Robert Stowe, M.D., F.R.C.P.C.—The author received an honorarium and travel support from Actelion, the pharmaceutical company that markets miglustat in North America, to attend an international conference on Niemann-Pick type C disease.

The following contributors to this book have indicated they have no competing interests or affiliations to declare:

Marie-Claire Baril, M.D., F.R.C.P.C.
Leon Berzen, M.B.B.Ch., F.F.Psych. (S.A.), F.R.C.P.C.
Catherine Chiles, M.D., D.F.A.P.A., F.A.P.M.
Marius Dimov, M.D., F.R.C.P.C.
Anthony Feinstein, M.B.B.Ch., M.Phil., Ph.D., F.R.C.P.C.
Omar Ghaffar, M.Sc., M.D., F.R.C.P.C.
Andrew K. Howard, M.D., F.R.C.P.C.
Trevor A. Hurwitz, M.B.Ch.B., M.R.C.P. (U.K.), F.R.C.P.C.
Magdalena Ilcewicz-Klimek, M.D., F.R.C.P.C.
Jennifer Klages, Ph.D., R.Psych.
Brenda Kosaka, Ph.D., R.Psych.
Warren T. Lee, M.D., Ph.D.
Aaron Mackie, M.D., F.R.C.P.C.
Scott McCullagh, M.D., F.R.C.P.C.

Sandra J. Mish, Ph.D., R.Psych.
William J. Panenka, M.Sc., M.D., F.R.C.P.C.
Robert M. Rohrbaugh, M.D.
Anton Scamvougeras, M.B.Ch.B., F.R.C.P.C.
David Sherman, M.Sc., M.D.
Vinod H. Srihari, M.D.
Joseph Tham, M.D., F.R.C.P.C.
Pieter Joost van Wattum, M.D., M.A., D.F.A.A.C.A.P.
Eugene Wang, M.D., F.R.C.P.C.

INTRODUCTION

Trevor A. Hurwitz, M.B.Ch.B., M.R.C.P. (U.K.), F.R.C.P.C.
Warren T. Lee, M.D., Ph.D.

Neuropsychiatry has reemerged as an important subspecialty of psychiatry and neurology. Jean-Martin Charcot, one of the preeminent neurologists of the nineteenth century, had a keen interest in neuropsychiatry before the field even formally existed. However, his student Sigmund Freud, another of the early pioneers, abandoned his neurological training to develop a disembodied field of psychoanalysis where mental functioning and pathology had a source and life of their own, disconnected from neuroanatomy and neurochemistry. Contemporary neuropsychiatry reasserts the intimate link between brain structure and function. Clinically, neuropsychiatry concerns itself with disorders due to structural brain injury, electrical malfunction (epilepsy), and extrinsic toxic-metabolic derangements. Neuropsychiatry also concerns itself with somatoform disorders, in which patients appear physically ill but organic causes cannot be uncovered. The conversion patient with psychogenic neurological signs is the best exemplar of such presentations.

The practice of neuropsychiatry requires clinical skills not usually acquired in general psychiatric and neurological training. These skills include a familiarity with neuroanatomy, neurophysiology, neuroimaging, and neuropsychology; knowledge of neurological diseases and their treatments; and a detailed understanding of the behavioral affiliations of the frontal, temporal, and parietal cortices, the limbic system, and the basal ganglia.

The field is moving rapidly, driven by the explosive growth of the basic and clinical neurosciences.

We take the clinical presentation as our starting point, focusing on common syndromes and cases where the history, mental status, and physical examination point strongly to an organic etiology. We use a specific clinical case to describe the approach to these patients, including the differential diagnosis, the diagnostic workup and the value of modern neurodiagnostic investigations, the neuroanatomical and neurochemical basis of psychopathology, and contemporary treatment options. The goal is to bring the subspecialty alive while demonstrating how experienced neuropsychiatrists wrestle with diagnostic dilemmas and treatment approaches, often where evidence-based guidance from literature is limited. Our audience is medical students, residents, and practicing generalist clinicians who would like to read stories rather than textbooks. By embedding the field of neuropsychiatry in real-life clinical problems, we hope to stimulate your interest and make it easier for you to update your knowledge and sharpen your skills. Our discussions take the reader to the mainstream of neuropsychiatric thinking and current knowledge, but not to the cutting edge of research or the most recent genetic or molecular discoveries.

A word about terminology: In most case reports authors have used the term *cognitive-intellectual* interchangeably with *cognitive* when referring to the patient's intellectual abilities as assessed by the Mini-Mental State Examination (Folstein et al. 1975), the Montreal Cognitive Assessment (Nasreddine et al. 2005), or bedside tests. This terminology is meant to emphasize that this domain of the mental status refers to the inborn higher-order computational abilities of the brain such as attention, memory, and calculation and not to thoughts and their content such as delusions and obsessions. To make this point clearer, when we do "cognitive" therapy, we do not teach the patient how to memorize or add or subtract; when neuropsychologists assess this domain, they report on the patient's IQ. Clinically the distinction is robust, with disorders of thought presenting as psychosis, obsessions, or thought disorder and disorders of cognitive-intellectual ability presenting as delirium, amnesia, dementia, or mental retardation. The other term that has been used to make this distinction is *neurocognitive*. The term *cognitive-intellectual* is a compromise that we hope lessens the confusion and emphasizes that we are referring to the inborn higher-order computational capacities of the brain.

It is important to note that this casebook is not a comprehensive textbook of neuropsychiatry. Readers looking for such a textbook are referred to, among other sources, *The American Psychiatric Publishing Textbook of Neuropsychiatry and Behavioral Neuroscience* (Yudofsky and Hales 2008) and *Lishman's Organic Psychiatry: A Textbook of Neuropsychiatry* (David et al. 2012).

References

David AS, Fleminger S, Kopelman MD, et al (eds): Lishman's Organic Psychiatry: A Textbook of Neuropsychiatry, 4th Edition. Hoboken, NJ, Wiley-Blackwell, 2012

Folstein MF, Folstein SE, McHugh PR: "Mini-mental state": a practical method for grading the cognitive state of patients for the clinician. J Psychiatr Res 12:189–198, 1975

Nasreddine ZS, Phillips NA, Bédirian V, et al: The Montreal Cognitive Assessment, MoCA: a brief screening tool for mild cognitive impairment. J Am Geriatr Soc 53(4):695–699, 2005

Yudofsky SC, Hales RE (eds): The American Psychiatric Publishing Textbook of Neuropsychiatry and Behavioral Neuroscience, 5th Edition. Washington, DC, American Psychiatric Publishing, 2008

ACKNOWLEDGMENTS

We would like to recognize Ms. Belinda Chen, M.Sc., for her tremendous and indefatigable efforts as editorial assistant for this book and for bringing this project to fruition. We would also like to express our sincere appreciation to Ms. Gillian Brangham for her tireless secretarial support.

This is an opportunity for us to express our gratitude to the Jemini Foundation, and to the Harris Family through the ERIN Fund, who have supported the research programs of the British Columbia Neuropsychiatry Program.

Last, and perhaps the most important of all, we would like to thank our patients, who have inspired us to greater heights of knowledge and discovery.

PSYCHOBEHAVIORAL DISINHIBITION

Psychobehavioral Disinhibition

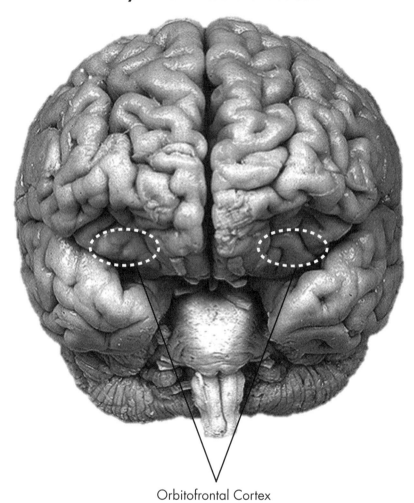

Orbitofrontal Cortex

Introduction

Psychobehavioral disinhibition following brain injury is a major management challenge and can only be addressed by grasping the underlying mechanisms. The first step is to clarify whether the behavior can be accounted for on the basis of a primary psychiatric disorder, especially mania. The orbitofrontal cortex is the critical neuroanatomical region and plays a fundamental role in inhibitory control. Multiple neurotransmitters are involved, but dopamine may be especially important.

Dopamine Excess in Parkinson's Disease

Andrew K. Howard, M.D., F.R.C.P.C.

A 62-year-old right-handed architect, married and with three adult sons, was referred for neuropsychiatric assessment by his neurologist. Eleven years prior to his assessment, he had experienced limited range of motion in his left shoulder and a postural tremor of his left hand, both of which were definitively responsive to levodopa. He developed constipation, progressive rigidity, bradykinesia, postural instability, and hypophonia. He was diagnosed with idiopathic Parkinson's disease with no evidence of a parkinson-plus syndrome. Computed tomography (CT) head scan 1 year following diagnosis was normal. After the original diagnosis he improved with benztropine, but this medication was discontinued because of memory difficulties 2 years prior to presentation. Early in his course, amantadine, trihexyphenidyl, ropinirole, and entacapone were tried; the last two medications were poorly tolerated.

He asserted repeatedly that the only intervention that helped him cope and enjoy a reasonable quality of life was levodopa (Sinemet). At one point, he was taking forty 100-mg tablets in a 24-hour period. He denied detrimental effects of levodopa excess. He disaffirmed any problem with gambling, substance abuse, excessive eating, picking, spending, or fire setting. However, notes from a brief psychiatric admission 7 years prior to his presentation indicated a change in personality, affect, and behavior, attributable to dopamine dysregulation syndrome. Over several months,

3

there were reports of uncharacteristic weight loss, anger outbursts, dia-phoresis, episodic tearfulness, compulsive masturbation, high-speed driv-ing (on one occasion he was chased by police), and hypersexuality. He indulged a fetish for female underwear and was sexually inappropriate with his niece and two female caregivers. These changes were curbed by a forced reduction in levodopa use. These behavioral complications of his condition and its treatment led to early retirement.

Four years prior to presentation, he began experiencing the feeling of bugs crawling and fluid moving over the skin of his abdomen, face, and ex-tremities. The sensation would, at times, migrate into his jaws, knees, shoul-ders, and feet. There was no association with medication times, but it was worse at night. He was convinced that an infestation of microscopic bugs, identifiable as spots on his skin, on the ground, and in his expectoration, caused this sensation. He performed frequent self-examination for the para-sites, attempting to remove them with a vacuum cleaner or mouthwash. He attributed floaters in his peripheral visual field to debris left by the bugs. Quetiapine was introduced, but he reported agitation as a result of taking it.

Three years prior to presentation, he complained of difficulty with sleep maintenance and an increased frequency of acting out his dreams (i.e., rapid eye movement [REM] sleep behavior disorder).

Two years prior to presentation, he started to develop more dyskine-sias, motor fluctuations, and cognitive-intellectual difficulties, described as problems with short-term recall and distractibility. His family indicated that he was becoming more disorganized, impulsive (surfing the Internet for pornography), perseverative, compulsive (assembling and disassem-bling electronics), and manipulative (spending money and leaving the family home without communicating his intentions to family members). These behavioral changes did not fluctuate with his motor state but were more consistently problematic in the evenings.

His past psychiatric history was otherwise negative, with no exposure to psychotropic drugs other than clonazepam, gabapentin, and trazodone, which were prescribed to help with sleep maintenance. There was no his-tory of depression, mania, psychosis, anxiety syndromes, or self-harm.

Past medical history was positive for childhood malaria and a tonsillec-tomy. Medications at assessment included eight tablets of Sinemet CR (200 mg of levodopa, 50 mg of carbidopa) per day and pramipexole 0.5 mg qid. He reported no drug allergies, and in terms of habits he was globally abstemious.

Family history was negative for any neurological, rheumatological, or psychiatric syndromes. His parents had both had complications of tuber-culosis. His mother died after a myocardial infarction, and his father died from respiratory failure.

He was the product of a normal pregnancy and delivery, and was born and raised in Thailand. His father worked in manufacturing and his mother in education. His paternal grandfather raised him. He was the oldest of three children. Other than long-standing shyness, he had a normal socialization pattern and temperament.

He did not manifest any academic or behavioral difficulties in school, completing a grade 12–equivalent education and enrolling in a university. He trained in architecture and joined a successful firm. One of his work placements led him to Canada, and he immigrated with his wife and three children. There was no history of marital disruption in his family of origin, and he himself disaffirmed a history of infidelity, violence, or marital separation. He had not incurred any legal charges. He described himself as conscientious, sending money to relatives back home regularly.

Mental status examination demonstrated an alert, oriented, and accessible historian. Reliability was limited because of impaired awareness of his behavior change. Rapport was superficial. There were multifocal dyskinesias. He was overly familiar in the interview. He expressed intermittent anger, grief, and frustration about his physical state. His speech was hypophonic, with no alteration in rate or prosody. No language disturbance was evident. Affect and mood were subjectively and objectively euthymic. He disaffirmed anhedonia, but he endorsed demoralization about his physical disability. There were no obsessions and no suicidal or homicidal thoughts. He expressed a delusion of infestation, but no other fixed false beliefs could be elicited. He reported tactile hallucinations in the absence of perceptual changes in any other modalities. He disaffirmed a feeling of a presence, passage hallucinations (visions of a person or animal passing on the sides of the visual field), or illusions. His judgment was clearly influenced by impulsivity and limited insight.

On a brief cognitive-intellectual screen, his digit span was 7 forward and 5 backward. On the Three Words–Three Shapes memory test, he was able to incidentally recall all six verbal and nonverbal stimuli and could freely recall six out of six after 5 minutes of distraction. Calculations, production of a three-dimensional cube, reading, writing, and a three-step command were all performed with ease. Trails A and B and phonemic fluency scores were in the normal range. On the Montreal Cognitive Assessment, he scored 27/30, losing 2 points for concrete interpretations of similarities and 1 point for verbal recall (although he benefited from a category cue). His Beck Depression Inventory scale score was 5 (not depressed).

Physical examination was completed 20 minutes following a dose of levodopa. While the patient was sitting, his pulse was 76 and regular, and his blood pressure was 100/70 mm Hg; while he was standing, his pulse was 84 and regular, and his blood pressure was 86/50 mm Hg. Cranial nerve examination was notable for impaired olfactory acuity and facial hypomimia but with normal pupillary reflexes, visual fields and acuity, extraocular movements, facial sensation, hearing, palate elevation, tongue protrusion, and neck strength. There was no neck rigidity.

Motor examination revealed a fine postural tremor in the upper extremities. No other involuntary movements were present at the time of the physical examination. Power, tone, and bulk were normal in all four extremities. Reflexes were within the normal range, and symmetrical and plantar responses were downgoing. There were no frontal release signs.

Sensory examination did not reveal any cortical sensory signs. He reported normal sensation to pinprick, light touch, temperature, position, and vibration. Romberg testing was negative.

The shoulder pull test was positive. There was no limb or truncal ataxia. He had decreased speed in finger tapping bilaterally and reduced rapid alternating movements in all four extremities. Gait, including turns, was smooth, with adequate arm swing.

The results of a complete blood count (CBC) and differential, electrolytes, and glucose, renal function, liver function, thyroid function, B_{12}, ferritin, and antinuclear antibody (ANA) tests were within normal range. An electroencephalogram (EEG) showed minor nonspecific (theta) slowing. A magnetic resonance imaging (MRI) scan of the head from 3 years prior to his presentation was reviewed; it showed minimal frontal ischemic changes in the periventricular white matter. No atrophy of the cortical or subcortical structures was evident. Single-photon emission computed tomography (SPECT) did not show any cerebral hypoperfusion.

He and his family were educated about his moderately advanced idiopathic Parkinson's disease with motor fluctuations and dyskinesias, his adjustment disorder with depressed mood (secondary to physical limitations), his history of dopamine dysregulation syndrome, his tactile hallucinations and consequent delusional parasitosis consistent with Parkinson's disease–associated psychosis, and his early frontal-subcortical cognitive and behavioral changes (executive dysfunction).

At his insistence, his psychosis became the focus of therapy because his preoccupation with the "bugs" troubled him the most, even though he truly believed that they were real. His family was more concerned about his impulsive behaviors and asked for help in managing them. Tapering and eventually discontinuing pramipexole reduced the time that he spent on the Internet and his preoccupation with electronics. Rasagiline 1 mg/day was introduced to help maintain mobility. Clonazepam 1 mg at bedtime helped with sleep maintenance, as did mirtazapine 15 mg qhs, which was also effective in limiting disinhibition, which had led to his unexplained absences from home. A trial of donepezil 5 mg/day caused insomnia, agitation, and gastrointestinal upset (abdominal pain and anorexia). A trial of rivastigmine 4.6 mg/day (transdermal patch) precipitated motor worsening, although it clearly improved his psychosis. Aripiprazole 2 mg/day caused insomnia and agitation, and worsened impulsivity.

Clozapine was started at 12.5 mg qhs and increased up to 200 mg qhs. However, this dose worsened postural dizziness (managed by fludrocortisone 0.2 mg/day) and caused afternoon sedation. After 3 weeks, no improvement was seen. He was then admitted to the neuropsychiatry ward, and within 5 weeks his psychosis remitted. He was persistently seeking levodopa and could not tolerate a levodopa dose of less than 1,600 mg/day. He struggled with motor disability following discharge. He required a reduction in his dose of clozapine and needed an increase in levodopa, with a consequent slight but not functionally impairing reemergence of hallucinations.

Discussion

Parkinson's disease–associated psychosis is confirmed when recurrent or continuous hallucinations, delusions, illusions, or the false sense of a presence occurs for at least 1 month after the onset of parkinsonism. The phenomena cannot be explained by delirium, a primary psychiatric disorder, or dementia with Lewy bodies, and they may be associated with retained insight, dementia, and antiparkinsonian medications (Ravina et al. 2007). Depression, sleep disturbance, and cognitive-intellectual decline are commonly comorbid. Approximately 25% of patients will report psychosis, and this increases to 75% with improved phenomenological discrimination (Diederich et al. 2009).

Psychosis in Parkinson's disease was once thought to be an exclusively medication-induced syndrome, but disease-related factors clearly contribute and explain why not all patients on antiparkinsonian medications experience psychosis. These disease factors include dysfunction of visual pathways, including a parkinsonian retinopathy and functional alterations of extrastriate visual pathways; disturbance of REM sleep; central dopaminergic hyperactivity; an imbalance in cholinergic neurotransmission; Lewy bodies in the ventral and medial temporal regions; and co-occurrence of visual association cortex and frontal executive dysfunction (Llebaria et al. 2010).

Patients with psychosis are at a higher risk of weight loss, caregiver burden, placement in a nursing home, and death. Management is limited to the reduction of antiparkinsonian medications to the lowest tolerable levels and the introduction of cholinesterase inhibitors and atypical antipsychotics, with clozapine demonstrating more robust evidence than quetiapine (Zahodne and Fernandez 2008) for reduction of psychotic symptoms. This patient subjectively reported agitation with quetiapine, more likely due to a coincidental rapid reduction in dopamine replacement therapy, which limited his willingness to undergo a repeat trial.

Hallucinations in Parkinson's disease have been classically described as visual, but emerging data are demonstrating that nonvisual hallucinations, including tactile hallucinations as seen in the case presented, as well as other so-called minor symptoms (e.g., visual illusions, false sense of a presence) are a far more important part of the spectrum of psychosis in Parkinson's disease than previously thought (Fénelon et al. 2010). This patient suffered from formication, a specific form of tactile misperception, which describes the feeling of insects crawling underneath one's skin and is seen in up to 21% of cocaine users (Brewer et al. 2008). *Ekbom syndrome*, another name for delusional parasitosis, is a fixed false belief (worse at night), often associated with formication, that an invisible bug is somehow able to live on inorganic materials such as furniture and then is able to convert to occupying the human body (Hinkle 2011).

Levodopa and other antiparkinsonian agents, like cocaine, upregulate the dopamine system. In Parkinson's disease, this results in improvement of the cardinal motor features, but it also contributes to dyskinesias, psychosis, impulse-control disorders, and compulsive behaviors (Fernandez 2008).

Dopamine plays a critical role in reward and addiction, so it is important to both educate patients about the risks and ask about the presence of impulse-control disorders, which occur in up to 25% of Parkinson's patients. These disorders include pathological gambling, hypersexuality, and excessive shopping, which are the most commonly described, but also intermittent explosive disorder, kleptomania, pyromania, binge eating, and trichotillomania (Ceravolo et al. 2010). The syndrome of hedonistic homeostatic dysregulation, now referred to as *dopamine dysregulation syndrome* (DDS), occurs in at least 4% of patients receiving dopamine replacement therapy. Patients with DDS take large doses of dopamine in excess of those required to control their motor symptoms. Features of addiction are present. These patients develop behavioral and social handicaps similar to those seen in psychostimulant disorders, such as the pattern of pathological use (patients feel like they are "on" only if they are dyskinetic or excessively medicated, and medication seeking is common) and interference with social and occupational functioning. Core clinical phenomena include affective instability (including hypomania when intoxicated and dysphoria when withdrawing), paranoia, anxiety about medication reductions, stereotypies, walkabouts, "punding" (continuous and repetitive handling, examining, and sorting of common objects), and sleep disturbance (O'Sullivan et al. 2009). Involvement of the ventromedial orbitofrontal cortex, the amygdala, and the ventral striatum/nucleus accumbens is likely.

The patient in this case demonstrated evidence of orbitofrontal dysfunction behaviorally, on mental status examination, and on examination of olfactory acuity. Like a subset of patients with idiopathic Parkinson's disease, these findings likely put him at risk for psychosis and dopamine dysregulation syndrome. The case also illustrates the perils of excessively self-medicating with dopamine replacement and the functional disability caused by psychosis in Parkinson's disease. As the focus of study, imaging, and therapies in Parkinson's disease shifts to a greater understanding of the nonmotor complications of this condition, these associated psychiatric syndromes promise to shed light on the pathophysiology of the disease as well as the pathophysiology of phenomena seen in general psychiatric syndromes.

Key Clinical Points

- Parkinson's disease–associated psychosis is common and associated with a poor prognosis, but it may be responsive to reduction in dopamine replacement and the introduction of cholinomimetics and atypical antipsychotics.
- Once considered a medication-induced phenomenon, psychosis in Parkinson's disease may also depend on changes in the balance of dopamine and acetylcholine, selective visual and cognitive dysfunction, Lewy body deposition in the medial and ventral temporal lobe, and interference with rapid eye movement sleep.
- Tactile hallucinations in Parkinson's disease may share a common underlying pathophysiological mechanism with formication seen in cocaine abuse.
- Dopamine excess contributes to dyskinesias, impulse-control disorders, and compulsive behaviors, and in some cases leads to a full-blown dopamine dysregulation syndrome.
- The loss of behavioral control due to dopamine replacement excess or in association with certain antiparkinsonian agents is potentially dangerous and clinically significant, and impulsive and compulsive behaviors must be discussed as part of the routine assessment.

Further Readings

Ceravolo R, Frosini D, Rossi C, et al: Spectrum of addictions in Parkinson's disease: from dopamine dysregulation syndrome to impulse control disorders. J Neurol 257:S276–S283, 2010

Diederich NJ, Fénelon G, Stebbins G, et al: Hallucinations in Parkinson disease. Nat Rev Neurol 5:331–342, 2009

Ravina B, Marder K, Fernandez H, et al: Diagnostic criteria for psychosis in Parkinson's disease: report of an NINDS, NIMH work group. Mov Disord 22:1061–1068, 2007

References

Brewer JD, Meves A, Bostwick JM, et al: Cocaine abuse: dermatologic manifestations and therapeutic approaches. J Am Acad Dermatol 59:483–487, 2008

Ceravolo R, Frosini D, Rossi C, et al: Spectrum of addictions in Parkinson's disease: from dopamine dysregulation syndrome to impulse control disorders. J Neurol 257:S276–S283, 2010

Diederich NJ, Fénelon G, Stebbins G, et al: Hallucinations in Parkinson disease. Nat Rev Neurol 5:331–342, 2009

Fénelon G, Soulas T, Zenasni F, et al: The changing face of Parkinson's disease–associated psychosis: a cross-sectional study based on the new NINDS-NIMH criteria. Mov Disord 25:763–766, 2010

Fernandez HH: What we have learned about sleep disorders and psychosis after nearly two centuries of Parkinson's disease. CNS Spectr 13:34–53, 2008

Hinkle NC: Ekbom syndrome: a delusional condition of "bugs in the skin." Curr Psychiatry Rep 13:178–186, 2011

Llebaria G, Pagonabarraga J, Martinez-Corral M, et al: Neuropsychological correlates of mild to severe hallucinations in Parkinson's disease. Mov Disord 25:2785–2791, 2010

O'Sullivan SS, Evans AH, Lees AJ: Dopamine dysregulation syndrome: an overview of its epidemiology, mechanisms and management. CNS Drugs 23:157–170, 2009

Ravina B, Marder K, Fernandez H, et al: Diagnostic criteria for psychosis in Parkinson's disease: report of an NINDS, NIMH work group. Mov Disord 22:1061–1068, 2007

Zahodne LB, Fernandez HH: Course, prognosis, and management of psychosis in Parkinson's disease: are current treatments really effective? CNS Spectr 13:26–33, 2008

Mania Associated With Brain Injury

Paul Dagg, M.D., F.R.C.P.C.
Jennifer Klages, Ph.D., R.Psych.

A 45-year-old man was admitted to the hospital with disinhibited behavior and impulsivity. He had been brought to the hospital by police after a verbal altercation at a local motel. He had become angry, accusing others of stealing a large amount of money, which he claimed he had previously hidden in the motel and which was no longer there. He demonstrated mood lability, increased sexual preoccupation, irritability, and mild pressure of speech. He complained of numerous physical problems, most of which he blamed on quetiapine, which he had been prescribed during a recent admission to the hospital. He did not feel that he had a mental illness. He did not think he needed to go to the hospital, because he had just signed a contract to purchase a house that he intended to live in with his son, even though he had not been able to work for the past 2 years and had no savings. His admission diagnosis was personality disorder and disinhibition secondary to an acquired brain injury.

He reported that he had been having episodes of increased energy starting 2 years previously and dating from a brain injury that he had sustained after the rupture of an aneurysm of his anterior communicating artery. He recalled complaining of vague headaches for several months prior to the aneurysm rupture. He then experienced a sudden loss of consciousness and required emergency neurosurgical intervention with coiling of the aneurysm. Although he did not report any neurological changes as a result of the aneurysm rupture, he acknowledged that for some months afterward he had had problems with irritability. His family had noted difficulties with his memory and attention immediately following the surgery. He misplaced objects and seemed to have difficulty with concentration. About 6 months after the surgery they first noticed a change in his personality, with more mood swings and impulsivity.

In the 2 years since the surgery, he moved from one small community to another, often quite impulsively. On one occasion, he was arrested and charged following a fight with the boyfriend of his ex-wife and was briefly incarcerated. He was on probation, but he had difficulty meeting the reporting conditions and was facing additional charges. He had been briefly hospitalized on several occasions, presenting with irritability and poor judgment. One hospitalization had been precipitated by a suicide attempt, with symptoms of depression that resolved after 10 days. He reported having had other periods of depression of longer duration since his brain injury. His treatment had varied, as had his diagnosis. On one occasion, he and his family were told that his symptoms were due to his brain injury and that no treatment would be helpful in changing his impulsivity and impaired judgment.

He was transferred to a tertiary facility for a more in-depth assessment. Based on his grandiosity, impulsivity, distractibility, and pressured speech, he was given a diagnosis of mania with an underlying bipolar disorder that had begun sometime after his aneurysm rupture and repair. He was started on divalproex sodium. The dose was slowly titrated upward to attain a serum blood level of 102 mcg/mL. He had previously been treated with quetiapine, with equivocal results. He was unhappy with the side effects from quetiapine, so he was switched to olanzapine and stabilized at 20 mg/day. Over the course of a few weeks, his symptoms resolved, other than some irritability and impairment of judgment. Once settled, he was able to acknowledge that he had experienced mood swings for much of his life, but that they had worsened since his brain injury.

He underwent detailed investigations, including neuroimaging and neuropsychological and functional assessments, so that the effect of his aneurysm rupture and repair on his current and recent symptoms and general functioning could be better understood.

The initial neuroimaging following his aneurysm rupture was reviewed. It demonstrated extensive bilateral subarachnoid and intraventricular hemorrhage. The temporal horns were dilated, in keeping with early hydrocephalus. Repeat MRI after coiling demonstrated bilateral mild spasm in the M1 segment of the middle cerebral arteries and mild-to-moderate spasm in the right M2 branch. MRI during his current admission demonstrated that the hemorrhage and hydrocephalus had fully resolved. An area of ischemic injury was now visible in the gyrus rectus of the right orbitofrontal cortex, representing either a vascular complication of the coiling procedure or the consequences of vasospasm in the territory of the right anterior cerebral artery (Figure 1–1). Nonspecific scattered bilateral frontal lobe white matter hyperintensities were also noted.

A full neuropsychological assessment was conducted once his mood symptoms had settled. On self-report he noted forgetting details like names, but overall he felt smarter and thought that his memory was better since his bleed. He denied any changes in his thinking other than that sometimes he "can't shut up."

In testing, he put forth good effort but responded impulsively and favored speed over accuracy. He had problems with tasks involving sustained attention, including erratic responding and becoming less consistent as the test progressed. There were no difficulties on measures of language or visuospatial skills, taking into account his variable attention and impulsive responses. Motor speed was in the average range. Immediate and delayed memory were impaired. He did better with visual information than with verbal information. Executive functioning was impaired, as reflected in a large number of perseverative errors and compromised mental flexibility and inhibition. Executive impairment was most clearly apparent with tasks of escalating complexity.

A comprehensive functional assessment done by occupational therapy showed overall good organization and planning, with some impulsive tendencies and some difficulties with problem solving.

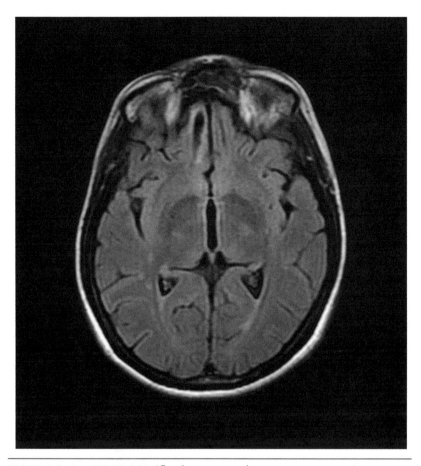

FIGURE 1–1. T2 FLAIR (fluid-attenuated inversion recovery) magnetic resonance image from a 45-year-old male, 2 years postinjury, demonstrating a linear area of encephalomalacia in the right gyrus rectus with increased signal in the surrounding white matter suggestive of postischemic gliosis.

Based on history, he likely had premorbid problems with attention and impulsivity, with some suggestion of a preexisting bipolar disorder. Since his brain injury from his ruptured aneurysm and coiling, he had developed an unequivocal bipolar disorder with psychobehavioral disinhibition, executive failure, and cognitive-intellectual difficulties. In this complex setting, it was not possible to determine the relative roles of brain injury and primary bipolar disorder in his now overt mood disorder—both were likely responsible. Similarly, both structural brain injury and an unstable mood could be inculpated in his disinhibition and executive failure. In contrast, his cognitive-intellectual problems, such as poor memory, were more likely related to his structural brain injury, although difficulties with attention and executive function can compromise memory encoding, consolidation, and retrieval.

Discussion

The challenge in this case is in determining the relative contributions of structural brain injury and primary psychiatric illness in the genesis of the patient's psychopathology. Premorbidly, he had cyclical mood patterns and risk-taking behavior but had never been formally diagnosed with nor treated for bipolar disorder.

Ruptured aneurysms of the anterior communicating artery have been associated with psychobehavioral dysfunction and pervasive cognitive-intellectual impairment, especially in those patients who have complicating vasospasm (Stenhouse et al. 1991). Deficits are varied and can include memory impairment, thought to be related to damage to the basal forebrain (Damasio et al. 1985), and increased risk-taking behavior, possibly associated with orbitofrontal damage (Mavaddat et al. 2000). Structural damage to the orbitofrontal lobes has been implicated in inappropriate social behaviors and impaired self-insight (Beer et al. 2006). These difficulties may result in poorly adjudicated and risky behavior, which may escalate to antisocial behavior and possible substance abuse and addiction (Bechara 2004). The right ventromedial prefrontal cortex (which extends into the orbitofrontal cortex) has been particularly associated with problems in social conduct and decision making (Tranel et al. 2002).

Determining the causation of mood symptoms in the setting of acquired brain injury is also complex, especially given that bipolar disorder can start relatively late in life and subtle symptoms may be present for many years before diagnosis. A review of patients with traumatic brain injury (TBI) concluded that bipolar disorder occurred in 4.2% of the subjects, which contrasts with a community lifetime prevalence of about 1% (van Reekum et al. 2000). Injury consistently preceded the onset of mood symptoms, but more severe injury was not always associated with a greater risk of developing bipolar disorder. Lesion laterality appears to be relevant, because the risk of developing mania correlates with right hemisphere injury (Rao and Lyketsos 2000). As in this case, the right orbitofrontal region has been implicated in many cases of secondary mania, with reports of right orbitofrontal lesions preferentially causing unipolar mania (Starkstein et al. 1991). Evidence in support of the importance of the orbitofrontal region in manic states can also be found in studies of primary bipolar disorder. Structural changes have been found in the orbito-frontal region in persons with familial bipolar disorder (Stanfield et al. 2009), and hypoactivity of the orbitofrontal region has been found in acute manic states using both positron emission tomography (Blumberg et al. 1999) and functional MRI (Altshuler et al. 2005).

Treatment of mania secondary to brain injury is similar to the treatment of primary mania, although Pope et al. (1988) reported a preferential response to valproate compared with lithium. This finding, along with the observation that seizures are frequent in bipolar disorder after brain injury (van Reekum et al. 2000), has led to a seizure hypothesis for secondary mania.

Psychiatric symptoms occurring after brain injury require careful assessment, because multiple causal mechanisms may be involved. Primary bipolar disorder can fully explain a mood disorder that surfaces after brain injury. However, many of the symptoms of hypomania or mania, such as impulsivity and impaired judgment, can also be manifestations of psychobehavioral disinhibition and executive failure caused by frontal lobe injury. In this case, symptoms were initially attributed to the patient's brain injury and the syndrome of mania was not recognized, contributing to the undertreatment of his bipolar disorder.

In the end, whether the patient's bipolar disorder arose as a result of his brain injury cannot be definitively determined. The visible damage on MRI was in a region that has been associated with bipolar disorder. Alternatively, injury in this critical limbic region may have simply exacerbated a preexisting bipolar disorder. What was important was recognizing the psychiatric syndrome and treating it effectively. Once the syndrome was treated, it became easier to justify the attribution of his remaining deficits to his brain injury. These deficits included poor attention, memory, and social judgment, but with his mood symptoms better controlled, there is an increased chance for the successful implementation of adaptive behavioral strategies and community rehabilitation.

Key Clinical Points

- The psychobehavioral consequences of ruptured anterior communicating artery aneurysm and its treatment can include persistent cognitive difficulties, such as impaired memory, and personality changes, such as increased risk-taking behavior.
- Persons with ruptured aneurysms of the anterior communicating artery can have persistent cognitive-intellectual problems, including difficulties with memory and executive functioning.

- Brain injury may be associated with an increased risk of developing bipolar disorder.
- The symptoms of bipolar disorder and of brain injury involving limbic structures may overlap and may be difficult to distinguish from each other.
- Bipolar disorder after brain injury may respond preferentially to anticonvulsant mood stabilizers.

Further Readings

Bechara A: The role of emotion in decision-making: evidence from neurological patients with orbitofrontal damage. Brain Cogn 55:30–40, 2004
van Reekum R, Cohen T, Wong J: Can traumatic brain injury cause psychiatric disorders? J Neuropsychiatry Clin Neurosci 12:316–327, 2000

References

Altshuler L, Bookheimer S, Proenza MA, et al: Increased amygdala activation during mania: a functional magnetic resonance imaging study. Am J Psychiatry 162:1211–1213, 2005
Bechara A: The role of emotion in decision-making: evidence from neurological patients with orbitofrontal damage. Brain Cogn 55:30–40, 2004
Beer JS, John OP, Scabini D, et al: Orbitofrontal cortex and social behavior: integrating self-monitoring and emotion-cognition interactions. J Cogn Neurosci 18:871–879, 2006
Blumberg HP, Stern E, Ricketts S, et al: Rostral and orbital prefrontal cortex dysfunction in the manic state of bipolar disorder. Am J Psychiatry 156:1986–1988, 1999
Damasio AR, Graff-Radford NR, Eslinger PJ, et al: Amnesia following basal forebrain lesions. Arch Neurol 42:263–271, 1985
Mavaddat N, Kirkpatrick PJ, Rogers RD, et al: Deficits in decision-making in patients with aneurysms of the anterior communicating artery. Brain 123:2109–2117, 2000
Pope HG Jr, McElroy SL, Satlin A, et al: Head injury, bipolar disorder, and response to valproate. Compr Psychiatry 29:34–38, 1988
Rao V, Lyketsos C: Neuropsychiatric sequelae of traumatic brain injury. Psychosomatics 41:95–103, 2000
Stanfield AC, Moorhead TW, Job DE, et al: Structural abnormalities of ventrolateral and orbitofrontal cortex in patients with familial bipolar disorder. Bipolar Disord 11:135–144, 2009
Starkstein SE, Fedoroff P, Berthier ML, et al: Manic-depressive and pure manic states after brain lesions. Biol Psychiatry 29:149–158, 1991
Stenhouse LM, Knight RG, Longmore BE, et al: Long-term cognitive deficits in patients after surgery on aneurysms of the anterior communicating artery. J Neurol Neurosurg Psychiatry 54:909–914, 1991

Tranel D, Bechara A, Denburg NL: Asymmetric functional roles of right and left ventromedial prefrontal cortices in social conduct, decision-making, and emotional processing. Cortex 38:589–612, 2002

van Reekum R, Cohen T, Wong J: Can traumatic brain injury cause psychiatric disorders? J Neuropsychiatry Clin Neurosci 12:316–327, 2000

Neuropsychiatric Manifestations of a Paraneoplastic Syndrome

Marie-Claire Baril, M.D., F.R.C.P.C.
Sandra J. Mish, Ph.D., R.Psych.

A 39-year-old married woman, who had worked as a receptionist in a busy medical clinic, was referred to a tertiary psychiatric facility for multidisciplinary assessment and recommendations for care planning. In particular, a neuropsychological assessment was recommended to better understand her current level of cognitive functioning and behavior as well as her capability to consent to or refuse care.

Five years previously she had been hospitalized following a 6-week history of progressive changes in her balance, numbness and tingling in her feet, and early-morning nausea and vomiting. On examination she had prominent vertical and horizontal nystagmus and an unsteady, broad-based gait. She had marked clubbing of her fingers and a history of heavy cigarette smoking since age 18. A computed tomography scan of the brain demonstrated prominent cerebellar vermis atrophy, with no evidence of any other intracranial abnormality. MRI showed similar findings. Paraneoplastic cerebellar degeneration (PCD) was strongly suspected.

Findings from bilateral mammograms and bone scans were normal. Lumbar puncture showed an elevated white cell count. Chest X ray identified a prominent left hilum. Chest CT showed left hilar adenopathy with at least two nodes in the 17-mm diameter range (Figure 1–2). There was a 5.5-mm well-defined nodule in the left upper lobe, too small to characterize but suggestive of a neoplastic nodule. Cytology of bronchial washings and lymph nodes, via endobronchial ultrasound-guided transbronchial needle aspiration, was negative for carcinoma. Subsequent lymph node biopsy, via anterior mediastinotomy, showed numerous clusters of malignant epithelial cells,

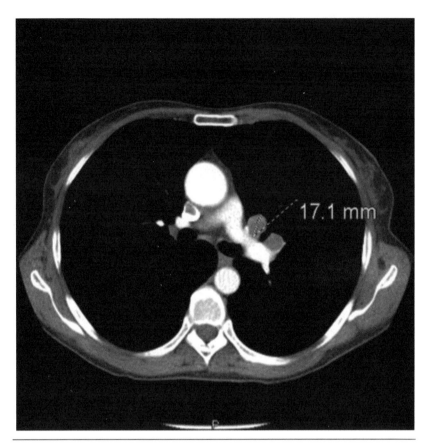

FIGURE 1–2.   Initial chest computed tomography scan, with two nodes
in the left hilum.

consistent with a small cell carcinoma confirmed by immunohistochemical
staining. Laboratory results were negative for antineuronal antibodies such as
anti-Yo (PCA-1), anti-Hu (ANNA-1), and anti-Purkinje cells. She was given
a clinical diagnosis of limited-stage small cell lung cancer with PCD.

She deteriorated during her hospital stay, with progressive ataxia necessitating a wheelchair. A neurological opinion was sought to clarify the
findings and to help assess her mental competence. On examination she
had marked limb ataxia but no frontal lobe release signs, unusual behavior, or resting tremor. There were no clinical features to suggest limbic encephalitis, and she was deemed competent to understand the risks and
benefits of treatment.

She received four courses of cisplatin-etoposide chemotherapy with
concurrent thoracic irradiation. Although treatment resulted in cancer

remission, her neurological symptoms failed to improve. She was transferred from the oncology service to an intensive physical rehabilitation program. When assessed by physiatry and neurology, she was noted to have horizontal nystagmus, a head and body tremor, and marked limb ataxia. A formal eye examination and cognitive screening were not attempted because of poor cooperation, although oscillopsia and memory problems were suspected.

Emotional dysregulation was a prominent feature of her clinical presentation. She was easily upset, often bursting into tears for no apparent reason. She was also easily frustrated, with periods of agitation and speaking in a loud voice, at times yelling. Her behavior proved challenging to manage. Her verbal outbursts were treated with lorazepam and quetiapine given as needed. Her behavior settled briefly with these medications, but irritability and emotional lability rapidly resurfaced soon after the medication effects wore off. For the most part, she refused medications and would not participate in rehabilitation activities. She was discharged because of lack of cooperation.

Neurological and psychiatric symptoms persisted at home, affecting her everyday functioning. She was unable to return to work. Her husband had to assume responsibility for most household chores. She was able to attend to most of her activities of daily living but required supervision for bathing. She became dependent on a manual wheelchair for mobility and needed floor-to-ceiling poles at her bed and grab bars in the bathroom for transfers.

Family and friends noted major changes in her personality and behavior. Her husband described emotional outbursts at home, with frequent irritability and episodes of screaming and yelling and occasional physical aggression (e.g., kicking, striking with her wheelchair). Her emotional lability led to strain within the marriage as well as in her other relationships. Premorbidly she was an intelligent, articulate, and outgoing individual with strong skills in decision making and organization at work. She had several friends and was a "loving and supportive" wife. She had no prior psychiatric history.

Home and community care had been asked to provide home services, but she had refused all help, stating that she was independent with self-care and household activities. She had no insight into her husband's burden. Home care workers felt uncomfortable providing services to a young woman who consistently declined their help. The only diagnoses, at that time, were small cell lung cancer (in remission) and functional issues due to PCD. Although cognitive, emotional, and behavioral issues were clearly recognized, she had no formal psychiatric diagnosis.

She was admitted to our tertiary facility for multidisciplinary assessment and recommendations for care planning. On admission she reported

ongoing visual problems. She had diplopia, particularly when there was
a great deal of information on a page. She had to rely on voice and hair
color to identify people. She struggled to read small print and required a
clock with large numbers. She acknowledged problems with speech, writing, and following multistep instructions. She had no concerns about her
attention, visuospatial skills, or memory. She described some emotional
changes, such as frequent crying and poor anger control.

On examination she exhibited cerebellar dysarthria. Her speech was
slurred and dysrhythmic, with irregularities in rate and loudness. She had
poor emotional control. Bursts of loud laughter and some "childlike" behavior were observed when she found something amusing. She often raised her
voice and yelled when frustrated. Angry outbursts were observed when she
experienced difficulty communicating with others, such as when she was
asked to repeat herself or to clarify or expand on her responses.

She underwent a comprehensive neuropsychological assessment. Cognitive measures were selected to reduce visual and motor demands. She
passed measures of effort, suggesting that she tried her best and that her
performance on other tests could be taken as a reliable indicator of her cognitive-intellectual abilities. Language, verbal abilities, and verbal memory
were unimpaired. Assessment of her visuospatial abilities was difficult because of visuomotor problems. On a task that required visual logical reasoning, she scored within the average range. Her attention was variable,
especially with more complex material and when she was required to direct attention in the face of distracting material. Executive functions were
impaired and included problems with verbal fluency, verbal abstract reasoning, and problem solving. Behavioral observations also suggested problems with cognitive flexibility.

An occupational therapy functional assessment concluded that she
was unable to safely use knives, scissors, or the stove. Cooking was unsafe
because of her motor and visual impairments as well as her inability to
concentrate or multitask. She was also noted to have poor insight and
judgment and was at risk for making impulsive and poorly reasoned
decisions.

A recent head CT scan (Figure 1–3) showed prominent cerebellar atrophy, which had developed since her initial CT scan. No other intracranial abnormalities were noted.

Discussion

Paraneoplastic neurological syndrome (PNS) is a neurological syndrome
due to the remote effect of a systemic carcinoma on the central and/or
peripheral nervous system. The term *paraneoplastic* is used to indicate

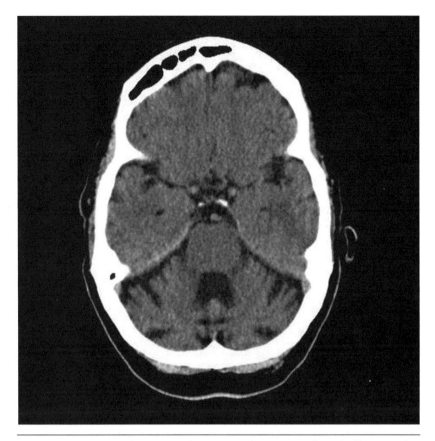

FIGURE 1–3.   Axial computed tomography image of cerebellar atrophy, 3 years after small cell lung cancer diagnosis.

that the neurological symptoms are not the direct result of tumor invasion or metastases, cancer therapy, malnutrition, or concurrent infection. These syndromes are rare compared with other neuro-oncologic diseases, such as a primary brain tumor or metastases. The same tumor can cause different paraneoplastic syndromes, and more than one PNS can be expressed in the same individual.

A PNS often precedes the diagnosis of the underlying cancer. Prompt recognition of a PNS is important because it directs a search for a potentially treatable cancer. However, even after successful treatment of the associated tumor, reversal of neurological symptoms is uncommon, although they may stabilize (Darnell and Posner 2003).

Subacute cerebellar degeneration has a paraneoplastic etiology in 50% of cases (Deangelis and Rowland 2010). PCD has been associated with a wide variety of neoplasms but is most common among patients with breast, gynecological, and small cell lung cancers. The incidence of cerebellar degeneration is about 2/1,000 cancer diagnoses (Braik et al. 2010). Patients display characteristic signs of cerebellar dysfunction, such as gait and truncal ataxia, oculomotor disturbances, dysarthria, and dysmetria. Symptoms usually develop rapidly over days to weeks (Bataller and Dalmau 2004).

Head MRI is a useful diagnostic tool for investigating PCD. Repeat testing is recommended, because patients usually show a normal scan in the initial stages but develop cerebellar atrophy (extensive loss of Purkinje cells) with disease progression (Braik et al. 2010). Functional neuroimaging such as positron emission tomography might also have diagnostic utility in PNS (Bataller and Dalmau 2004).

Antineuronal antibodies should be measured in all patients suspected to have a PNS (Bataller and Dalmau 2004). There is increasing evidence that PNS result from autoimmunity. The tumor may contain antigens normally found in the nervous system, provoking an immune response against both the tumor and the nervous system. Antineuronal antibodies can be markers of the neurological syndrome as well as the underlying neoplasm. For example, high titers of antibodies such as anti-Hu can be found in the serum and cerebrospinal fluid in some patients with small cell lung cancer and PCD (Bataller and Dalmau 2004). However, in many patients with PNS, antineuronal antibodies may not be detectable. Diagnosis will then depend on exclusion of other etiologies of similar neurological syndromes and a thorough search for the underlying cancer (Braik et al. 2010).

The patient presented with subacute cerebellar dysfunction, which developed over a period of 6 weeks. As is often the case, her neurological symptoms preceded the diagnosis of the underlying malignancy. Lung cancer was suspected because of her history of smoking, signs of clubbing, and abnormal chest X ray. Her diagnosis of small cell lung carcinoma was confirmed by chest scan and biopsy. A second PNS, limbic encephalitis, was suspected and ruled out. Limbic encephalitis presents with rapid onset of psychiatric symptoms and short-term memory impairments, which may progress to dementia (Kayser et al. 2010). Small cell lung cancer is also commonly associated with this disorder. Brain MRI often shows abnormalities in the medial region of one or both temporal lobes (Kayser et al. 2010).

In addition to cerebellar motor impairments, the patient had striking cognitive and affective disturbances, consistent with the literature on cerebellar damage. Schmahmann and Sherman (1998) introduced the concept of *cerebellar cognitive-affective syndrome* to describe a spectrum of cognitive deficits (e.g., language, visuospatial, executive functions) and behavioral-affective disturbances (e.g., emotional blunting or disinhibition) associated with cerebellar disease. This syndrome has been observed in both congenital and acquired cerebellar damage (Baillieux et al. 2010). Diversity in clinical presentation likely depends on several factors, such as functional lateralization of the cerebellum. As a result of strong crossed cerebello-cerebral connections, patients with right-sided cerebellar damage might show a typical pattern of left hemisphere dysfunction, with impaired language skills such as poor naming, verbal fluency, and verbal working memory (Baillieux et al. 2010).

In this patient, prompt and effective treatment resulted in cancer remission. However, as is typical in PNS, she continued to exhibit neurological and neuropsychiatric symptoms. She has been left with major functional and psychobehavioral impairments that have required intensive community supports. She had poor insight into her illness and was unable to cooperate with assessments while in the hospital and thus did not benefit from rehabilitation.

Key Clinical Points

- Paraneoplastic neurological syndromes, although uncommon, should be included in the differential diagnosis of middle-aged and elderly patients with neuropsychiatric symptoms and without a psychiatric history.
- The development of neurological symptoms often precedes the diagnosis of cancer. Early detection may allow for diagnosis and treatment when the primary tumor is small and localized, potentially improving survival rate.
- Antineuronal antibodies may point to the underlying malignancy and a PNS. However, a negative result does not preclude the diagnosis of a paraneoplastic syndrome.
- Neurological and neuropsychiatric manifestations of cancers often persist even after cancer remission.
- Cognitive and behavioral-affective manifestations may undermine a patient's capability to appreciate the nature of the illness and its sequelae, compromising treatment and rehabilitation.

Further Readings

Breitbart WS, Lederberg MS, Rueda-Lara MA, et al: Psycho-oncology, in Kaplan & Sadock's Comprehensive Textbook of Psychiatry, 9th Edition. Edited by

Sadock BJ, Sadock VA, Ruiz P. Philadelphia, PA, Lippincott Williams & Wilkins, 2009, pp 2314–2353

Collinson SL, Anthonisz B, Courtenay D, et al: Frontal executive impairment associated with paraneoplastic cerebellar degeneration: a case study. Neurocase 12:350–354, 2006

Darnell RB, Posner JB: Paraneoplastic Syndromes. New York, Oxford University Press, 2011

References

Baillieux H, De Smet HJ, Dobbeleir A, et al: Cognitive and affective disturbances following focal cerebellar damage in adults: a neuropsychological and SPECT study. Cortex 46:869–879, 2010

Bataller L, Dalmau JO: Paraneoplastic disorders of the central nervous system: update on diagnostic criteria and treatment. Semin Neurol 24:461–471, 2004

Braik T, Evans AT, Telfer M, et al: Paraneoplastic neurological syndromes: unusual presentations of cancer—a practical review. Am J Med Sci 340:301–308, 2010

Darnell RB, Posner JB: Paraneoplastic syndromes involving the nervous system. N Engl J Med 349:1543–1554, 2003

Deangelis LM, Rowland LP: Paraneoplastic syndromes, in Merritt's Neurology, 12th Edition. Edited by Rowland LP, Pedley TA. Philadelphia, PA, Lippincott Williams & Wilkins, 2010, pp 468–472

Kayser MS, Kohler CG, Dalmau J: Psychiatric manifestations of paraneoplastic disorders. Am J Psychiatry 167:1039–1050, 2010

Schmahmann JD, Sherman JC: The cerebellar cognitive affective syndrome. Brain 121:561–579, 1998

Aggression and Brain Injury

Jennifer Klages, Ph.D., R.Psych.
Paul Dagg, M.D., F.R.C.P.C.

A 48-year-old man sustained an anoxic brain injury after a cardiac arrest. He was found unconscious and was successfully resuscitated. Since he was alone at the time of the incident, the duration of the cardiac arrest and subsequent hypoxia was unknown. In the emergency room he had a seizure, and his Glasgow Coma Scale rating was 3/15. His urine was positive for cocaine. At 48 hours post–cardiac arrest, his brain stem reflexes were intact and he was responsive to pain. Seven days post-arrest, primary medical concerns were agitation and wandering. Head CT scans 1 and 5 days post-arrest showed evidence of a hypodense lesion in his left internal capsule. An EEG showed a diffuse slowed dysrhythmic pattern suggestive of moderate anoxic encephalopathy. A head CT scan 5 months later showed an increased prominence of the ventricles and gyri globally, compatible with atrophy secondary to anoxic injury.

He had a ventricular septal defect at birth that did not close and required surgical intervention. Ten years prior to the cardiac arrest, he developed third-degree atrioventricular block and had a pacemaker implanted. He had a diagnosis of cardiomyopathy with decreased left ventricular ejection fraction, which was felt to have precipitated ventricular arrhythmias leading to an anterior myocardial infarction. He was described by his father as having been an oppositional and impulsive child, but he did not receive any mental health assistance as a child or as an adult. He had a history of mixed substance abuse (alcohol, marijuana, and cocaine), with periods of incarceration for drug-related charges. He had a brother with schizophrenia.

His placement following his anoxic injury was a challenge due to significant aggression and cognitive difficulties requiring one-to-one care. He had no insight into his injury and frequently insisted that he needed to see his wife and children, from whom he had been estranged for years. He did not tolerate limits well and could become threatening if he did not get his way. He became more physically aggressive toward his environment and, 7 months after his injury, was admitted to our specialized inpatient unit for further assessment and treatment.

His Mini-Mental State Examination score was 22/30, with deficiencies in recall and orientation. Formal neuropsychological testing showed preserved verbal and visuospatial functioning. He was profoundly impaired on measures of memory and executive functioning, including mental flexibility and inhibition. A family rating scale of his behavior before and after the anoxic brain injury showed premorbid problems with disinhibition and executive functioning, with a severe worsening of apathy and executive functioning after his anoxic injury. Disinhibited behavior, while previously a problem, was not seen by his family as being any worse.

At the time of admission, he was taking risperidone 6 mg/day in split dosing and divalproex sodium 500 mg/day. He had had no other psychotropic medication trials. He was also taking the beta-blocker carvedilol 6.25 mg bid for his cardiomyopathy and impaired left ventricular function. Over the first 2 weeks, his behavior was relatively settled. When confused, he would still respond to redirection and reorientation by staff. After this initial period, his behavior became more difficult to manage. He demonstrated a pattern of settled behavior interspersed with episodes of severe threatening and aggressive behaviors. These episodes were often accompanied by a suspicious demeanor and usually occurred when he was confused about where he was and what he was doing. For example, he would insist that he wanted to go to work or that he wanted to see his wife and children, who he believed were in the building. During these times he would threaten staff physically, kick windows and doors, and throw objects at windows. On one occasion he picked up a large chair/table combination and threw it through a window; another time he punched the glass separating the nursing unit from the ward. These episodes occurred several times per week and could last for 1–2 hours. Use of benzodiazepines or risperidone on an as-needed basis had minimal effect.

Behavioral tracking showed that the trigger was often confusion, so memory aids were used. For example, he would forget that he had recently had a cigarette, and his demands for more cigarettes would trigger an aggressive outburst. He was asked to sign a sheet to indicate that he had received his cigarette at a specific time. However, later he would simply insist that he had not signed anything and that the staff had forged his signature. A trial of donepezil was initiated based on some evidence that cholinesterase inhibitors may help attention and memory-related difficulties after a TBI (Griffin et al. 2003). However, he obtained no benefit, and there was no noticeable improvement in his performance on neuropsychological testing or in his behaviors. De-escalation techniques were also ineffective.

The severity of his behavior put staff and co-patients at significant risk and prevented future care anywhere other than in a specialized high-security facility. For this reason, medication trials were initiated that targeted his aggression. The first trial involved an increase in carvedilol, given the evidence supporting the role of beta-blockers in treating aggression (Fleminger et al. 2006). This had no effect, so the dose was reduced to the admission dose. Because his admission dose of divalproex sodium was subtherapeutic, it was gradually increased to 750 mg bid, which resulted in a valproate blood level of 98 mcg/mL (therapeutic range for treatment of epilepsy is 50–100 mcg/mL and for mania is 85–125 mcg/mL), but again without effect. Over the next several months, he had trials of olanzapine, with a maximal dose of 20 mg/day, citalopram 20 mg/day, and buspirone 45 mg/day in split dosing. None of these treatments resulted in any improvement. Demands for cigarettes were triggers for agitation and aggression. Consequently, he was given a trial of bupropion to see if this medication would reduce the urge to smoke and decrease the frequency of the behaviors, but this medication also had no effect.

After 4 months in the hospital, he was given a trial of cyproterone acetate, an antiandrogen medication that blocks androgen receptors and suppresses luteinizing hormone, thus reducing testosterone levels (Huertas et al. 2007). This appeared to have a modest effect on his aggression and agitation at a dosage of 100 mg bid. Outbursts were reduced in frequency but remained severe in intensity and difficult to manage safely.

Finally, 6½ months after admission, he was started on clozapine based on some limited evidence of efficacy in the treatment of aggression in brain injury (Michals et al. 1993) and in schizophrenia, where the anti-aggressive effects are independent of controlling psychotic symptoms (Citrome et al. 2001). At 250 mg/day in split dosing, we began to see a substantial reduction in intensity and frequency of agitation and aggression. The aggression gradually disappeared, and he began to respond much more easily to redirection by staff. At a dose of 300 mg/day, his serum clozapine level was 411 ng/mL and his norclozapine level was 224 ng/mL (therapeutic range for treatment of schizophrenia is 100–700 ng/mL, with refractory symptoms requiring more than 350 ng/mL). He was still taking divalproex sodium and cyproterone, but all other psychotropic medications had been discontinued.

Over the next month, divalproex was discontinued without problems and the cyproterone dose was reduced. Once the dose of cyproterone fell below 150 mg/day, staff again noticed an increase in the intensity of his anger and a greater resistance to their interventions. His behavior improved when the dose was returned to 150 mg/day. Six weeks later, out of concern about the side effects and the lack of clarity regarding its benefit, the dose was again reduced. Within a few weeks his intense anger resurfaced, and the cyproterone dose was returned to 150 mg/day. Thereafter he remained stable and free of substantial aggression and agitation. He had some periods of apathy and occasional agitation, but these were easily managed by staff redirection. Throughout this period of stability, he received infrequent benzodiazepine doses as needed, averaging two to four doses per month.

He was successfully discharged to a group home specializing in the care of persons with brain injury. His discharge medications were clozapine, cyproterone, and carvedilol.

Discussion

Every year in the United States, over 1.5 million individuals sustain a TBI. Of those hospitalized, 43.3% experience a long-term disability (Langlois Orman et al. 2011). Estimates of the frequency of aggression after brain injury vary. Tateno et al. (2003) found aggressive behavior in one-third of patients in the first 6 months after TBI, a frequency three times that of their comparator group—patients with multiple traumas but no TBI. Risk factors for aggression after brain injury include greater injury severity, frontal lesions, pre-injury aggression, pre-injury substance abuse, and more than one injury with loss of consciousness (Kim et al. 2007). The patient in our case had many of these factors, including a severe brain injury, pre-injury aggression (suggested by his criminal involvement), and pre-injury substance abuse. His premorbid difficulties with inhibition and executive functioning (as identified by his family and suggested by his criminal history) were likely exacerbated by his post-injury memory impairment, which resulted in his having greater confusion and misconstruing his circumstances and thus led to more pronounced and destructive behavioral outbursts.

Aggression is a complex behavior that can involve lesions in multiple areas of the brain (e.g., frontal lobe, especially the orbitofrontal region; temporal lobe; limbic system) and many different neurotransmitter systems (e.g., increased norepinephrine, decreased serotonin, increased dopamine). It is therefore unsurprising that it has been difficult to find a class effect in medication trials. A Cochrane review (Fleminger et al. 2006) found that there was consistent evidence of efficacy only for beta-blockers, but they are often difficult to tolerate. Finding an effective pharmacological treatment for aggression is thus challenging. Clinicians must rely on limited evidence and balance anticipated medication side effects against the risks posed by the individual's behaviors.

The first step in treating aggression is a clear analysis and documentation of the aggression and its phenomenology. This can include the antecedents, timing, intensity, frequency, and effect of staff interventions. Many behaviors can be labeled as aggression, so specific descriptions are vital in terms of treatment planning and response assessment, especially when the behavior is relatively infrequent. Standardized and consistent behavioral interventions and care approaches are essential, because aggression may be understandable in terms of poorly managed interpersonal interactions or environmental cues that are misconstrued. A multidisciplinary team approach is vital, with all team members applying the agreed-upon approach to care and behavioral interventions. Since memory deficits can often result in agitation or aggression, use of various memory cues and aids can be effective.

Despite best efforts and good intentions, nonpharmacological approaches may fail to fully treat the aggressive behavior, and medications then become an important part of treatment. The term *chemical restraint* is often used when describing the use of medications for the management of aggression. This term is often misused, is poorly defined, and can stigmatize the treatment of aggression. Treatment involves targeting complex behaviors such as aggression. By contrast, chemical restraint is the nontargeted use of medications to impede mobility. Our facility, like others, has a policy of minimal restraint, which includes chemical restraint. However, when faced with persistent aggression and violence that have failed to respond to nonpharmacological approaches, we advocate an evidence-based approach to the use of medications, targeting specific symptoms and behaviors and tracking the effect of the medications with clear documentation.

Our patient showed a robust response to clozapine but an equivocal response to cyproterone and divalproex. His response to clozapine occurred in the absence of overt psychosis and was likely due to clozapine's antiaggressive effect, which is independent of its antipsychotic effect (Citrome et al. 2001). Clozapine is superior to other antipsychotics when aggression occurs in the setting of psychosis (Volavka et al. 2004). Our patient's tendency to suspicion could possibly reflect a paranoid psychosis, although his history of incarceration would also predispose to suspicion of authority figures. Additionally, his family history of schizophrenia indicated a genetic vulnerability to psychosis. In our view, neither of these reflected clinically important variables to account for his response to clozapine.

We also attempted withdrawal of both cyproterone and divalproex. We were able to withdraw the latter without impact. We attempted withdrawal of the cyproterone on two occasions. However, within 2 weeks of cyproterone at a dosage below 150 mg/day, previously observed patterns of aggression returned. His benefit from cyproterone was sufficiently convincing to justify its continued use in combination with the clozapine, even though the evidence for the use of cyproterone in nonsexual aggression is weak.

Our approach in the absence of evidence-based guidelines is to methodically work through a variety of medications with a reported role in the management of aggression. This approach involves treating every medication trial as an experimental intervention with careful observation for effect, and withdrawal of medication if the evidence of efficacy is not clear. In this way, we were able to identify the optimal medication treatment that allowed our patient to return to community living.

Key Clinical Points

- Traumatic brain injuries are common, and aggression is a frequent psychobehavioral consequence of severe TBI.
- Careful description and documentation of behaviors described as aggressive is an important first step in their treatment.
- Behavioral interventions and care approaches are essential, be-

cause aggression may be understandable in terms of environmental cues or interpersonal interactions.

- Medication approaches to the treatment of aggression should be designed as single-case experiments with measurement of pre- and post-behaviors, and consideration should be given to an on-off-on approach to treatment. This is especially important when results are equivocal, medication side effects are substantial, or there is little evidence for the treatment used.

- The term *chemical restraint* should be reserved for use of medication that is not targeted to specific symptoms, illnesses, or behaviors and that is primarily focused on limiting mobility. As such, it is a strategy whose use should be limited in the same way that physical restraint is limited.

Further Readings

Kim E, Lauterbach EC, Reeve A, et al: Neuropsychiatric complications of traumatic brain injury: a critical review of the literature (a report by the ANPA Committee on Research). J Neuropsychiatry Clin Neurosci 19:106–127, 2007

Silver JM, Yudofsky SC, Anderson KE: Aggressive disorders, in Textbook of Traumatic Brain Injury, 2nd Edition. Edited by Silver JM, McAllister TW, Yudofsky SC. Washington, DC, American Psychiatric Publishing, 2011, pp 225–238

Tateno A, Jorge RE, Robinson RG: Clinical correlates of aggressive behaviour after traumatic brain injury. J Neuropsychiatry Clin Neurosci 15:155–160, 2003

References

Citrome L, Volavka J, Czobor P, et al: Effects of clozapine, olanzapine, risperidone, and haloperidol on hostility among patients with schizophrenia. Psychiatr Serv 52:1510–1514, 2001

Fleminger S, Greenwood RRJ, Oliver DL: Pharmacological management for agitation and aggression in people with acquired brain injury. Cochrane Database of Systematic Reviews. Issue 4, Art. No.: CD003299, 2006 DOI: 10.1002/14651858.CD003299.pub2

Griffin SL, van Reekum R, Masanic C: A review of cholinergic agents in the treatment of neurobehavioral deficits following traumatic brain injury. J Neuropsychiatry Clin Neurosci 15:17–26, 2003

Huertas D, López-Ibor Aliño JJ, Molina JD, et al: Antiaggressive effect of cyproterone versus haloperidol in Alzheimer's disease: a randomized double-blind pilot study. J Clin Psychiatry 68:439–444, 2007

Kim E, Lauterbach EC, Reeve A, et al: Neuropsychiatric complications of traumatic brain injury: a critical review of the literature (a report by the ANPA Committee on Research). J Neuropsychiatry Clin Neurosci 19:106–127, 2007

Langlois Orman JA, Kraus JF, Zaloshnja E, et al: Epidemiology, in Textbook of Traumatic Brain Injury, 2nd Edition. Edited by Silver JM, McAllister TW, Yudofsky SC. Washington, DC, American Psychiatric Publishing, 2011, pp 3–22

Michals ML, Crismon ML, Roberts S, et al: Clozapine response and adverse effects in nine brain-injured patients. J Clin Psychopharmacol 13:198–203, 1993

Tateno A, Jorge RE, Robinson RG: Clinical correlates of aggressive behaviour after traumatic brain injury. J Neuropsychiatry Clin Neurosci 15:155–160, 2003

Volavka J, Czobor P, Nolan K, et al: Overt aggression and psychotic symptoms in patients with schizophrenia treated with clozapine, olanzapine, risperidone, or haloperidol. J Clin Psychopharmacol 24:225–228, 2004

Disinhibition Mistaken for Mania

Andrew K. Howard, M.D., F.R.C.P.C.

A 58-year-old right-handed man approached the left-hand turn lane. His wife expected that he would wait for the intersection to clear before cautiously proceeding with the turn, just as he had done for the last 35 years. This time was different. Despite a large moving van barreling toward them from the opposite direction, he thought that he could beat the oncoming traffic and proceeded through the intersection. This decision resulted in a collision, and the man and his wife were taken to the emergency room.

The emergency room physician was comfortable sending the couple home with their minor injuries. Significant concerns remained, however, about the husband's mental state. His family doctor had prescribed gabapentin 300 mg bid as a mild sedative the week prior after observing the man behaving strangely and being told by the man's wife about other behavior occurring over the preceding months that had concerned her. For example, the man had laughed childishly while getting his blood pressure checked, and he confabulated about recent world events. He had been more irritable with his wife and tireless in his sexual advances toward her. He had bitten the family dog. He had appeared more indifferent about work and hobbies.

The emergency psychiatry service referred him for neuropsychiatric evaluation for possible poststroke mania. He disclosed surfing Internet pornography sites, engaging the services of prostitutes, and consuming more alcohol than usual. He also endorsed a new habit of gambling in the casino. A reliable employee for 25 years, he had been encouraged to take early retirement from work after making inappropriate jokes with colleagues.

He was well educated and well respected. He endorsed three premorbid lapses of judgment. The first was an affair early in his marriage that lasted 3 months. The second was smoking for 20 years until he had a heart attack 10 years prior to referral. The third was driving while intoxicated on a number of occasions. On average, he had consumed 4–6 pints of beer per week until 2 years prior to presentation. At that time, he had suffered his first stroke, which manifested suddenly with a left hemiparesis (involving face, arm, and leg). Computed tomography demonstrated an infarction in the posterior limb of the right internal capsule, felt to be due to hypertensive small vessel disease. After several months, he had returned to work. When carefully questioned, he reported that he had begun using the Internet to solicit prostitutes a year prior to his first stroke.

One year prior to presentation, he had suffered his second stroke. He slumped over in the living room, reportedly without losing consciousness. There was some associated facial twitching, and his mild residual left-sided weakness was exacerbated. A new lesion was seen in the genu of the right internal capsule.

Noting a loss of motivation, his family physician prescribed paroxetine 3 months after this stroke, without any perceived benefit. This apathy was unaccompanied by low mood or anhedonia, sleep disturbance, or appetite disturbance. In fact, he affirmed feeling better than he had ever felt, but he denied ideomotor pressure, a decreased need for sleep, or an increase in energy or productivity. He was periodically irritable, but never grandiose, and he denied any acute or subacute alteration in his mental content. There was no history of violence, illicit drug use, psychosis, or anxiety.

Neurological and psychiatric review of systems was otherwise negative. General review of systems revealed intermittent abdominal cramping and a weight gain (presumed due to increased alcohol intake) of 20 pounds over the previous year.

His health history included one myocardial infarction, long-standing hypertension, hypercholesterolemia, gastroesophageal reflux disease, and asthma. He had recently been diagnosed with iron deficiency anemia (colonoscopy negative) due to hemorrhoidal bleeding. He was hepatitis B and C negative and HIV negative. He had never had a seizure, thyroid irregularity, or TBI.

Medications on admission to the neuropsychiatry unit included quetiapine 400 mg qhs, valproic acid 250 mg qam and 1,000 mg qhs, ferrous gluconate 300 mg/day, atorvastatin 20 mg qhs, rabeprazole 20 mg qhs, quinapril

10 mg/day, salbutamol and Symbicort (budesonide/formoterol fumarate dihydrate) inhalers, clopidogrel 75 mg/day, and aspirin 81 mg/day. The patient had smoked a quarter of a pack of cigarettes a day for 20 years.

Family history was negative for psychiatric and neurological conditions, including alcohol dependence. The patient's father had had asthma and died of heart disease at the age of 65. His mother lived well into her 80s and died 6 months after his first stroke.

He had been born in Sri Lanka, the youngest of six children. One-half of the sibship eventually immigrated to North America. Birth and development were reportedly normal. His father was a politician, a stern but compassionate man. He described his mother as an affectionate, soft-spoken homemaker. He disaffirmed a history of physical, emotional, or sexual abuse. He perceived himself as the spoiled youngest child in the family, but did not describe any persisting maladaptive personality traits. He performed well in school and did not experience attention or learning difficulties. After completing high school, he enrolled in a postgraduate business program, leaving before graduation to pursue a new direction overseas. He was an avid soccer player and athlete. He met his wife, also Sri Lankan, at his first work placement upon arriving in Canada. There was no reported sexual dysfunction in the marriage. He disaffirmed a personal history of irregular sexual drive and altered sexual functioning. He had never had problems with the law.

On mental status examination, he presented as an alert, oriented, and accessible historian. The reliability of his history was questionable due to limited insight into his personality change. Rapport was established with ease. He was aloof but not strikingly apathetic. He demonstrated interpersonal disinhibition with loud laughter and periodic belching. He was organized in his responses and actions. There was appropriate eye contact and no involuntary movements. Speech was normal in rate and prosody but overly loud. He disaffirmed subjective psychomotor acceleration. Thought form was coherent and goal oriented. He demonstrated inappropriate jocularity given the circumstances and the potential impact on his career and family. There was no pathological laughing or crying. He was not objectively anxious, depressed, or irritable. He scored 10/63 on the Beck Depression Inventory—Second Edition (minimal depression), with fatigue, worries about his physical condition, and shame being prominent responses. Mental content was negative for delusions, somatizations, obsessions, and suicidal and homicidal ideation. There were no perceptual abnormalities. Judgment and self-control were grossly impaired. He minimized responsibility for his actions, citing an involuntary increased need for sexual contact with women, and endorsing disbelief over some of his behaviors while grinning fatuously.

On a screen of cognitive-intellectual functions, his digit span was 6 forward and 5 backward. He scored 15/20 on the Brief Test of Attention, putting him in the 25th–74th percentile for his age. On the Three Words–Three Shapes memory test, uncued recall at 5 minutes was 3/3 shapes and 2/3 words, increasing to 3/3 with forced choice. He could double numbers up to 1,024, but he made impulsive errors during calculations and while drawing a three-dimensional cube. He produced the names of 14 animals in 1 minute, with two perseverative errors. Comprehension, naming, reading, writing, repetition, and fluency were intact. There was no apraxia. He scored 16/18 on the Frontal Assessment Battery, losing 2 points for concrete interpretations of similarities.

On neurological examination, his cranium was normocephalic and atraumatic. Neck was supple. Cranial nerve examination was unremarkable with the exception of bilateral arcus senilis and left central facial weakness, characterized by widening of the palpebral fissure and deepening of the nasolabial fold. Motor examination revealed a mild left pronator drift and decreased fine motor movements and rapid alternating movements of the left hand, in the absence of any pathological change in bulk or power. Tone was mildly spastic on the left. Reflexes were brisk on the left. Plantar responses were flexor. Results of sensory examination, including cortical sensory signs and visual fields, were unremarkable. Testing of station and coordination yielded normal findings. Gait was characterized by mild left hip flexion delay and circumduction of the left leg.

General examination revealed normal vital signs and an absence of head and neck, cardiorespiratory, abdominal, musculoskeletal, and dermatological findings.

Serology included CBC and differential, electrolytes, fasting blood sugar, renal function, thyroid function, liver function, liver enzymes, calcium, magnesium, ammonia, vitamin B_{12}, prolactin, free testosterone, rapid plasma reagin (RPR) and fluorescent treponemal antibody–absorption (FTA-ABS) for syphilis, and HIV. All results were unremarkable.

An electroencephalogram showed normal findings, as did single-photon emission computed tomography (SPECT) brain scans 2 and 3 years after his behavior change. Computed tomography head scans at 1, 2, 3, 4, and 7 years following the behavior change showed progressive enlargement of frontal sulci and the frontal horns of the lateral ventricles (see Figure 1–4). Unequivocal frontal atrophy was first detected in the third scan.

Magnetic resonance imaging (MRI) head scan 4 years following the behavior change demonstrated infarcts in the right posterior limb of the internal capsule, extending into the anterior thalamus, and a lacunar infarct in the right cerebellar hemisphere. There were multiple areas of T2-weighted hyperintensity in the deep and superficial white matter,

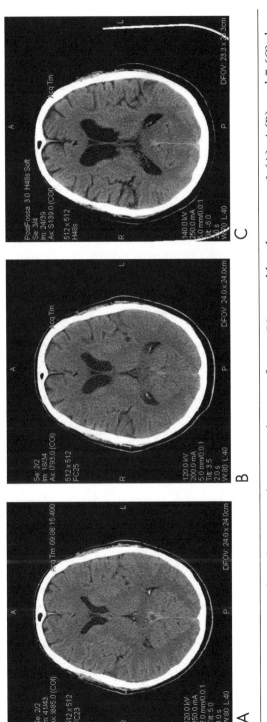

FIGURE 1–4. Sequential axial computed tomography scans from a 58-year-old male at years 1 (A), 4 (B), and 7 (C) demonstrating progressive volume loss with widening of the frontotemporal sulci and expansion of the frontal horns of the lateral ventricles.

Wallerian degeneration of the right cerebral peduncle and pons, and moderate frontotemporal cortical tissue loss, also involving mesial temporal regions (see Figure 1–5).

Neuropsychological data acquired 3 years following the behavior change are presented in Figure 1–6. A comprehensive battery revealed a significant decline from estimated premorbid intelligence. Executive functioning was severely impaired, as were some aspects of memory and language, but visuospatial functioning appeared relatively preserved.

Behavioral stabilization was attempted with antimanic agents. Lithium caused asterixis and concentration difficulties and did not improve impulsivity. Valproic acid was similarly ineffective. Clonazepam caused ataxia. Antipsychotics (risperidone, ziprasidone) led to worsening of agitation, although quetiapine later in the course of his illness had helpful calming and antilibidinal effects. Unfortunately, he gained 60 pounds over 3 years on quetiapine, increasing his risk of morbidity. He was consequently maintained with the minimum effective dosage of quetiapine (400 mg/day) after topiramate and sibutramine were ineffectual in promoting weight loss. Citalopram was introduced to limit erections and libido after paroxetine and sertraline failed at low doses and caused adverse effects at higher doses. Nabilone, dextroamphetamine, and naltrexone were all ineffective for behavioral control. Cyproterone was unequivocally successful in reducing unwanted sexual behaviors. Behavioral strategies, such as rewarding self-control and negatively reinforcing inappropriate behaviors, were ineffective. The most effective interventions for behavioral problems were the provision of a 1:1 caregiver in the home and the appointment of a power of attorney to control his finances.

Shortly after discharge from the neuropsychiatric unit, following an inpatient stay of 4 months, he resumed smoking and escalated his alcohol consumption. He also managed to engage in premeditated indiscretions, despite having lost access to a driver's license and a car. He gambled excessively, losing up to $70,000. The couple was forced to remortgage their home. He was almost left behind on a cruise while drinking at a bar in one of the ports. On one occasion, he nearly fell off a balcony while trying to elope from his home. He repeatedly attempted to secure funds through obtaining credit cards or lines of credit, often successfully. He would then buy items on impulse, such as a laptop computer. He admitted to stealing chocolates and eating them in the store. He experienced hyperphagia not solely attributable to medication effects.

His interpersonal conduct deteriorated. He solicited his wife's friends to go on dates and phoned her colleagues for sex. He blew kisses at professionals and neighbors, asked women if he could rape them, and masturbated in front of his tenant and on one occasion his grandchildren. He frequently im-

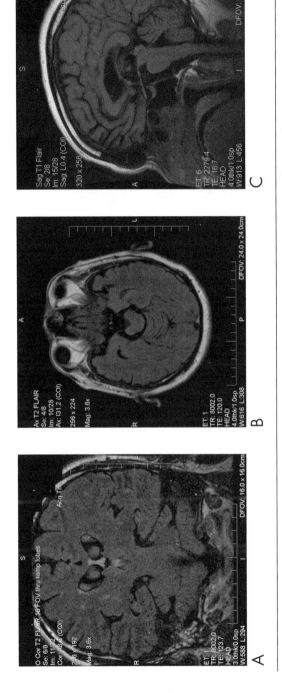

FIGURE 1-5. FLAIR (fluid-attenuated inversion recovery) coronal (A), axial (B), and sagittal (C) magnetic resonance images from the patient whose scan is shown in Figure 1–4 demonstrating multiple areas of hyperintensity in the deep and superficial white matter (A) and moderate frontotemporal cortical tissue loss (B, C), also involving mesial temporal regions.

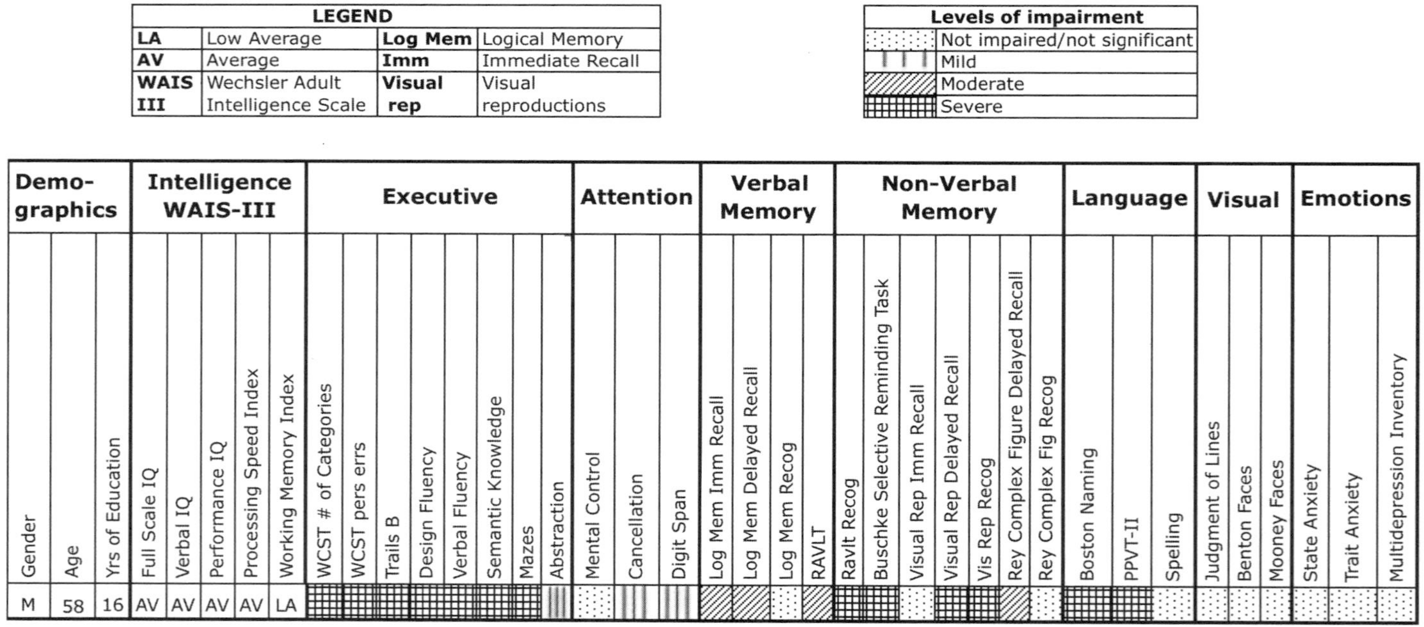

LEGEND

LA	Low Average	Log Mem	Logical Memory	
AV	Average	Imm	Immediate Recall	
WAIS	Wechsler Adult	Visual	Visual	
III	Intelligence Scale	rep	reproductions	

Levels of impairment

	Not impaired/not significant
	Mild
	Moderate
	Severe

Demo-graphics			Intelligence WAIS-III					Executive								Attention			Verbal Memory					Non-Verbal Memory						Language			Visual			Emotions		
Gender	Age	Yrs of Education	Full Scale IQ	Verbal IQ	Performance IQ	Processing Speed Index	Working Memory Index	WCST # of Categories	WCST pers errs	Trails B	Design Fluency	Verbal Fluency	Semantic Knowledge	Mazes	Abstraction	Mental Control	Cancellation	Digit Span	Log Mem Imm Recall	Log Mem Delayed Recall	Log Mem Recog	RAVLT	Ravlt Recog	Buschke Selective Reminding Task	Visual Rep Imm Recall	Visual Rep Delayed Recall	Vis Rep Recog	Rey Complex Figure Delayed Recall	Rey Complex Fig Recog	Boston Naming	PPVT-II	Spelling	Judgment of Lines	Benton Faces	Mooney Faces	State Anxiety	Trait Anxiety	Multidepression Inventory
M	58	16	AV	AV	AV	AV	LA																															

FIGURE 1–6.   Data from a neuropsychological test battery for the patient whose scans are shown in Figures 1–4 and 1–5.

portuned his caregiver to take him to see prostitutes. Eventually, the combination of an antiandrogen, an antipsychotic, an antidepressant, and progressive apathy limited his desire to pursue sexual relations.

He became more inflexible and distractible, unable to sit at the dinner table for short periods. There was no major short-term memory failure (making the frontal variant of Alzheimer's disease improbable), although he reported more forgetfulness in terms of misplacing items. He developed urinary urge incontinence. He had a third strokelike episode, manifesting with vertigo and ataxia, and worsening of left hemiparesis. A new lesion in the right superior cerebellar hemisphere was imaged on CT scan. This event did not significantly impact his behavioral presentation. Three elopements associated with high-risk behavior precipitated short involuntary psychiatric hospitalizations. During one of these, he managed to escape from a locked ward.

The profile of early, persistent, progressive, and predominant behavioral features (especially social disinhibition, but also elation and altered eating behavior), progressive frontotemporal atrophy on neuroimaging, and severe compromise of executive functions on neuropsychological testing supported the diagnosis of behavioral variant frontotemporal dementia (bvFTD).

Discussion

This case illustrates, among other issues, the challenge in dissociating hypomania and disinhibition in neuropsychiatric conditions. Hypomania and disinhibition may represent overlapping syndromes involving the same neural circuitry (Nagaratnam et al. 2006). Lesions involving the subcortical-orbitofrontal and basotemporal-amygdala circuits, particularly in the right hemisphere, are more often associated with mania after stroke (Shulman 1997). The patient's lesion location in the right internal capsule extending into the thalamus could have potentially resulted in mania or disinhibition by disrupting these orbitofrontal-subcortical-limbic circuits. However, sexually disinhibited behaviors had surfaced a year prior to his first stroke and then progressed insidiously, which is more in keeping with a neurodegenerative process than a mood disorder. It is still likely that the stroke was an exacerbating factor. Subjective mood elevation (endorsed by this patient) has been observed in bvFTD (Piguet et al. 2011), which is considered one of the causes of secondary mania (Mendez 2000). Grandiosity and a decreased need for sleep were absent in this case.

Recent studies suggest that determining the presence of apathy and assessing social cognition, such as limited empathy and theory of mind ability, may aid in an earlier diagnosis of frontotemporal dementia. The incapacity to attribute mental states to oneself and to others or to represent others' intentions and beliefs may correlate with early degeneration of anterior medial frontal lobe structures or ventromedial frontopolar cortex (Adenzato et al. 2010). Neuroimaging (Toney et al. 2011) and neuropsychological data may help establish the diagnosis, but these data may become definitively abnormal only after several years of behavior change.

Treatment of bvFTD remains largely supportive at present, using environmental modifications, education, and symptom-based pharmacotherapy (serotonergic antidepressants for aggression, apathy, rigidity, "hypersexuality," and obsessive-compulsive behaviors such as hoarding; and antipsychotics for delusions, aggression, and disinhibition). However, there is active research into potential disease-modifying therapies, such as those that modulate tau protein (Rabinovici and Miller 2010). Several trials of memantine are also under way. Hypersexuality in neuropsychiatric conditions (Krueger and Kaplan 2000) can be a challenge to treat, but numerous options are available to clinicians (Guay 2008), as demonstrated in this case.

Key Clinical Points

- Hypomania and disinhibition may be challenging presentations to dissociate. Key discriminating features of hypomania typically include acute or subacute onset and episodic nature of mental status changes, and the presence of psychomotor acceleration, grandiosity, and a decreased need for sleep.
- Hypomania and disinhibition are both dangerous to the affected individual, who is often unable to appreciate what is happening, and to caregivers and others.
- Disinhibition and impulsive behavior may be very difficult to control with medications and behavior modification approaches, and may respond more reliably to environmental modifications.
- Pharmacological interventions in behavioral variant frontotemporal dementia may help with specific symptoms such as hypersexuality, attentional failure, and agitation.
- Frontotemporal dementia remains predominantly a clinical diagnosis during life, with neuroimaging and neuropsychological data assisting with diagnostic confidence.

Further Readings

Krueger RB, Kaplan MS: Disorders of sexual impulse control in neuropsychiatric conditions. Semin Clin Neuropsychiatry 5:266–274, 2000

Piguet O, Homberger M, Mioshi E, et al: Behavioural-variant frontotemporal dementia: diagnosis, clinical staging, and management. Lancet Neurol 10:162–172, 2011

Shulman K: Disinhibition syndromes, secondary mania and bipolar disorder in old age. J Affect Disord 46:175–182, 1997

References

Adenzato M, Cavallo M, Enrici I: Theory of mind ability in the behavioural variant of frontotemporal dementia: an analysis of the neural, cognitive, and social levels. Neuropsychologia 48:2–12, 2010

Guay DR: Inappropriate sexual behaviors in cognitively impaired older individuals. Am J Geriatr Pharmacother 6:269–288, 2008

Krueger RB, Kaplan MS: Disorders of sexual impulse control in neuropsychiatric conditions. Semin Clin Neuropsychiatry 5:266–274, 2000

Mendez M: Mania in neurological disorders. Curr Psychiatry Rep 2:140–145, 2000

Nagaratnam N, Wong K, Patel I: Secondary mania of vascular origin in elderly patients: a report of two clinical cases. Arch Gerontol Geriatr 43:223–232, 2006

Piguet O, Homberger M, Mioshi E, et al: Behavioural-variant frontotemporal dementia: diagnosis, clinical staging, and management. Lancet Neurol 10:162–172, 2011

Rabinovici GD, Miller BL: Frontotemporal lobar degeneration: epidemiology, pathophysiology, diagnosis and management. CNS Drugs 24:375–398, 2010

Shulman K: Disinhibition syndromes, secondary mania and bipolar disorder in old age. J Affect Disord 46:175–182, 1997

Toney LK, McCue TJ, Minoshima S, et al: Nuclear medicine imaging in dementia: a practical overview for hospitalists. Hosp Pract 39:149–160, 2011

APATHY

Apathy

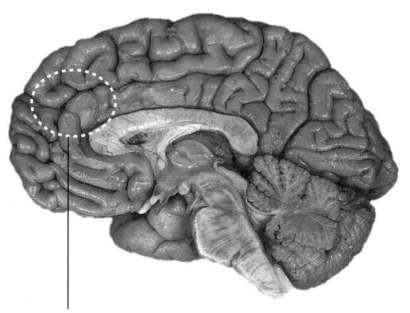

Medial Prefrontal
Region

Introduction

Psychomotor slowing is a common neuropsychiatric presentation seen within the context of depression. More profound states present with gross motivational failure and a seeming absence of all, or almost all, self-initiated motor activity, a psychobehavioral state known as *apathy*. The extreme form is termed *abulia*. In the presence of known brain injury, depression should always be considered diagnostically and treated energetically. The critical neuroanatomical structure is the medial prefrontal region. Multiple neurotransmitters systems are involved.

Apathy in Frontal Lobe Injury

Marius Dimov, M.D., F.R.C.P.C.

A 45-year-old right-handed man was referred for neuropsychiatric assessment regarding his ongoing issues with apathy, irritability, and difficulties with cognitive-intellectual functions after a resection of a central neurocytoma, which was done 1 year before the assessment. Before the onset of his illness, he worked as a computer engineer and software programmer for a construction business. He had a stable family environment (with three school-age children) and a supportive wife.

Two years prior to neuropsychiatric assessment, he was seen by a neurologist for new onset of headaches. Workup eventually led to magnetic resonance imaging (MRI) of the head, which demonstrated the presence of a mass arising in the body of the left lateral ventricle, consistent with a central neurocytoma causing obstructive hydrocephalus. He was seen by a neurosurgeon, who performed an endoscopic biopsy and placed two ventriculoperitoneal shunts. Pathology confirmed the diagnosis of a low-grade central neurocytoma. After surgery he had a complete resolution of his headaches and had no cognitive-intellectual or motor problems.

Later that year, his headache returned. He was assessed by another neurosurgeon, and the decision was made to resect the tumor. His postoperative course was difficult and complicated by hypothalamic and thalamic infarcts, bilateral frontal hygromas, and a postoperative central nervous system infection leading to a comatose state. He required a 2-week stay in an intensive care unit and a prolonged hospitalization. His postoperative course was complicated by seizures, which were controlled by anticonvulsants. He gradually improved and 2 months later was able to ambulate, communicate, and feed himself. He underwent 1 month of rehabilitation in a specialized setting. At discharge he was able to function at home under supervision. Before rehabilitation his Montreal Cognitive Assessment (MoCA) score was 13/30; this eventually improved to 21/30. Ongoing problems included difficulties with attention and orientation and severe deficits with short-term recall.

One year after surgery, his main issues were his behavioral and cognitive-intellectual deficits. Premorbidly he was a very energetic person. After surgery he was slow and looked uninterested in the tasks that he was performing. The most disturbing change for his wife was his lack of interaction with his children. He was less spontaneous and much less engaging in his interactions with them. For instance, he would only help the children with their morning routines if asked. He was also notably less verbal, using only short sentences and "yes/no" answers. He showed an atypical short temper, with a lowered threshold for yelling at the children. Although there was no physical violence, his anger outbursts were very sudden and completely out of character and very disturbing for his family.

He was conscious of his anger outbursts and experienced remorse after the fact. He was also more emotional than he used to be. However, he denied depressive symptoms, stating that he did not experience low energy, anhedonia, or suicidal thoughts. He also disaffirmed any changes in his appetite, weight, or sleep. He was not excessively anxious and did not endorse any psychotic experiences. He spent hours on the computer, and although he was not being productive, he found the activity enjoyable. His short-term memory was impaired. He often forgot new faces and new images. He had a scheduler but would often forget to consult it. He used an alarm on his wrist to remind him to take his medications.

His previous medical history was significant only for hypertension, a phenytoin allergy, and a cefazolin allergy. There was no psychiatric history or history of alcohol or substance abuse, and there was no family history of psychiatric illness. His mother died at age 74 from colon cancer. His father was alive and had Parkinson's disease.

On physical examination his blood pressure was 120/80 mm Hg. Cranial nerve examination findings were unremarkable. He had mild right-sided weakness. Strength was grade 5/5 on the left and 4+/5 on the right. He had no pronator drift. Tone and reflexes were mildly increased in the right upper and lower extremities. Coordination was within normal range. His gait was normal.

On mental status examination, he presented as a calm male, looking his stated age. He demonstrated bradykinesia and bradyphrenia. There was no evidence of agitation or disinhibition. He did not initiate conversation and spoke only when addressed. His speech showed a small but significant delay in response, with decreased prosody. His affect was restricted but not dysphoric. Overall his affect appeared flat and he appeared apathetic. Thought form was concrete but goal directed. Thought content showed no delusional thinking and no suicidal or homicidal ideation. There was no report of auditory or visual hallucinations. His insight about his apathy was partial, but he was fully aware of his memory problems. When asked why he was not engaging with his children, he said, "I don't want to interrupt their game."

A cognitive-intellectual examination using the MoCA yielded a score of 21/30, with 0/5 on delayed verbal recall (3/5 with cues, suggesting, at least in part, a problem with retrieval rather than encoding), and a digit span of 6 forward and 3 backward. He had no difficulty with abstraction or visuospatial function, but he reversed the hands of a clock on the subtest for executive functioning. His naming, repetition, reading, comprehension, and writing tasks displayed no obvious deficits. Severe impairments in executive function and verbal and nonverbal memory were noted on formal neuropsychological examination (Figure 2–1).

Results of laboratory studies, including complete blood count and differential, electrolytes, liver and renal chemistries, thyroid testing, fasting blood sugar, and urinalysis, were normal. Postoperative follow-up computed tomography and MRI showed no changes over time and demonstrated postsurgical encephalomalacia within the right frontal lobe and stable calcification along the lateral aspect of the left lateral ventricle (Figures 2–2 and 2–3). There was also increased T2/FLAIR (fluid-attenuated inversion recovery) signal intensity along the medial aspect of the left thalamus (not shown) consistent with his known intraoperative injuries.

He was started on dextroamphetamine 5 mg qam, which was progressively increased to 20 mg. This helped his apathy and bradyphrenia. He became more motivated and interactive with his family. He was able to make and then follow lists of regular activities involving his children and of household chores that were his responsibility. His wife was needed initially to assist with compliance, but later he required no help. His functioning improved, but he was not capable of returning to any form of work. Approximately 6 months later he had a generalized tonic-clonic seizure lasting 2–3 minutes. He was started on levetiracetam 500 mg bid and remained seizure free subsequently.

Discussion

Prefrontal lobe injuries and the associated deficits are well described in the literature. The medial frontal cortex, orbitofrontal cortex, and dorso-

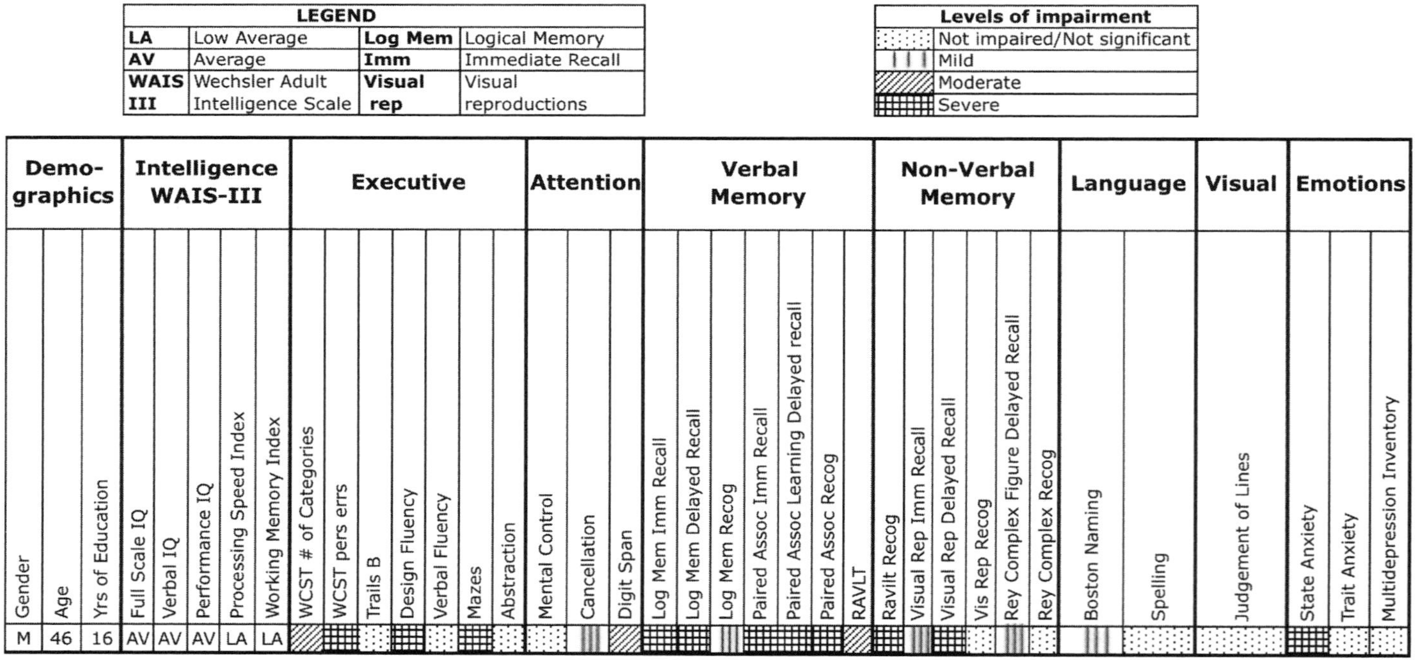

FIGURE 2–1. Data from a neuropsychological test battery for a 46-year-old male with apathy.

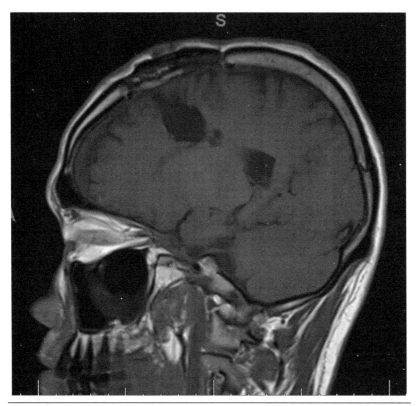

FIGURE 2–2. T1-weighted sagittal magnetic resonance image showing area of postsurgical encephalomalacia in the medial aspect of the right frontal lobe.

lateral prefrontal cortex are three main anatomical areas associated with specific syndromes (Lichter and Cummings 2001; Miller and Cummings 1999). Damage to the medial frontal cortex can lead to apathetic states, whereas damage to the orbitofrontal cortex is characterized by interpersonal disinhibition, poor social judgment, impulsive decision making, lack of consideration for the impact of behavior on others, and lack of empathy. Executive functioning deficits are commonly associated with injury to the dorsolateral prefrontal cortex (Lichter and Cummings 2001; Miller and Cummings 1999).

Apathy is the most prevalent neuropsychiatric presentation in patients with acquired brain injury (ABI). In a recent study, 43% of ABI patients suffered from apathy (Ciurli et al. 2011). Other symptoms of ABI (and their prevalence) include irritability (37%), dysphoria (29%), disinhibition (28%), appetite/eating disturbance (27%), and agitation/aggression

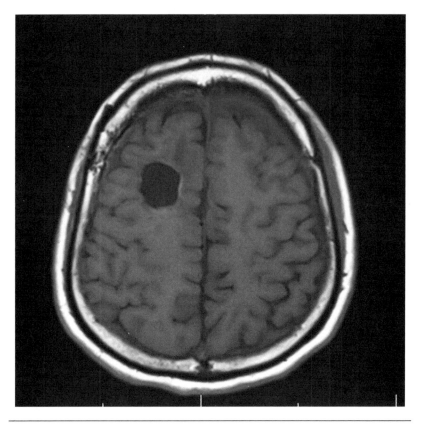

FIGURE 2–3. T1-weighted axial magnetic resonance image showing area of postsurgical encephalomalacia in the medial aspect of the right frontal lobe.

(24%) (Ciurli et al. 2011). Severe apathy is categorized as *abulia*. When the abulia is extreme, movement and speech cease, producing akinetic mutism, which is characterized by a total absence of spontaneous behavior and speech but preserved visual tracking (Marin and Wilkosz 2005).

The differential diagnosis of an apathetic state includes delirium, dementia, depression, demoralization, akinesia, catatonia, and aprosodia. Delirium is primarily due to an acute failure of attention and is associated with an abnormal electroencephalogram. Dementia usually follows a slowly progressive course, which may ultimately end in a state of apathy but the etiology is understood (Chase 2011; Marin and Wilkosz 2005). By contrast, the possibility of depression in patients with known brain injury is always a diagnostic challenge since it is frequently difficult to determine whether a state of apathy is due to the known intrinsic and irreversible structural brain injury or to a reversible failure of brain function as a result of a primary mood disorder.

Several clinical features may help with this distinction. Depression usually includes an affective component (including tearfulness, sadness, and an inhibited capacity for pleasure and joy) and a negative view of oneself and one's present and future. In comparison, affective symptoms are typically absent in patients with an apathetic syndrome (Marin and Wilkosz 2005). Patients with apathy in the absence of depression tend to be motivated when activities are suggested to them, whereas depressed patients are more globally apathetic. The combined use of an apathy scale, such as the Apathy Evaluation Scale (AES) (Glenn 2005), and a standardized depression scale (Andersson et al. 1999) can be helpful, because higher scores on the AES with lower scores on a depression scale point toward the separate phenomenon of apathy. Another useful scale to differentiate between apathy and depression is the Neuropsychiatric Inventory (Cummings et al. 1994); this scale is beneficial in assessing functional deficits and includes apathy items.

The conditions associated with apathy, abulia, and akinetic mutism form an extensive list (Chase 2011; Marin and Wilkosz 2005). Neurological diseases that injure cortico-striato-pallido-thalamic circuits are common causes of apathy and include traumatic brain injury, frontotemporal dementia tumors, infarcts, movement disorders, and multiple sclerosis.

Pharmacological approaches to improve motivation target the dopaminergic, glutamatergic, noradrenergic, and cholinergic systems. In contrast, serotonin and gamma-aminobutyric acid (GABA)–enhancing medications may have a negative effect and worsen apathy (Chase 2011; Lichter and Cummings 2001; Marin and Wilkosz 2005; Miller and Cummings 1999). There are no approved medications for apathetic syndromes and no proof of efficacy for any of the drugs in current use. Benefit has been obtained from various dopaminergic agents (amantadine, bromocriptine, selegiline, carbidopa-levodopa, pergolide, and pramipexole), cholinergic compounds (donepezil, galantamine, rivastigmine), stimulants (dextroamphetamine, methylphenidate, modafinil), and activating antidepressants (bupropion, tranylcypromine, protriptyline, venlafaxine, and sertraline) (Chase 2011; Lichter and Cummings 2001; Marin and Wilkosz 2005). Depression, if present, needs to be treated, but one should bear in mind that some antidepressants (selective serotonin reuptake inhibitors [SSRIs]) will worsen organically based apathy. It is also important to limit or reduce doses of antipsychotics because they also may worsen apathy (Marin and Wilkosz 2005). Finally, any medical conditions that could exacerbate fatigue (e.g., anemia or endocrine dysfunction) should be optimally treated.

Family and caregivers need to be involved in the care of these patients. They require education about the patient's condition so that they do not accuse the patient of lacking effort. Behavioral strategies and environmental changes should be implemented to promote and facilitate motivation. Strategies include specific and clear instructions, a system of rewards, positive stimulation, and persistent cuing and redirection. Socialization should be encouraged, and new sources of pleasure, interest, and stimulation should be introduced because novelty and positive outcomes promote the initiation of activity. For many patients, returning to the familiar personal and physical circumstances of their homes may be the fastest way to a healthier physical and social environment. Attention must also be paid to sensorimotor deficits, which can be minimized by adaptive devices such as motorized wheelchairs, voice-activated computers, and other methods of enhancing autonomy.

The diagnostic formulation in this case was that the patient had an organically caused apathetic state with cognitive-intellectual compromise arising from brain injuries sustained intraoperatively. There was no evidence of a confounding depression. The psychobehavioral affiliations of the visualized lesions, which included the right prefrontal cortex and cingulum, provided an explanatory anatomical substrate for his problems with apathy, irritability, and deficits in attention, memory, and executive functioning. The role of amphetamines in provoking his seizure was raised. The risk is, however, mostly theoretical, with very little evidence in the literature, and was outweighed by the substantial benefit that he had obtained from dextroamphetamine. Moreover, he had been taking dextroamphetamine for 6 months before he had the breakthrough seizure, a fact that casts doubt on its role (if any) in causing the seizure.

Key Clinical Points

- Frontal lobe injury frequently presents as an apathetic syndrome.
- Depression may be a comorbid factor and should be treated. The differentiation of depression from organically based apathy can be aided by a detailed clinical assessment and use of the Apathy Evaluation Scale (or another apathy scale) and a standardized depression scale.
- Treatment of apathy involves a combination of nonpharmacological strategies and the use of dopaminergic and other activating psychotropic medications.
- Antipsychotics and selective serotonin reuptake inhibitors should be avoided because they may make apathy worse.

Further Readings

Chase TN: Apathy in neuropsychiatric disease: diagnosis, pathophysiology, and treatment. Neurotox Res 19:266–278, 2011

Lichter DG, Cummings JL: Frontal-Subcortical Circuits in Psychiatric and Neurological Disorders. New York, Guilford, 2001

Marin RS, Wilkosz PA: Disorders of diminished motivation. J Head Trauma Rehabil 20:377–388, 2005

References

Andersson S, Krogstad JM, Finset A: Apathy and depressed mood in acquired brain damage: relationship to lesion localization and psychophysiological reactivity. Psychol Med 29:447–456, 1999

Chase TN: Apathy in neuropsychiatric disease: diagnosis, pathophysiology, and treatment. Neurotox Res 19:266–278, 2011

Ciurli P, Formisano R, Bivona U, et al: Neuropsychiatric disorders in persons with severe traumatic brain injury: prevalence, phenomenology, and relationship with demographic, clinical, and functional features. J Head Trauma Rehabil 26:116–126, 2011

Cummings JL, Mega M, Gray K, et al: The Neuropsychiatric Inventory. Neurology 44:2308–2314, 1994

Glenn M: The Apathy Evaluation Scale, 2005. Available at: http://www.tbims.org/combi/aes. Accessed August 11, 2012.

Lichter DG, Cummings JL: Frontal-Subcortical Circuits in Psychiatric and Neurological Disorders. New York, Guilford, 2001

Marin RS, Wilkosz PA: Disorders of diminished motivation. J Head Trauma Rehabil 20:377–388, 2005

Miller BL, Cummings JL: The Human Frontal Lobes: Functions and Disorders. New York, Guilford, 1999

DEPRESSION

Depression

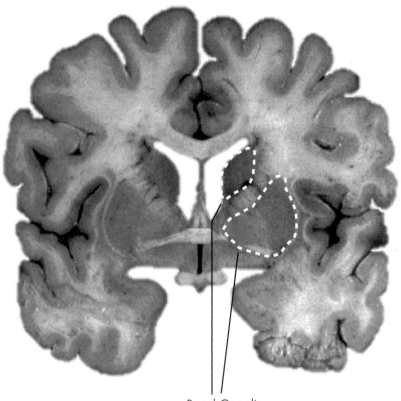

Basal Ganglia

INTRODUCTION

Depression is a frequent occurrence after brain injury of any kind. Depression following brain injury has multiple determinants, which include the location and extent of injury and the psychosocial burden of the underlying neurological condition. In the case of multiple sclerosis, the psychosocial burden is unpredictable, with the ever-present threat of progressive neurological decline or a catastrophic episode of demyelination. Neuroanatomical structures involved include the basal ganglia and anteriorly placed limbic networks. The effect of laterality is now unclear, with recent evidence no longer supporting a higher risk after left-sided injury. Multiple neurotransmitters are involved but include noradrenergic and serotonergic systems, given the response of organic depression to standard antidepressants.

Major Depression and Panic Disorder Following Epilepsy Surgery

Leon Berzen, M.B.B.Ch., F.F.Psych. (S.A.), F.R.C.P.C.
Eugene Wang, M.D., F.R.C.P.C.

A 40-year-old married man with two sons, ages 8 and 11 years, presented for a neuropsychiatric assessment on the advice of his treating epileptologist. The diagnosis of epilepsy had been made approximately 10 years previously while he was on holiday in Florida; the first symptom of epilepsy was a complex partial seizure after he became ill with infectious mononucleosis. He began to experience complex partial seizures approximately once a month, characterized by an initial epigastric aura, followed by behavioral arrest ("stop and stare"). He had occasional secondary generalization with tonic-clonic seizures. Despite numerous trials of anticonvulsants and excellent medication compliance, his seizure control remained suboptimal.

At the time of his assessment, he had not worked for 6 months; he was on recovery leave, having undergone epilepsy surgery 6 months previously. He worked in a senior management position in a private business but had been unable to return to work because his functioning had not yet returned to baseline following the surgery. He had worked in the same position for the preceding 13 years. He had a degree in building technology and was highly regarded by his employers.

He had been seeing his epileptologist on a regular basis following a right anterior temporal lobe resection for the management of his epilepsy. Histologically, there was evidence of cortical dysplasia in the resected brain tissue. His recovery was lagging despite excellent seizure control since his surgery. His epileptologist noted that he was becoming increasingly anxious, irritable, and depressed.

He stated that within a few weeks postoperatively he noted emotional changes, including more irritability and poor motivation. He also felt physically exhausted almost all of the time. He was sleeping excessively but found that he was not refreshed on awakening. He derived little to no pleasure from activities that he had once enjoyed. He was becoming increasingly withdrawn from his wife and children, and his libido had declined markedly.

Prior to his surgery, he had been an active person who kept busy most of the time with work and with numerous outside interests. Although he had worked long hours, he had always made time for his family and had engaged enthusiastically in his sons' extracurricular sporting activities. Postsurgery, all such enthusiasm disappeared. His appetite decreased, and he lost 25 pounds. His concentration was markedly reduced. He reported that he was unable to follow simple television programs, read the newspaper, or attend to his financial affairs. He felt that his memory had also deteriorated.

He was experiencing an increasing sense of demoralization despite having been seizure free since the surgery. At times he would become so discouraged that he contemplated committing suicide by carbon monoxide poisoning.

He also reported experiencing recurrent anxiety attacks up to once or twice a day since the surgery. His description was typical of a classic panic attack, with overwhelming fear and depersonalization lasting up to 20 minutes. He noted that these panic episodes were clearly different from his prior seizure aura experiences.

He had no past psychiatric history, and specifically no prior problems with depression or panic.

His past medical and surgical history was negative. His family history was negative for panic disorder, generalized anxiety disorder, and depression.

He was taking carbamazepine CR 600 mg bid. Serum levels for carbamazepine were therapeutic.

He was a nonsmoker. He consumed alcohol occasionally. There was no history of illicit drug use.

He was born in rural British Columbia. He was the second youngest of four children. He had an older sister who was adopted, a younger biological sister, and an older biological brother. Both his parents were still living. His father was a construction worker and ran his own business.

His birth, early development, and health in childhood were normal. He stated that he was motorically and intellectually advanced for his age. In school he was well socialized and was accomplished in sports. He was involved in junior hockey for 8 years. Following high school he worked with his father for a few years and then attended college, where he studied building technology.

He had never experienced any employment problems and typically made a positive impression on his employers. He married at the age of 27. Although he believed that his marriage of 13 years' duration had always been good, he was concerned that his recent poor health had been putting extra strain on his wife. He believed that she was withdrawing more and becoming increasingly resentful of the extra obligations imposed on her by his incapacity.

Mental status examination at the time of the assessment revealed a healthy-looking male who appeared his stated age. He made good eye contact. He was a reliable informant, and a good rapport was established from the start.

He endorsed a depressed mood, anxiety, excessive sleep, decreased appetite with weight loss, decreased libido, and suicidal ideation. The examination was negative for psychotic symptoms.

Examination of his cognitive-intellectual functions revealed impaired attention. His digit span was 6 forward and 4 backward. He had great difficulty doing the serial 7s test but was able to complete the task. He had no problems with recent verbal and nonverbal memory as assessed by the Three Words–Three Shapes test. He scored 30/30 on the Montreal Cognitive Assessment.

He was diagnosed as having symptoms of a major depression and panic disorder. These symptoms were occurring 6 months after his right temporal lobectomy (Figure 3–1) and in the absence of any breakthrough seizures. There was no evidence of cognitive-intellectual decline, but his functioning had not returned to baseline as would be expected 6 months postsurgery. Carbamazepine was an unlikely cause of his somnolence and anergy, since he had been on this medication before surgery without similar effects. Clinically undetected seizures contributing to his presentation were also excluded as a causal or contributory mechanism after a 72-hour ambulatory electroencephalogram (EEG) revealed no evidence of

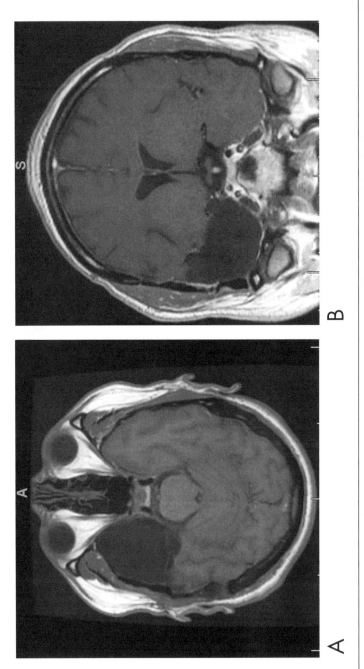

FIGURE 3–1.   T1 axial (A) and coronal (B) magnetic resonance images from a 40-year-old male demonstrating extent of right temporal lobectomy.

ongoing seizure activity. Environmental stressors, which included mild marital strain, were present, but these were viewed as secondary to his protracted and poor postoperative course.

A decision was made to treat him with escitalopram 15 mg/day and to provide supportive psychotherapy weekly. Within 2 months his depressive and anxiety symptoms abated, and within 6 months he had returned to his previous employment without incident. At his last follow-up visit, he reported that he had been successfully weaned off his anticonvulsant, was driving a motor vehicle again, and, in comparison to before surgery, had been working even more productively. He had made a full recovery from his epilepsy and the postoperative complications of major depression and panic disorder.

Discussion

The surgical procedure most commonly performed for epilepsy is an anterior temporal lobe resection, which was done in this case. Following surgery, 60%–70% of patients become seizure free. Other less commonly performed procedures include selective amygdalohippocampectomy and neocortical resections to remove the epileptogenic areas from the lateral temporal neocortex and extratemporal neocortex. Disconnective surgical procedures such as corpus callosotomy are even less common, while functional hemispherectomy is very rarely done in adults.

Persons with epilepsy have a lifetime prevalence of psychiatric morbidity of up to 50% (Altshuler et al. 1999; Kanner and Palac 2000). Those patients with temporal lobe epilepsy have the highest prevalence (Glosser et al. 2000). There is also an approximately 12% increased risk for suicide among patients with epilepsy compared with the general population (Jones et al. 2003).

Patients with temporal lobe seizures are at a higher risk of depression than those with other types of epilepsy. The role of gender is uncertain because higher rates have been reported in both males and females. Neither the age at onset of epilepsy nor the duration of epilepsy appears to influence the risk of developing depression. Evidence for the lateralization of the temporal epileptic focus in depression is inconclusive, with reports supporting both a left and right focus or demonstrating no laterality effect. Antiepileptic medications such as barbiturates, vigabatrin, topiramate, and tiagabine may contribute to depression.

Blumer (1991) found that depressive disorders may be atypical in some patients with epilepsy and that their phenomenology is not captured by the standard classification systems. In epileptic patients with depression that is characterized by intermittent depressed mood, irritability, anxiety, anergia, and insomnia, a more appropriate diagnostic label may be intermittent dysphoric disorder (Blumer et al. 2004).

As in this case, psychiatric symptoms can develop for the first time after surgery. Preexisting depression and anxiety symptoms can also be exacerbated following surgery, raising the question of whether preexisting psychiatric symptoms should be considered a contraindication to surgery. Reassuringly, almost all postoperative psychiatric complications remit when treated with psychotropic medication (Blumer et al. 1998).

The most commonly reported psychiatric complications following epilepsy surgery are mood disorders, with symptoms such as emotional lability and depression. These symptoms are often transient and usually occur in the first 3 months following surgery (Ring et al. 1998). Devinsky and colleagues (2005) conducted a prospective multicenter study of 358 patients who had epilepsy surgery. The patients were followed for up to 2 years using the Beck Depression Inventory, the Beck Anxiety Inventory, the Composite International Diagnostic Interview, and a structured interview schedule. The authors found that the rate of depression decreased significantly by 3 months following surgery and was further reduced to about half the presurgical rate (22.1%) by the end of the 2-year follow-up (11.7%).

Depression has been reported in 24%–38% of patients undergoing epilepsy surgery. Preoperative depression is the strongest predictor of postoperative depression. Persistent seizures postsurgery represent a risk factor for postoperative depression. Thus, improvement of depression is associated with improved seizure control after surgery (Macrodimitris et al. 2011).

Whether patients undergoing left versus right temporal lobe resection are at greater risk of postoperative depression remains controversial. The severity of depressive symptomatology in epilepsy patients who have undergone corrective surgery is correlated with the extent of hippocampal and amygdala resection. This association appears to be more evident in left-sided resections, but overall, psychiatric complications seem to occur more frequently following right temporal lobectomies.

Anxiety may also occur following epilepsy surgery, with prevalence rates between 17% and 54% (Bladin 1992; Wrench et al. 2004). Anxiety is most severe in the first 3 months postoperatively but is significantly reduced by 12–24 months postsurgery. Patients with a past history of affective disorders, including anxiety disorders, are likely to be more susceptible to postoperative anxiety. Patients with temporal lobe epilepsy with ictal fear may be at greater risk of postoperative anxiety and panic attacks despite becoming seizure free.

This case illustrates some of the psychiatric complications associated with temporal lobe epilepsy surgery. Surgical treatment is now a viable option for an increasing number of patients with epilepsy, especially in cases of temporal lobe epilepsy. Psychiatric input will often be needed both pre- and postoperatively to advise about psychiatric risks and to provide treatment.

Key Clinical Points

- Surgical treatment is now a viable option for an increasing number of patients with epilepsy, and in particular those with temporal lobe epilepsy.
- Preoperative depression is the strongest predictor of postoperative depression.
- Improvement of depression is associated with improved seizure control after surgery.
- Anxiety is a common symptom after surgery for seizure control, with prevalence rates between 17% and 54%.
- Postoperative psychiatric complications respond well to treatment with appropriate psychotropic medications.

Further Readings

Blumer D, Wakhlu S, Davies K, et al: Psychiatric outcome of temporal lobectomy for epilepsy: incidence and treatment of psychiatric complications. Epilepsia 39:478–486, 1998

Glosser G, Zwil AS, Glosser DS, et al: Psychiatric aspects of temporal lobe epilepsy before and after anterior temporal lobectomy. J Neurol Neurosurg Psychiatry 68:53–58, 2000

Kanner AM, Palac S: Depression in epilepsy: a common but often unrecognized comorbid malady. Epilepsy Behav 1:37–51, 2000

References

Altshuler L, Rausch R, Delrahim S, et al: Temporal lobe epilepsy, temporal lobectomy, and major depression. J Neuropsychiatry Clin Neurosci 11:436–443, 1999

Bladin PF: Psychosocial difficulties and outcome after temporal lobectomy. Epilepsia 33:898–907, 1992

Blumer D: Epilepsy and disorders of mood. Adv Neurol 55:185–195, 1991

Blumer D, Wakhlu S, Davies K, et al: Psychiatric outcome of temporal lobectomy for epilepsy: incidence and treatment of psychiatric complications. Epilepsia 39:478–486, 1998

Blumer D, Montouris G, Davies K: The interictal dysphoric disorder: recognition, pathogenesis, and treatment of the major psychiatric disorder of epilepsy. Epilepsy Behav 5:826–840, 2004

Devinsky O, Barr WB, Vickrey BG, et al: Changes in depression and anxiety after resective surgery for epilepsy. Neurology 65:1744–1749, 2005

Glosser G, Zwil AS, Glosser DS, et al: Psychiatric aspects of temporal lobe epilepsy before and after anterior temporal lobectomy. J Neurol Neurosurg Psychiatry 68:53–58, 2000

Jones JE, Hermann BP, Barry JJ, et al: Rates and risk factors for suicide, suicidal ideation, and suicide attempts in chronic epilepsy. Epilepsy Behav 4:S31–S38, 2003

Kanner AM, Palac S: Depression in epilepsy: a common but often unrecognized comorbid malady. Epilepsy Behav 1:37–51, 2000

Macrodimitris S, Sherman EMS, Forde S, et al: Psychiatric outcomes of epilepsy surgery: a systematic review. Epilepsia 52:880–890, 2011

Ring HA, Moriarty J, Trimble MR: A prospective study of the early postsurgical psychiatric associations of epilepsy surgery. J Neurol Neurosurg Psychiatry 64:601–604, 1998

Wrench J, Wilson SJ, Bladin PF: Mood disturbance before and after seizure surgery: a comparison of temporal and extratemporal resections. Epilepsia 45:534–543, 2004

Poststroke Depression

Magdalena Ilcewicz-Klimek, M.D., F.R.C.P.C.

A 35-year-old married man and father of two young children was referred for assessment of depression. He had a very busy life as a manager in a small company. He was involved in skiing, surfing, and rock climbing and went to the gym regularly. He had pushed himself physically because his plan was to become a personal trainer and open up his own business to provide greater opportunities for his family. He was in very good health, and there was no history of any psychiatric diseases. He was a nonsmoker and denied substance abuse. He drank alcohol socially. One day, after completing his training routine, which included numerous strenuous exercises, he experienced a sudden headache as he walked out of the gym. He then developed difficulty with his speech and right-sided muscle weakness, which progressed to full hemiparesis and confusion. His friends drove him immediately to the emergency room. When he arrived at the hospital, his vital signs, including blood pressure, were normal. Cranial CT showed a hemorrhage involving the left basal ganglia with extension to the corona radiata and a smaller right caudate and putamen bleed.

Because of his young age, extensive investigations were ordered to rule out any underlying causes. All results were negative, including a screen for vasculitis and hematological abnormalities. A conventional cerebral angiogram was reported as normal, with no evidence of arteriove-nous malformation or aneurysms. He later admitted to regularly taking a supplement with a small amount of ephedrine, purchased from a health food store. The final diagnosis was postexercise hypertensive intracranial hemorrhages, potentially linked to the use of ephedrine.

On examination his initial findings included an expressive aphasia and right-sided hemiplegia. Neurologically his motor recovery was excellent, but despite extensive speech and language therapy, he was left with some deficits in expressive language. Almost immediately after the stroke, he started to experience severe fatigue and problems with cognitive-intellec-tual functioning. He had problems with multitasking, planning, problem solving, and short-term memory. For instance, he reported a compromised ability to organize his tools or to do household repairs. He also found it ex-tremely difficult to play with his children, finding it too exhausting and overstimulating. He had a 3- to 4-hour period of productivity per day and needed to rest or nap for the remainder of the day. He tried to return to his previous managerial work through a gradual return-to-work program but quickly realized that he was unable to function adequately. His wife also noticed a change in his personality, such as his need for considerable en-couragement to initiate tasks and focus on his goals.

At approximately 4 months poststroke, he began to experience a loss in enjoyment of most activities. His mood was low, with no diurnal vari-ation. He became easily tearful and was more irritable, having less pa-tience with his family. He had moderate insomnia but his appetite was unchanged. He lost hope that his life would return to normal and had passive suicidal thoughts that life was not worth living.

He was also trying to deal with the loss of his premorbid function and his dreams for the future, continually comparing himself with his friends. He began to feel inadequate as a husband and a father, blaming himself for his low level of function. Because he showed no overt physical signs of a stroke, his friends and family members thought he had fully recovered and could not understand why he was unable to return to work, continue with his previous activities, or help more with the children at home. His self-esteem was very low. Attempts to push himself to do more simply pro-voked severe exhaustion and the need to rest for the next several days. His family doctor made a diagnosis of depression and prescribed fluoxetine and later sertraline. At 6 months poststroke, with no benefit from either anti-depressant, he was referred for neuropsychiatric assessment.

He presented as a well-groomed man with a mild degree of psychomo-tor retardation. He was frequently tearful during the interview, and his affect was depressed. He reported low mood, anhedonia, and a decreased motivation to participate in activities. He continued to struggle with prominent fatigue and cognitive-intellectual problems. His speech was slow and soft, with goal-directed thought processing. There was no evidence of suicidal ideation or psychosis. He described occasional panic attacks, coupled with anxiety about his family's future due to financial stressors. Neuropsychological testing revealed decreased psychomotor speed, impaired complex executive function, impaired verbal memory, markedly impaired performance on verbal fluency testing, word-finding difficulties with paraphrasic errors, and problems with spelling and reading comprehension. His MRI brain scan showed a large area of left-sided basal ganglia encephalomalacia (Figure 3–2).

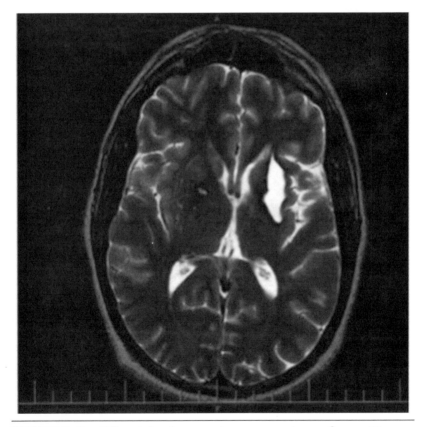

FIGURE 3–2.   T2-weighted magnetic resonance image from a 35-year-old male showing left striatum posthemorrhage encephalomalacia.

Investigations were ordered to rule out causes of his overwhelming fatigue, and included hormonal studies and screens for anemia, vitamin deficiencies, and metabolic disturbances; all results were normal. A sleep study did not show any significant periods of desaturation. His serum ferritin level and fasting iron saturation levels were unexpectedly elevated, which led to further investigations and ultimately confirmed a diagnosis of familial hemochromatosis on the basis of a positive DNA test for the hemochromatosis gene (*HFE*) mutation. There was no evidence of any organ damage due to deposition of excess iron, and he was treated with regular phlebotomies.

A diagnosis of poststroke depression (PSD) was made. He initially had difficulties accepting this diagnosis. The initial intervention was focused on extensive education about depression and its relationship to stroke. Information was also provided about the cognitive-intellectual deficits associated with stroke and their impact on daily function. Understanding the nature of the neuropsychiatric complications due to stroke was a very important step in his treatment. A meeting with his wife was arranged to discuss his diagnosis and treatment plan. He had tried antidepressants before without benefit but admitted to poor compliance with the prescribed medications. He agreed to another trial with an antidepressant, and citalopram was prescribed. The dosage was gradually increased to 40 mg/day. By 8 weeks he reported a significant improvement in his depressive symptoms.

During follow-up appointments, treatment focused on helping him adjust to his functional limitations and improving his self-esteem. He learned to set more realistic goals and to incorporate regular frequent rest periods during his daily schedule. He continued to have problems with motivation, and having a daily structured routine proved helpful. Once he started to accomplish some tasks, his confidence level improved. His wife became more supportive when she better understood the nature of his problems, and their relationship improved significantly.

Despite great improvement in his mood, anxiety, and self-esteem, he continued to experience executive dysfunction with prominent difficulties with problem solving, planning, and organization of tasks. He continued to have severe fatigue and problems with task initiation. Further increases in the dose of citalopram had no effect on these symptoms. Repeat neuropsychological testing done 10 months after the initial evaluation showed no evidence of improvement. Possible causes of his persistent symptoms included residual PSD, poststroke fatigue, fatigue related to hemochromatosis, and poststroke apathy and executive dysfunction.

Discussion

Apathy is a debilitating complication of cerebrovascular disease (CVD) or stroke, with prevalence rates of up to 25% (Bhatia and Marsden 1994; Jorge et al. 2010; Robinson and Starkstein 2010). Apathy occurs independently or in the context of depression and is linked, as in this case, to injury to the frontal-subcortical circuits. Apathy is more frequent in patients who also present with some degree of cognitive-intellectual impairment. Bilateral basal ganglia strokes in particular can be associated with the presence of apathetic depression (Hama et al. 2007). This patient's bilateral basal ganglia injury thus provided an anatomical structural explanation for at least some of his persistent apathy.

Fatigue has also been frequently reported as a consequence of stroke (Christensen et al. 2008; Tang et al. 2010). This patient's fatigue appeared to be a problem independent of his depression. Fatigue surfaced abruptly poststroke, preceded the onset of depression and anxiety, and was not altered by the effective treatment of his other neuropsychiatric symptoms. Although hemochromatosis may cause fatigue, there was no evidence to suggest it was playing any role in his symptoms. There was no evidence of any organ involvement and no improvement after 2 years of regular treatment with phlebotomies. All factors considered, the strokes and their location were felt to be the most likely mechanism for his persistent fatigue. This is consistent with a report of fatigue following basal ganglia strokes. In this study, fatigue was demonstrated to be independent of overt depression (Tang et al. 2010).

There is limited evidence regarding the treatment of fatigue and apathy in the stroke population (Christensen et al. 2008). The patient underwent trials of augmentation with bupropion and venlafaxine without benefit. With his informed consent, a trial of low-dose dextroamphetamine was undertaken, and his condition carefully monitored, but had to be abandoned because his blood pressure began to rise. Trials of dopamine agonists, pramipexole, and amantadine were unhelpful.

The pattern of his cognitive-intellectual deficits, including expressive aphasia, executive dysfunction, and verbal memory difficulties, was consistent with the known complications of basal ganglia injury (Fromm et al. 1985; Su et al. 2007). Depression may have also contributed to his cognitive-intellectual problems (the dementia syndrome of depression) but is a less likely explanation given that these difficulties were apparent immediately post–acute stroke and prior to the development of depression.

Poststroke depression is a very common consequence of CVD; it occurs in up to 50% of patients, depending on the population studied. It has been associated with poor rehabilitation outcomes, longer hospital stays, increased cognitive-intellectual impairment, and increased mortality (Robinson and Spalletta 2010; Robinson and Starkstein 2010). The relationship between lesion location and depression has been controversial. The original observation of the correlation between depression and CVD affecting left anterior brain regions has been disputed. Strokes affecting basal ganglia, especially on the left side, as in this case, have been implicated in the etiology of PSD in some studies (Robinson and Spalletta 2010; Robinson and Starkstein 2010; Vataja et al. 2004). Placebo-controlled studies in PSD, although limited, have demonstrated positive treatment response to the antidepressants citalopram and nortriptyline. Citalopram was used in this case. Psychosocial interventions are always part of comprehensive treatment and were provided to this patient, but the benefit of psychotherapy remains unproven (Hackett et al. 2008; Robinson and Spalletta 2010; Robinson SE and Starkstein 2010).

This case illustrates the complexity of neuropsychiatric symptoms following striatal injury linked to the extensive connectivity involved, which goes beyond well-known motor pathways and includes prefrontal, parietal, and limbic networks. Via connections to the prefrontal network, the basal ganglia play a role in cognitive-intellectual processes, and via their limbic connections, they play a role in the regulation of emotions and motivational drives.

Key Clinical Points

- Common neuropsychiatric complications of stroke include depression, generalized anxiety disorder, apathy, pathological affect, fatigue, and cognitive-intellectual impairment.
- Poststroke depression is the most frequent psychiatric complication of stroke.
- Depressive symptoms after cerebrovascular disease have been associated with poor functional recovery and increased mortality. Hence prompt diagnosis and treatment are important to optimize recovery.
- Most studies in PSD have demonstrated positive response to antidepressants, with the most evidence for citalopram and nortriptyline.
- Poststroke apathy and fatigue may occur independently or together with depression. There are currently no recommendations for treatment. Some studies report the use of stimulants, dopamine agonists, and cholinesterase inhibitors.

Further Readings

Robinson RG: The Clinical Neuropsychiatry of Stroke: Cognitive, Behavioral, and Emotional Disorders Following Vascular Brain Injury. Cambridge, UK, Cambridge University Press, 2006

Robinson RG, Starkstein SE: Neuropsychiatric aspects of cerebrovascular disorders, in Essentials of Neuropsychiatry and Behavioral Neurosciences, 2nd

Edition. Edited by Yudofsky SC, Hales RE. Washington, DC, American Psychiatric Publishing, 2010, pp 299–322

References

Bhatia KP, Marsden CD: The behavioural and motor consequences of focal lesions of the basal ganglia in man. Brain 117:859–876, 1994

Christensen D, Johnsen SP, Watt T, et al: Dimensions of post-stroke fatigue: a two year follow up study. Cerebrovasc Dis 26:134–141, 2008

Fromm D, Holland AL, Swindell CS, et al: Various consequences of subcortical stroke: prospective study of 16 consecutive cases. Arch Neurol 42:943–950, 1985

Hackett ML, Anderson CS, House A, et al: Interventions for preventing depression after stroke. Cochrane Database of Systematic Reviews. Issue 3, Art. No. 2008: CD0003689

Hama S, Yamashita H, Shigenobu M, et al: Post-stroke affective or apathetic depression and lesion location: left frontal lobe and bilateral basal ganglia. Eur Arch Psychiatry Clin Neurosci 257:149–152, 2007

Jorge RE, Starkstein SE, Robinson RG: Apathy following stroke. Can J Psychiatry 55:350–354, 2010

Robinson RG, Spalletta G: Poststroke depression: a review. Can J Psychiatry 55:341–349, 2010

Robinson RG, Starkstein SE: Neuropsychiatric aspects of cerebrovascular disorders, in Essentials of Neuropsychiatry and Behavioral Neurosciences, 2nd Edition. Edited by Yudofsky SC, Hales RE. Washington, DC, American Psychiatric Publishing, 2010, pp 299–322

Su CY, Chen HM, Kwan AL, et al: Neuropsychological impairment after hemorrhagic stroke in basal ganglia. Arch Clin Neuropsychol 22:465–474, 2007

Tang WK, Chen YK, Mok V, et al: Acute basal ganglia infarcts in poststroke fatigue: an MRI study. J Neurol 257:178–182, 2010

Vataja R, Leppavuori A, Pohjasvaara T, et al: Poststroke depression and lesion location revisited. J Neuropsychiatry Clin Neurosci 16:156–162, 2004

Psychiatric Aspects of Multiple Sclerosis

Joseph Tham, M.D., F.R.C.P.C.

A 40-year-old married, right-handed woman was admitted to a neurology ward. She was described by her husband as being previously "upbeat," dynamic, and fun loving. However, over the preceding 5 years, he had noted more frequent episodes of irritability lasting hours, with days of uncharacteristic sadness. During the preceding 2 years, she had seen a general psychiatrist and received a diagnosis of major depression. She attended group therapy and took the antidepressant citalopram, resulting in some improvement in mood. Although she vaguely recalled brief periods (days) of numbness or limb weakness over the years, these symptoms had not affected day-to-day functioning and she had not felt the need to consult a neurologist.

Six months prior to hospitalization, she started noticing "strange electrical sensations" throughout her body lasting a day or two at a time. On a few occasions, she noticed right-sided weakness of her legs affecting exercise tolerance. She was referred to a community neurologist. An MRI brain scan showed a number of white matter lesions, numerous enough to satisfy radiographic criteria for multiple sclerosis (MS). Beta-interferon medications were being considered.

One morning over breakfast, 2 weeks prior to hospitalization, she told her husband, "I'm pregnant," and started making statements with religious references to being able to conceive through miraculous intervention. Over the next four nights and despite a negative home pregnancy test, she continued to talk about her pregnancy. Her sleep gradually diminished and her rate of speech became elevated. At presentation to the hospital, she was floridly delusional, believing that she was empowered by God with the ability to "change the world for peace" and that "this pregnancy represents the birth of a new religion."

She appeared physically disheveled and had psychomotor acceleration. She was sleeping only 3–4 hours per night. Her mood was now primarily irritable—angry about being "unjustly hospitalized." She demonstrated a severe formal thought disorder with circumstantial speech, tangentiality, and loosening of association. She was newly religious, and her thought content consisted of illogical and poorly systematized religious delusions incorporating elements of Judeo-Christian religious material. She described auditory perceptual disturbances, including hearing the voice of God speaking, but denied visual hallucinations.

Over the next few days, nursing staff noticed brief disorientation to place and time. On the Mini-Mental State Examination (MMSE) done within 48 hours of admission, she scored 20/30, likely due to her poor concentration and delusional thought content. Cranial nerve examination demonstrated bilateral nystagmus on lateral gaze with no internuclear ophthalmoplegia or relative afferent pupillary defect. There were no facial sensory or motor deficits. She demonstrated bilateral hyperreflexia in the lower extremities. Babinski responses were present bilaterally. Her gait was very unsteady, with relative right-sided leg weakness.

The results of laboratory studies done in the emergency room (complete blood count and differential, electrolyte panel, thyroid screen, renal and hepatic function tests, and urinalysis) were all normal. A repeat MRI brain scan showed a significant increase in white matter lesions when compared with her prior MRI scan (Figure 3–3). A lumbar puncture to look for elevated white cells and oligoclonal banding in her cerebrospinal fluid—findings typical of MS—was not, however, done during this admission.

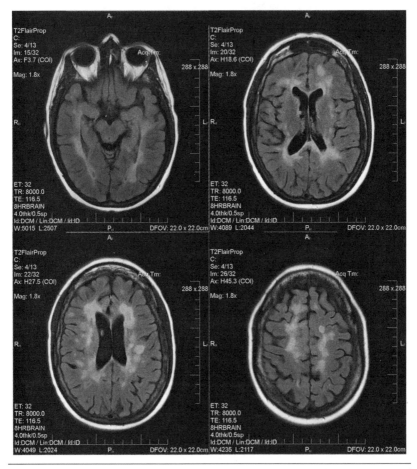

FIGURE 3–3. Magnetic resonance imaging FLAIR (fluid-attenuated inversion recovery) noncontrast sequences from a 40-year-old female demonstrating extensive cerebral white matter lesions throughout representative axial images.

Because of her fluctuating orientation, an EEG was done; it showed bilateral intermittent generalized slowing of 1–3 seconds for every 5–10 seconds. This was consistent with nonspecific cerebral dysfunction. No epileptiform activity was observed.

She was immediately started on a course of intravenous (IV) steroids to treat the severe acute white matter disease responsible for her psychiatric, cognitive-intellectual, and motor symptoms. She was given methylprednisolone 1 g over 2 hours on 3 consecutive days. The psychiatric clinical picture resembled a manic episode with psychotic features. Psychiatric treatment involved withdrawing citalopram and introducing risperidone 1 mg hs with lorazepam 2 mg hs to control psychotic symptoms and normalize sleep, respectively.

She tolerated the methylprednisolone well. Over the next 2 weeks, her delusional beliefs started to settle, sleep duration lengthened to about 8 hours per night, and psychomotor acceleration diminished to almost normal. In the third week of admission, she was started on IV mitoxantrone (an MS disease–modifying agent) because of the severity of her white matter disease.

Her hospitalization lasted for 6 weeks. At the time of discharge she was essentially euthymic, sleeping 8 hours per night. Her thought form was logical, but she still, at times, admitted to a vague subjective sensation of "feeling something spiritual happening." She no longer believed that she was pregnant or that she had any direct communication with the spiritual realm.

Over the next 3 years, she was followed at the MS clinic and neuropsychiatry outpatient program. She received IV mitoxantrone over 18 months (dosed as 8 mg/m^2 every 2 months). A repeat MRI brain scan about 1 year after her admission demonstrated an obvious reduction in her white matter disease burden (Figure 3–4).

Her psychiatric condition over these 3 years consisted of symptoms of generalized anxiety mixed with moderate depression. She was hypervigilant around her two children and obsessed over unlikely catastrophic scenarios. For example, once she was almost convinced that her son would die in a plane crash when he went on a school trip to Europe. Citalopram 40 mg/day was restarted about 6 months after her hospital stay, with no manic provocation. Her delusional symptoms completely dissipated within a year after the hospital stay, and so the risperidone was discontinued.

Despite clear improvement in physical and emotional symptoms, she continued to complain of chronic memory problems, decreased concentration, and general cognitive fatigue. Two years after the acute admission, her Montreal Cognitive Assessment score was 26/30, demonstrating deficits in verbal fluency and limitations in delayed spontaneous verbal recall of five words. Her MMSE score by contrast was 30/30. Formal neuropsychological testing showed evidence of poor memory (Wechsler

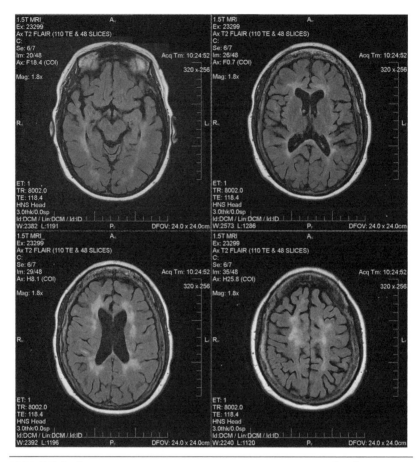

FIGURE 3–4. Magnetic resonance imaging T2/FLAIR (fluid-attenuated inversion recovery) sequences from the patient whose scan sequence is shown in Figure 3–3 one year later, demonstrating the reduction in disease burden, with axial slices at levels similar to those in Figure 3–3.

Adult Intelligence Scale—Third Edition [WAIS-III] Working Memory Index, 5th percentile), slowed processing speed (WAIS-III Processing Speed Index, 3rd percentile), and subtle deficits in problem solving, abstraction ability, and executive functioning.

A number of pharmacological agents were tried to help alleviate fatigue and improve cognitive functioning. Amantadine up to 100 mg bid and modafinil up to 200 mg bid were tried but did not appear helpful. The best result was obtained with long-acting dextroamphetamine 10 mg in the morning combined with regular moderate exercise (low-impact aerobics and pool exercises at the local community center three times a week). Despite some improvement in energy level, she has continued to complain of memory deficits, partially compensated for by making lists and setting reminders through her PDA or smartphone. During waking hours, she has enough energy to perform light household duties; she otherwise occupies her time with crafts, reading, and brief social activities.

Discussion

Multiple sclerosis is the most common type of demyelinating autoimmune disorder of the central nervous system. This disorder can affect numerous neurological systems, including sensory, motor, and autonomic, as well as cognitive-intellectual, behavioral, and psychiatric functioning. Although the prevalence of the disorder varies, the lifetime risk has been commonly quoted as approximately 1 in 400 in the white population, potentially making it the most common cause of neurological disability starting in young adulthood.

Multiple sclerosis is fundamentally an autoimmune disease, although the pathogenesis is not fully understood and multiple factors have been implicated (e.g., genetics, HLA type, environmental factors, infections). Immune-mediated activation of T cells triggers a lymphocytic attack against the myelin sheath surrounding neuronal axons. The oligodendrocytes producing myelin become damaged. Depending on the severity of the immune response, the neurons themselves may also suffer damage. As expected, demyelination compromises saltatory signal conduction down axons, causing the various neurological symptoms depending on the localization and extent of the lesions. Improved neuroimaging using MRI criteria now permits an earlier diagnosis of MS (McDonald et al. 2001). The basic diagnostic principle has, however, remained and is based on the confirmation of two or more episodes of demyelinating illness demonstrating dissemination of lesions in time (well-defined episodes of neurological impairment at least 1 month apart) and space (symptoms suggesting that a different region of the central nervous system has been affected).

The most common longitudinal course of MS is the relapsing-remitting form, in which the patient experiences episodic "attacks" of disease interspersed with periods of remission when symptoms and signs may be completely absent. More aggressive forms of MS can appear that are gradually progressive in nature, with a gradual buildup of neurological deficits over the years.

Patients with MS are at increased risk for developing psychiatric disorders. Historically, mood disorders (primarily depression) have been associated with MS; an early study by Surridge (1969) demonstrated higher rates of depression in patients with MS compared with patients with muscular dystrophy with similar levels of physical dysfunction. The life-time prevalence of a depressive disorder is approximately 50% for MS patients (Patten and Metz 1997). The increased risk of depression is mul-tifactorial. Potential causes include the psychological impact of the dis-ease and organic factors due to the lesion load.

In comparison to depression, mania has not been nearly as well stud-ied in MS, but the prevalence is believed to be higher than in the general population. In the author's experience, except for patients with a pre-morbid history of bipolar disorder, most cases of new-onset manic-like psychosis in MS have been in the context of insomnia and sensory misper-ceptions due to severe demyelination with encephalopathy.

Empirical data on treatment of mood disorders in MS are limited. Psychological treatments like cognitive-behavioral therapy have been re-ported to be successful for MS depression (Mohr et al. 2001). Antide-pressants with proven efficacy in MS depression include desipramine, paroxetine, sertraline, and moclobemide. There are no controlled studies of specific treatment of psychosis, mania, or the various forms of anxiety disorders in MS patients. On occasion, patients may require a benzodiaz-epine or hypnotic agent to help reduce anxiety and promote sleep.

The treatment of an acute MS attack often involves corticosteroids such as oral prednisone or IV methylprednisolone to suppress the active inflammatory response. These medications are well known to increase risk for mood instability, and vigilance for this effect is appropriate. Sev-eral disease-modifying medications, such as the beta-interferons, have been available since the mid-1990s, but there are concerns that these agents may worsen mood disorders. Although there have been cases of depression and suicide potentially correlated with beta-interferon treat-ment, pooled medication trial data have so far not shown an association between interferon use, depression, and suicide (Patten et al. 2005). It is therefore reasonable to not withhold interferon treatment when indi-cated but to closely monitor those patients with a history of severe de-pression. Psychiatric side effects of newer disease-modifying agents such as the monoclonal antibodies have not been well described.

Over time, especially with increasing white matter lesion load, 40%–60% of MS patients will experience cognitive-intellectual problems (Rao et al. 1991). Cognitive-intellectual disorder is recognized as being a ma-jor factor leading to occupational difficulties and lower quality of life in patients with MS. A characteristic pattern of cognitive-intellectual dys-function may not exist, because the white matter lesions are generally sub-cortical and idiosyncratic in location for each patient. However, the two most common cognitive-intellectual difficulties in MS patients are slowed

information processing (Archibald and Fisk 2000) and difficulty with episodic memory recall and recognition (DeLuca et al. 1998). In later stages
of the illness, executive functioning, motor learning, and "cortical" features such as apraxia, agnosia, and aphasia may develop.

Over the years, specialized cognitive-intellectual tests have been published for use in MS. One of the earliest and most influential is the Brief
Repeatable Battery of Neuropsychological Tests for Multiple Sclerosis (Rao
1991). As the importance of cognitive-intellectual deficits became recognized, cognitive-intellectual tasks such as the Paced Auditory Serial
Addition Task began to be included in measures like the Multiple Sclerosis Functional Composite (Cutter et al. 1999).

A number of medication trials have addressed the cognitive difficulties
in MS. Some benefit in domains such as improving attention or enhancing
performance on memory rating scales has been found for potassium
channel blockers (e.g., 4-aminopyridine), stimulants (methylphenidate,
amphetamine), and acetylcholinesterase inhibitors (e.g., donepezil, rivastigmine). Unfortunately, the studies tend to be small and lack replication.
As a result, clinical use of these agents remains off-label until further study.

The patient in this case may have relapsing-remitting disease, because
there were complaints of vague physical symptoms during the 5 years
preceding her hospitalization, and her emotional problems may also have
reflected symptomatic demyelination presenting as depression. A very
severe attack of demyelination then precipitated her hospitalization. At
the time of her admission to the hospital, she was clearly psychotic with
evidence of manic symptoms. Despite what appears to have been successful treatment with little evidence of new lesions on MRI over the subsequent 3 years, she has continued to complain of what likely will remain
permanent cognitive-intellectual deficits.

This case demonstrates the complex interaction between the MS disease process and psychiatric phenomenology. There was a clear deterioration in her mood state during her acute MS attack, and she continues
to demonstrate challenges due to cognitive-intellectual impairment. Correctly attributing symptoms to demyelination, whether acute or chronic,
is often not straightforward. Diagnostic difficulties arise as a result of
the disseminated nature of the central nervous system lesions in time and
space intersecting with variable disease activity. Physical symptoms can
range from the subtle (e.g., vague fluctuating sensory changes) to the obvious (e.g., hemiplegia or visual impairment). This principle extends to
mental phenomena as well, where the disease can give rise to various
types of emotional disturbances, thought disorders, and cognitive-intellectual compromise representing different symptomatic brain regions.
Psychopathology, similar to physical symptoms, will also fluctuate over

time in parallel with disease activity or surface because of increasing disease burden. And then, as in all psychiatric conditions, emergent psychopathology can only be accurately attributed and correctly treated by factoring in the unique patient in front of you, caught up in an unpredictable, potentially catastrophic neurological disease and a personal psychosocial environment with its own vicissitudes.

Key Clinical Points

- Multiple sclerosis is the most common chronic neurological disorder affecting young adults and should be considered in patients with fluctuating neurological symptoms.
- Psychiatric and cognitive-intellectual effects of MS do not necessarily correlate with the physical symptoms but may worsen during acute attacks of illness.
- There is an increase in the lifetime prevalence of mood disorders, especially depression, in MS patients. Although there are few medication trials, a number of antidepressants have been found to be effective.
- Cognitive-intellectual disorder is common in MS and may worsen over time with disease progression.
- Cognitive-intellectual symptoms commonly present as slowed processing speed and difficulty with episodic memory. Treatment options are limited, but some patients may benefit from medications such as stimulants.

Further Readings

Compston A, McDonald I, Noseworthy J, et al: McAlpine's Multiple Sclerosis, 4th Edition. London, Churchill Livingstone, 2005

Ghaffar O, Feinstein A: The neuropsychiatry of multiple sclerosis: a review of recent developments. Curr Opin Psychiatry 20:278–285, 2007

Wilken JA, Sullivan C: Recognizing and treating common psychiatric disorders in multiple sclerosis. Neurologist 13:343–354, 2007

References

Archibald CJ, Fisk JD: Information processing efficiency in patients with multiple sclerosis. J Clin Exp Neuropsychol 22:686–701, 2000

Cutter GR, Baier MS, Rudick RA, et al: Development of a multiple sclerosis functional composite as a clinical trial outcome measure. Brain 122:101–112, 1999

DeLuca J, Gaudino EA, Diamond BJ, et al: Acquisition and storage deficits in multiple sclerosis. J Clin Exp Neuropsychol 20:376–390, 1998

McDonald WI, Compston A, Edan G, et al: Recommended diagnostic criteria for multiple sclerosis: guidelines from the International Panel on the Diagnosis of Multiple Sclerosis. Ann Neurol 50:121–127, 2001

Mohr DC, Boudewyn AC, Goodkin DE, et al: Comparative outcomes for individual cognitive-behavior therapy, supportive-expressive group psychotherapy, and sertraline for the treatment of depression in multiple sclerosis. J Consult Clin Psychol 69:942–949, 2001

Patten SB, Metz LM: Depression in multiple sclerosis. Psychother Psychosom 66:286–292, 1997

Patten SB, Francis G, Metz LM, et al: The relationship between depression and interferon beta-1a therapy in patients with multiple sclerosis. Mult Scler 11:175–181, 2005

Rao SM: Neuropsychological Screening Battery for Multiple Sclerosis. New York, National Multiple Sclerosis Society, 1991

Rao SM, Leo GJ, Ellington L, et al: Cognitive dysfunction in multiple sclerosis, II: impact on employment and social functioning. Neurology 41:692–696, 1991

Surridge D: An investigation into some psychiatric aspects of multiple sclerosis. Br J Psychiatry 115:749–764, 1969

ANXIETY

Anxiety

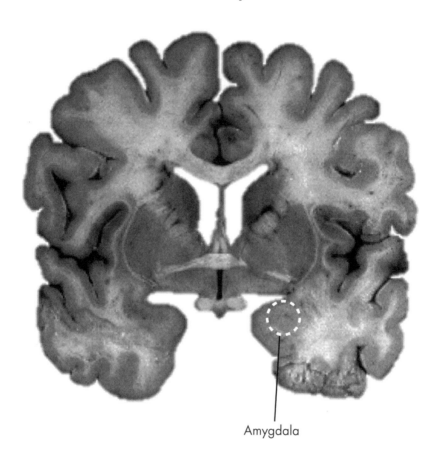

Amygdala

Introduction

Anxiety is not often attributed to intrinsic focal brain disease. Temporal lobe epilepsy (TLE) is the one exception that can present exclusively as panic attacks. Thus TLE highlights the centrality of the amygdalae in the experience of anxiety and the "fear network." The specific neurotransmitters that are involved are unknown.

Obsessive-compulsive disorder (OCD) is classically regarded as an anxiety disorder. Brain lesion models cast doubt on this categorization, given the ability of focal nonanxiogenic injuries to produce OCD. One model focuses on the cortico-striato-pallido-thalamo-cortical (CSPTC) circuit, with OCD resulting from a disinhibited and consequently reverberating corticothalamic pathway. The neurotransmitters involved include gamma-aminobutyric acid (GABA), glutamate, and serotonin (5-HT).

Temporal Lobe Epilepsy Presenting as Panic Attacks

Scott McCullagh, M.D., F.R.C.P.C.

A 37-year-old right-handed woman was referred by a neurologist for "atypical anxiety." She had been treated for presumed epilepsy for many years, although findings from recent sleep-deprived electroencephalography and head magnetic resonance imaging (MRI) were normal.

She was married with one daughter, was college educated, and worked as an administrative assistant. She was the product of a healthy pregnancy and delivery, with normal development, satisfactory school performance, and a supportive family upbringing. She had been healthy, without early febrile convulsions or head trauma, prior to a nocturnal seizure at age 26. Her husband had described generalized shaking with unresponsiveness. Results of an initial workup, including an electroencephalogram (EEG) and head computed tomography scan, were negative. One year later she had a similar nocturnal event. Although a second EEG showed normal findings, she was started on valproic acid and had no further episodes. She recalled having fluctuating mild anxiety and a tendency to worry since her

83

teens, with a possible depressive episode and increased anxiety at the age of 24. She did not recall any panic attacks. Symptoms improved with a course of supportive psychotherapy. Family history was negative for neurological or psychiatric disorders.

At her initial neuropsychiatric assessment, she described a 6-month history of awakening at night in terror, as if "from a nightmare that I couldn't remember." She recalled palpitations, shortness of breath, and tremulousness, all of which seemed to improve relatively quickly, although it took her some time to fall back to sleep. The episodes occurred about twice per week, but never during the day. She denied agoraphobic anxiety, obsessions, or social phobia. Her mood had recently been more dysphoric, with reduced enthusiasm and energy, disrupted sleep, and frequent self-critical thoughts.

Her family physician had ordered a 24-hour Holter monitor study, which showed normal findings, and prescribed citalopram 20 mg/day, which she took for about 3 weeks. Her mood and sleep were slightly improved. Response to inquiry regarding perceptual abnormalities was negative. She denied snoring, headaches, or other neurological or general medical symptoms. She did not smoke or use illicit drugs, and her alcohol and caffeine intake were minimal. Her medications included valproate 1,000 mg/day and citalopram 20 mg/day.

The mental status examination revealed a neatly dressed woman with a mildly anxious and dysphoric affect. Her speech and thought form were normal. There were no psychotic features. The results of screening cognitive-intellectual and neurological examinations were normal.

The provisional diagnoses included a partially treated major depressive episode and probable generalized anxiety. The nature of her nocturnal anxiety was not entirely clear, yet her description seemed most compatible with panic attacks, suggesting a diagnosis of primary panic disorder without agoraphobia. Although a presentation with *exclusively* nocturnal attacks is uncommon, this diagnosis was consistent with her prior history of fluctuating anxiety and the tentative response to a selective serotonin reuptake inhibitor (SSRI). The differential diagnosis included secondary panic attacks due to a general medical condition such as active seizures, or to a coincident cardiac or endocrine cause, but the recent negative investigations were reassuring. A primary sleep disorder such as apnea was possible, but it was considered less likely given her age and body habitus. Night terrors, a childhood parasomnia with intense fear, confusion, and autonomic arousal, was also unlikely given the absence of prior history or characteristic amnesia for the events.

Continuation of the SSRI and intermittent follow-up were recommended. One month later, further improvement in her mood was noted. The nocturnal attacks had not occurred for 2 weeks. Laboratory results included normal glucose, electrolytes, thyroid-stimulating hormone, vitamin B$_{12}$, calcium, and liver/renal chemistries, and a therapeutic valproate level.

Her depression soon resolved and her sleep normalized. Yet after several months, mild anxiety returned, with brief periods of "apprehension" that seemed to occur at random. She was asked to carefully monitor her symptoms. She subsequently reported a "severe panic attack" that started after an argument with her spouse and persisted for almost an hour. An abrupt increase in anxiety accompanied palpitations, shortness of breath, dizziness, and numbness in her face and extremities. She felt as if she were "going crazy" and recalled muscle spasms in her hands and feet. At a local emergency room, she was diagnosed with hyperventilation and carpopedal spasm. A similar incident 1 week later lasted about 30 minutes. At follow-up, education regarding the nature of hyperventilation was provided, along with cognitive-behavioral strategies to regulate her breathing.

Over the next year, her anxiety attacks occurred intermittently. At times they seemed to start with a feeling of warmth in her feet, which rose upward toward her stomach and chest and was accompanied by mild nausea. Palpitations and panic abruptly followed. Awareness remained intact, and she attempted to focus on slowing her breathing. The episodes were short, lasting for 1–2 minutes. She later became aware of a vague perception, as if she "had been in a situation before, or dreamt about it," which coincided with some of the episodes. In retrospect she recalled experiencing déjà vu many years earlier, although it was infrequent and occurred in isolation.

Her attacks slowly increased over time to a rate of several per week and now frequently began with a feeling of rising warmth and déjà vu. Her neurologist attempted treatment with different anticonvulsants. She felt discouraged and more forgetful and took leave from work. Depression returned, despite antidepressant optimization and supportive psychotherapy. A second sleep-deprived EEG was unrevealing, and she was referred for video-electroencephalographic monitoring at a specialized epilepsy center. During 48 hours of recording, one of her attacks was captured and was accompanied by medium-amplitude sharp and slow wave discharge over the right frontotemporal area. Clinical observation confirmed a simple partial seizure (SPS).

Additional anticonvulsant combinations had little impact on episode frequency, and she was referred for possible neurosurgical intervention. In the interim, her depression persisted and she became socially withdrawn. She avoided walking alone for fear of having another seizure. She now seemed "confused" during some of the episodes and less aware of what was happening around her.

A year after the referral she was admitted for a comprehensive evaluation. Five days of video-electroencephalographic monitoring captured four seizures, all confined to the anterior, mid, and basal regions of the right temporal lobe, as well as interictal electroencephalographic changes (see Figures 4–1 and 4–2). Concurrent behavioral features included an anxious facial expression, tachycardia, and hyperventilation. Two attacks progressed to a complex partial seizure (CPS), with cessation of activity, a blank stare, and unresponsiveness, followed by lip smacking and fumbling movements of her hands. The events lasted approximately 90 seconds and were followed by lethargy. High-resolution MRI with thin coronal cuts showed "subtle evidence of right mesial temporal sclerosis," with mild atrophy of the hippocampus and increased signal on T2-weighted images within the hippocampus and amygdala.

She underwent right anterior temporal lobectomy (amygdalohippocampectomy). The pathological report confirmed neuronal loss and gliosis of the right hippocampus, with mild involvement of the amygdala. She recovered well after surgery and was continued on lamotrigine 350 mg/day, which she had been taking preoperatively. Of note, she experienced no further seizures or paroxysmal anxiety/panic episodes during subsequent follow-up. Although depressive symptoms reemerged at about 6 months postoperatively, they responded to escitalopram 10 mg/day. After 18 months, lamotrigine was tapered to 200 mg/day and was continued along with the SSRI as maintenance treatment. Two years after surgery she returned to work.

Discussion

Panic disorder and TLE are both prevalent conditions that are not often confused. Yet when the latter presents with paroxysmal episodes of intense anxiety or fear, and an absence of characteristic motor activity, diagnostic difficulties may arise (Kanner 2011; Sazgar et al. 2003; Spitz 1991). This woman's diagnosis of TLE and auras of "ictal fear" were only decisively confirmed after a lengthy period of follow-up; the delay in confirming the diagnosis was largely due to the absence of electroencephalographic or neuroimaging abnormalities until her condition had sufficiently progressed. The diagnosis had been suspected earlier, yet was confounded by the fact that many of her early episodes appeared virtually identical to idiopathic or primary panic attacks. Adding to the diagnostic challenge is the fact that higher rates of *interictal* anxiety disorders are observed in epilepsy patients relative to the general population (Kanner 2011). Her paroxysmal attacks remained refractory to treatment until her temporal lobectomy. This suggests that virtually all of her panic-like episodes were in some way associated with ictal activity within the anterior mesial temporal region.

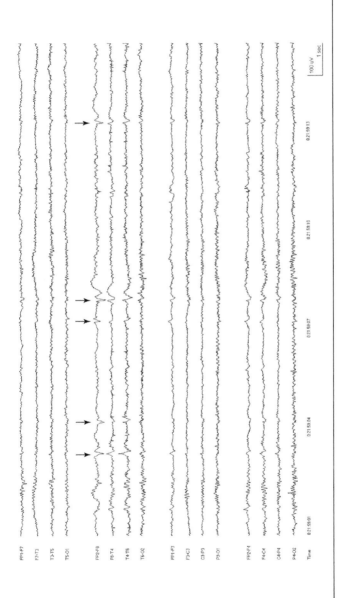

FIGURE 4–1. Electroencephalogram showing sharp and slow-wave interictal discharges (arrows) in right anterior temporal region (channels Fp2-F8, F8-T4, T4-T6).

C=central; Fp=frontal pole scalp electrode; F=frontal; O=occipital; P=parietal; T=temporal. Even numbers indicate right-sided electrodes.

Source. Courtesy of Dr. Richard Wennberg, Toronto Western Hospital Epilepsy Clinic.

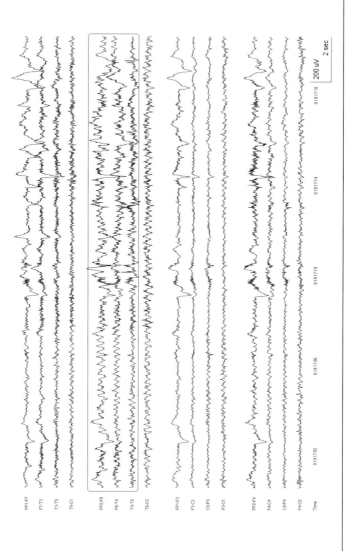

FIGURE 4–2. Electroencephalogram during a right temporal seizure with predominant fear, showing rhythmic ictal activity in the theta frequency range (outlined).

Source. Courtesy of Dr. Richard Wennberg, Toronto Western Hospital Epilepsy Clinic.

TLE is the most common epilepsy syndrome in adults (Engel and Williamson 2008). In its most frequent form, mesial TLE (MTLE), seizures arise from limbic structures, including the hippocampus, amygdala, and parahippocampal region—regions that are inherently epileptogenic and also uniquely susceptible to mesial temporal sclerosis (MTS), the principal lesion in MTLE. MTS is characterized by neuronal loss, gliosis, and heightened neuronal excitability. There is a strong association between MTS and early developmental insults such as febrile seizures, as well as evidence for a genetic or familial contribution. In individual cases, however, no such factors may be apparent. Although childhood onset is typical, presentation in adulthood is not uncommon. As in this patient, a period of quiescence typically follows an initial response to anticonvulsants (about 10 years on average), before seizures recur and eventually become refractory to treatment. Fortunately, MTLE is among the most surgically remediable of the epilepsy syndromes, with success rates of 60%–80% (Engel and Williamson 2008).

Features unique to MTLE may confound or delay a diagnosis of epilepsy. MTLE is characterized by both subjective auras with preserved conscious awareness (i.e., SPS) and auras followed by impairment of consciousness or with impaired consciousness at onset (i.e., CPS). In CPS, impairment of consciousness is typically accompanied by a motionless stare and oroalimentary automatisms (a "stop and stare" episode with lip smacking, chewing, or swallowing). Of note, a majority of individuals (about 75%) experience isolated auras that occur separately from their observable, "behavioral" seizures (Engel and Williamson 2008). Isolated auras are often more frequent than CPS and at times may be the only manifestation of seizures. It is possible that this woman's very early difficulties with anxiety resulted from early, mild SPS; however, this remains unknown. The pattern of ictal features often evolves over time, with auras becoming increasingly elaborate before finally presenting as a "behavioral" CPS. Additionally, progression to generalized tonic-clonic seizures is uncommon in MTLE—again placing limits on "objective" data that might otherwise support a diagnosis of seizures.

The most common MTLE seizure aura is an epigastric/substernal visceral sensation, with a rising, rolling feeling, and often nausea. Other frequent auras include a variety of autonomic symptoms, "psychic" phenomena such as mnemonic illusions of familiarity or strangeness (déjà vu or jamais vu), and affective symptoms—particularly anxiety and fear, which may occur in up to one-third of individuals. Although associated with MTLE, olfactory and gustatory auras are actually quite rare. Other pure sensory illusions or hallucinations (e.g., auditory, complex visual, or vertigo) suggest seizure activity within lateral temporal regions.

The link between fear and epilepsy has long been recognized. In 1880, John Hughlings-Jackson first stressed that fear can represent an intrinsic part of a seizure itself, rather than merely a reaction to its onset (Hughlings-Jackson 1880). Subsequent authors have noted that ictal fear can range in intensity from a slight feeling of apprehension to intense terror, and it may highly resemble a natural state of fear or panic. It typically appears in isolation or out of context, but at other times it may accompany a frightening memory or hallucination (Daly 1958).

Hughlings-Jackson was also the first to link ictal fear to lesions of the anterior mesial temporal lobe. Much evidence has since confirmed the importance of this region in both the generation of seizures and the mediation of fearful emotion (Davis 1997; Gloor 1992). Fear is the most frequent emotional response elicited by spontaneous seizures or stimulation with depth electrodes placed in the anterior mesial temporal lobes (e.g., during presurgical investigation). Pierre Gloor, a pioneer in this work, noted that fear was typically elicited by direct stimulation of the amygdala, whereas stimulation of the hippocampus and parahippocampal region produced fear much less often (Gloor 1992). Stimulation of the amygdala also elicited a wide range of autonomic responses (often sympathetic).

Ictal fear can also result from seizures/stimulation of mesial frontal regions (orbitofrontal and anterior cingulate cortex) and the insula, which is the principal site of cortical viscerosensory representation. This suggests that ictal fear may result from recruitment of a broader limbic network linking structures within prefrontal, insular, and mesial temporal regions. Extensive study of the fear response in animals has revealed a widespread neural "fear network" that is centered around the amygdala (Davis 1997). Gorman and colleagues (2000) subsequently proposed that primary panic disorder might reflect an underlying "hyper-reactivity" within the brain's fear network—possibly resulting from insufficient "top-down" regulation by control areas such as the medial prefrontal cortex, or perhaps from heightened reactivity to specific stimuli, such as internal bodily sensations registered by the insula. Thus, while TLE and panic disorder represent distinct disorders, the at-times striking overlap in phenomenology suggests that shared neurobiological mechanisms may underlie the two conditions (Kanner 2011).

Certain clinical features can aid in differentiating primary panic attacks from episodes of ictal fear. The latter tend to be very brief (30–120 seconds), repetitive, and highly stereotyped (i.e., the same pattern of symptoms with each occurrence). In contrast, panic attacks last substantially longer—peaking in severity over several minutes before slowly subsiding—and show greater variation from one attack to another. Patients and observers should be questioned about factors surrounding the onset of an attack, its duration, and the precise sequence of events. The presence of other TLE-associated phenomena, such as an epigastric aura or déjà vu—especially if occurring prior to the onset of fear or as part of a stereotyped sequence—points toward a diagnosis of partial seizures. Dyscognitive symptoms such as aphasia or amnesia, frank hallucinations (in any modality), and unilateral sensory changes are considered atypical for primary panic attacks. Although anticipatory anxiety can be observed in TLE, episodes that occur in more typical agoraphobic situations strongly suggest panic disorder. Both may occur at night and are worsened with sleep deprivation, although panic rarely presents with attacks that are solely nocturnal.

Neurodiagnostic investigations are critical when seizures are among the diagnoses being considered. Interictal epileptiform activity (spikes or sharp waves) may be observed on a routine scalp EEG, which supports a diagnosis of epilepsy (Figure 4–1). It is important to note that some healthy adults may show epileptiform activity on a routine EEG (about 1%), and the rate increases in nonepileptic psychiatric populations. In contrast, such abnormalities are found in about 50% of single awake recordings in adults with epilepsy; this statistic rises to over 90% with the inclusion of sleep deprivation, multiple recordings, and additional anterior and basal temporal leads (Devinsky 2003). However, only a seizure recorded *during* an EEG can confirm the diagnosis (Figure 4–2). Continuous video-electroencephalographic monitoring remains the gold standard for the diagnosis of episodic events, because the relationship between electrical and clinical activity can be carefully examined. MRI is also essential to evaluate for focal pathology that could give rise to seizures, such as MTS. The MRI requisition should specify that TLE is under consideration. This will ensure that the appropriate study is done; the study should always include a coronal FLAIR (fluid-attenuated inversion recovery) sequence. A coronal FLAIR study offers the best view of the medial temporal region and maximizes the chance of identifying pathology there. Although such pathology helps support a diagnosis of TLE, it cannot differentiate between *interictal* panic attacks occurring comorbidly with epilepsy and episodes of seizure-related ictal fear.

Key Clinical Points

- Increased rates of anxiety disorders are observed in epilepsy patients.
- Temporal lobe epilepsy can also present as paroxysmal episodes of ictal fear, at times with autonomic symptoms that mimic primary panic attacks.

- A detailed history is necessary to distinguish primary panic attacks from ictal fear. The latter is suggested when episodes are very brief, highly stereotyped, and out of context with preceding cognitions and events.

- Electroencephalographic studies are essential in the evaluation of suspected epilepsy, but a "normal" scalp EEG does not rule out epilepsy. Continuous video-electroencephalographic monitoring remains the gold standard for differentiating episodic events.

- Although ictal fear and primary panic attacks are distinct clinical entities requiring different approaches to diagnosis and treatment, the overlap in phenomenology suggests that shared neurobiological mechanisms may underlie the two conditions.

Further Readings

Davis M: Neurobiology of fear responses: the role of the amygdala. J Neuropsychiatry Clin Neurosci 9:382–402, 1997

Kanner AM: Ictal panic and interictal panic attacks: diagnostic and therapeutic principles. Neurol Clin 29:163–175, 2011

References

Daly D: Ictal affect. Am J Psychiatry 115:97–108, 1958

Davis M: Neurobiology of fear responses: the role of the amygdala. J Neuropsychiatry Clin Neurosci 9:382–402, 1997

Devinsky O: A 48-year-old man with temporal lobe epilepsy and psychiatric illness. JAMA 290:381–392, 2003

Engel J Jr, Williamson PD: Limbic seizures, in Epilepsy: A Comprehensive Textbook, 2nd Edition. Edited by Engel J Jr, Pedley TA, Aicardi J, et al. Philadelphia, PA, Lippincott-Raven, 2008, pp 541–552

Gloor P: Role of the amygdala in temporal lobe epilepsy, in Neurobiological Aspects of Emotion, Memory and Mental Dysfunction. Edited by Aggleton J. New York, Wiley-Liss, 1992, pp 505–538

Gorman JM, Kent JM, Sullivan GM: Neuroanatomical hypothesis of panic disorder, revised. Am J Psychiatry 157:493–505, 2000

Hughlings-Jackson JH: On right or left-sided spasm at the onset of epileptic paroxysms, and on crude sensation warnings, and elaborate mental states. Brain 3:192–206, 1880

Kanner AM: Ictal panic and interictal panic attacks: diagnostic and therapeutic principles. Neurol Clin 29:163–175, 2011

Sazgar M, Carlen PL, Wennberg R: Panic attack semiology in right temporal lobe epilepsy. Epileptic Disord 5:93–100, 2003

Spitz MC: Panic disorder in seizure patients: a diagnostic pitfall. Epilepsia 32:33–38, 1991

Secondary Obsessive-Compulsive Disorder Associated With Pallidal Lesions[1]

Robert Stowe, M.D., F.R.C.P.C.

A 63-year-old right-handed man was admitted to a neurobehavioral unit for investigation and management of intractable obsessive-compulsive disorder (OCD), which had begun 17 years earlier following accidental carbon monoxide poisoning. The poisoning was treated in an emergency room with oxygen, and he was released several hours later. Over the next several weeks, his wife observed decreased spontaneity and motivation and new episodes of "odd behavior," including repetitive buttoning and unbuttoning of his clothes, repeated tapping, and compulsive reading from right to left. He was admitted to a psychiatric unit, where choreiform movements of the orofacial region, trunk, and limbs were noted. Chlordiazepoxide, thiamine, and papaverine hydrochloride were administered. Soon thereafter, he developed a prominent compulsion to twirl objects.

Twelve years after his first admission to the psychiatric unit, he was readmitted for worsening of twirling compulsions, and received haloperidol and thioridazine without significant improvement. One year thereafter, he was briefly readmitted because of worsening choreiform movements, bradykinesia, postural instability, masklike facies, and intermittent gait hesitancy. Carbidopa-levodopa, imipramine, and alprazolam were prescribed. There was some improvement in extrapyramidal signs but minimal benefit for compulsions. Four years later, haloperidol was discontinued, and clonazepam (0.5 mg bid) was started.

One month thereafter, he was referred for neuropsychiatric assessment and was admitted to the neurobehavioral unit because of further deterioration in activities of daily living and personal hygiene and his ir-

---

[1]This case was previously published in abstract form in *Biological Psychiatry* (Stowe et al. 1991). The author wishes to acknowledge the contributions of David Barnas, C.R.N.P, and Michael S. Diamond, M.D., to the case summary, and of Karen Galin, Ph.D., who performed the neuropsychological evaluation.

resistible compulsion to twirl any available objects, including ashtrays, plates, and cigarette lighters. He had repeatedly burned himself by twirling hot stovetop burner rings and lit cigarettes (which he smoked compulsively, averaging 50 a day). Before switching a light or a stove burner on or off, he felt compelled to toggle the control at least 20 times. He admitted to continuous moderate anxiety, touching and counting rituals, and compulsive hand washing after touching money.

Upon his admission to the neurobehavioral unit, all medications were discontinued for 7 days, during which he was frequently incontinent of urine and feces. Once in a bathroom, he twirled his dentures, his toothbrush, his hairbrush, or the toilet paper continuously, unable to put them down to remove his pants. He took over 2 hours to shower or shave. He had to be fed because of his compulsion to twirl utensils. He was mostly unable to relinquish twirled objects on request.

His wife described him as premorbidly "hardworking, hyperactive, and charming," with a good sense of humor, and free of anxiety, ritualistic thoughts, and compulsions. He had worked as a chef, and he played the accordion. After the poisoning, he lacked spontaneity and became more withdrawn and socially isolated.

There was a past history of several depressive episodes and of heavy alcohol use (up to six beers a day). Ten years prior to admission, he stopped drinking, following several admissions for substance abuse treatment.

Past medical history included bilateral lower-extremity cellulitis and left shoulder surgery for bursitis; the surgery was followed by occasional ticlike movements of that shoulder, attributed to chronic discomfort. No other tics were reported or observed.

Family history was negative for tic disorders, as well as neurological and psychiatric illness.

Mental status examination revealed an alert, oriented, pleasant, and cooperative but mildly abulic man with reasonable hygiene and grooming. Self-reported mood was euthymic; affect was mildly restricted. The Beck Depression Inventory score was 7/63 (no depression). On the Maudsley Obsessional Compulsive Inventory, he endorsed 4/9 checking-, 3/10 cleaning-, 4/7 slowness-, and 5/7 doubting-related items. Speech was hypophonic and at times palilalic, terse, and mostly aspontaneous, but fluent and grammatical, without paraphasias or word-finding difficulty. Thought processes were logical, coherent, and goal directed, but mildly impoverished. Depression, delusions, and disturbances of cognitive-intellectual abilities were denied. Intellectual insight into his compulsions, which were ego-dystonic, was intact.

Digit span was 7 forward and 3 backward. Months of the year backward were recited quickly and accurately. Naming was normal. Letter fluency was 12 words beginning with *f* and 13 with *s*, over 1 minute each. Category fluency was normal. Writing was micrographic and dysgraphic (Figure 4–3), as were constructions, which were poorly planned (Figure 4–4). The Three Words–Three Shapes memory test revealed moderately severe impairment of encoding (immediate recall of one word and one shape, improving to six items following three study periods). He recalled none of the stimuli without cues after 5 and 30 minutes of distraction but recognized all six on multiple choice. Perseveration and micrographia were seen on alternating graphomotor sequences and Luria loops (Figure 4–5). Interpretation of similarities was moderately concrete.

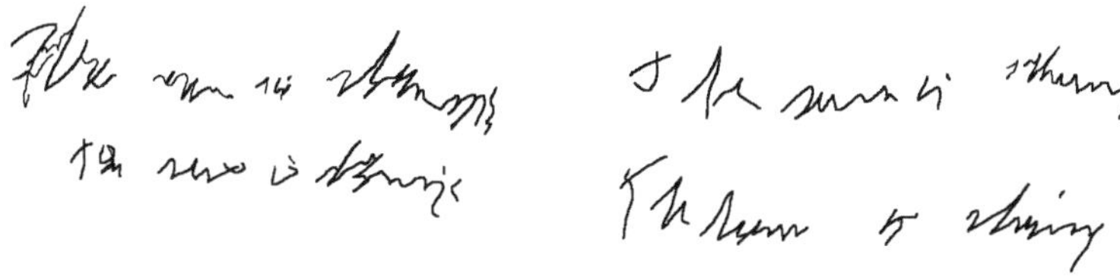

FIGURE 4–3.   Micrographia.
The patient was instructed to write "the sun is shining" four times.

General neurological examination showed multiple extrapyramidal abnormalities, including saccadic ocular pursuit; facial hypomimia and hypophonia; an intermittent left dystonic head tilt; choreiform movements of the tongue, lips, jaw, and fingers, and left shoulder athetosis; an intermittent resting tremor, accompanied by marked cogwheel rigidity (left greater than right); and mild bradykinesia. Power and reflexes were unremarkable. The left plantar response was equivocal, whereas the right was flexor. There were snout and glabellar, but no grasp, reflexes. Sensory examination was normal. There was bilateral limb dysmetria on the finger-to-nose test (no worse with eyes closed) and dysdiadochokinesis, left greater than right. Gait showed mild start hesitancy despite surprisingly good arm swing, with a normal base and stride length. He was able to perform a tandem gait.

Neuropsychological testing revealed a Wechsler Adult Intelligence Scale—Revised Verbal IQ of 103, Performance IQ of 86, and Full Scale IQ of 94. Wide Range Achievement Test subtest percentiles ranged from the 47th (Arithmetic) to the 84th (Reading). Naming was unimpaired, but visuospatial ability and recent memory (nonverbal worse than verbal) were impaired, especially uncued retrieval. Executive capacity as mea-

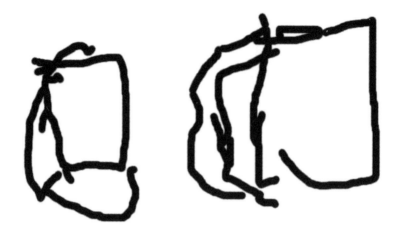

FIGURE 4–4.   Cube drawing.

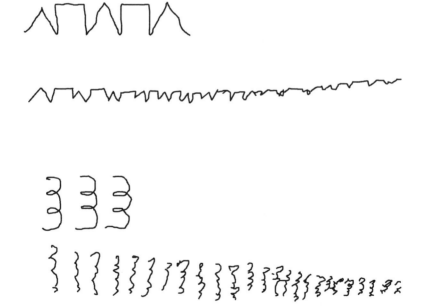

FIGURE 4–5.   Graphomotor sequences (upper two traces) and Luria loops (lower two traces) demonstrating perseveration and akinesia.
The patient was asked to "copy and continue" the first sequence and to "make a whole row of these designs, with the same number of loops as I've drawn here."

sured formally was variably mildly impaired. Grip strength and rapid automatized finger movements were moderately impaired, with severely impaired fine finger dexterity.

The results of routine laboratory studies, thyroid function tests, serum ceruloplasmin level, and serum calcium and phosphate tests were normal.

MRI revealed cerebellar atrophy and bilateral medial globus pallidus cavitation. A small left subdural hematoma, without mass effect or shift, was also present and was judged clinically insignificant by a neurosurgeon. There were no epileptiform abnormalities on sleep-deprived EEG. A sleep study showed very frequent arousals, during which the patient twirled his pillow for several minutes in a semiawake state.

Fluoxetine was started and titrated up by 20 mg every 4 days. On day 6, buspirone 5 mg tid was added for worsening anxiety. At 80 mg of fluoxetine per day, a dystonic "stare" and more sustained head deviation were noted. Blood pressure rose to 174/84 mm Hg, despite reduced anxiety. Specific features of serotonin syndrome such as myoclonus and diarrhea were absent. Fluoxetine was lowered to 60 mg/day, with improvement. By day 16, for the first time, twirling behavior stopped reliably on command, and he no longer required assistance with meals. Over the next few weeks, improved spontaneity and a further decrease in compulsions were evident. Bathing and dressing were done independently, and incontinence became very infrequent. A repeat sleep study showed marked reduction in twirling-related arousals. He was discharged home.

Several months later, recurrent chain-smoking exacerbated twirling behaviors, occasioned by his wife's hospitalization with breast cancer and systemic lupus erythematosus. Another relapse associated with depression responded to partial cross-titration to clomipramine (25 mg qam and 50 mg qhs), with optimization of fluoxetine at 40 mg qd.

Discussion

OCD is a relatively common disorder, with an estimated incidence of between 1% and 3% worldwide. This disorder is now broadly conceptualized as a neurobiological disorder, given converging evidence from structural and functional imaging studies, neurological "soft signs" research, psychiatric genetics, animal models, neuroimmunology, and psychopharmacology, all suggesting abnormalities in cortico-striato-thalamic circuits, including state-dependent hyperactivity of the orbitofrontal cortex (OFC) and the ventral striatum. Whether or not OFC hyperactivity is primary or secondary (given activation when subjects try to suppress obsessions and compulsions during functional imaging procedures) is debated. Other sites of possible involvement include the anterior cingulate cortex, thalamus, insula, superior temporal gyrus, amygdala, and hippocampus (Maia et al. 2008). Improvement following functional neurosurgical procedures (stereotactic anterior capsulotomy, subcaudate tractotomy and/or cingulotomy, and deep brain stimulation of the ventral caudate and anterior internal capsule), which anatomically or functionally disconnect prefrontal cortical and paralimbic areas from striatal and thalamic targets, is consistent with the broad hypothesis of abnormally increased activity and/or connectivity in CSPTC or corticothalamic circuits (Greenberg et al. 2010).

Although in the majority of cases an underlying neurological disorder or structural lesion will not be readily identifiable in unselected patients with OCD (as in Tourette's disorder, which is not infrequently associated), the well-documented association between striatal damage and the development of obsessive-compulsive symptomatology motivated neurobiologically oriented research into this disorder. Etiologies of "secondary" OCD associated with basal ganglia damage are pathologically diverse and include the following:

- Vascular (lacunar) strokes and occasionally neoplasms (Chacko et al. 2000)
- Disorders of parathyroid hormone metabolism causing pathological basal ganglia calcification
- Anoxic pallidal insults from anaphylaxis, asphyxiation, pulmonary embolism, or metabolic toxins such as carbon monoxide (Laplane et al. 1989)
- Degenerations (e.g., Huntington's disease, frontotemporal degenerations with striatal involvement, Wilson's disease, non-Wilsonian hepatolenticular degeneration, Hallervorden-Spatz disease/neuroferritinopathy, and neuroacanthocytosis)
- Infectious and immunological insults (e.g., postencephalitic parkinsonism/tic disorders and streptococcal autoimmunity, as in Sydenham's chorea and PANDAS [pediatric autoimmune neuropsychiatric disorders associated with streptococcal infections] syndrome)

When OCD presents acutely, a search for streptococcal infection—including a throat culture and antistreptolysin O and anti-DNase B titers—should be performed.

Structural neuroimaging and other appropriately targeted investigations should be performed in the face of neurological findings or neurocognitive dysfunction. MRI is generally more sensitive than computed tomography (CT), except for basal ganglia calcification.

Carbon monoxide has a 225-fold higher affinity for hemoglobin than oxygen; hence it displaces oxygen from hemoglobin and alters the oxyhemoglobin dissociation curve, resulting in tissue hypoxia. Carbon monoxide also binds to other intracellular proteins and inhibits mitochondrial cytochrome oxidase, thus poisoning oxidative phosphorylation. The heart and brain are particularly vulnerable because of their high oxygen requirements.

Following carbon monoxide poisoning, loss of pyramidal neurons in neocortical layers 3 and 5 (especially in striate and peristriate cortices) may produce field defects and even cortical blindness, as well as higher-order visuoperceptual impairments such as achromatopsia, visual agnosia, and prosopagnosia; executive dysfunction; aphasia, apraxia, and agnosia; akinetic mutism; and incontinence. Loss of Purkinje cells in inferior olivary and dentate nuclei contributes to ataxia and anoxic myoclonus. Sommer's sector of the hippocampus is exquisitely sensitive to anoxia, and memory is often the most affected neurocognitive function in milder cases.

Basal ganglia damage is associated with movement disorders and contributes to the neurocognitive and behavioral deficits seen after carbon monoxide poisoning. The globus pallidus, especially its internal segment (GPi), and the anatomically and functionally related substantia nigra pars reticulata (SNpr) are particularly susceptible to anoxia-induced excito-toxic neuronal injury and apoptosis following carbon monoxide poisoning. Neuroimaging evidence of damage has been reported in up to 32%–86% of cases in a meta-analysis of case series of predominantly retrospectively studied patients, but in only 1 of 73 patients studied prospectively with MRI (Hopkins and Fearing 2006). Differences across series in imaging modality (e.g., MRI vs. CT), severity of poisoning, timing of postexposure imaging, and retrospective bias likely account for this high variability in incidence. The putamen is less frequently affected than the pallidum. In a Korean series of 242 patients poisoned by carbon monoxide (Choi and Cheon 1999), 13.2% developed delayed movement disorders, over two-thirds of whom manifested parkinsonism, with smaller numbers manifesting dystonia (presenting with an average latency of almost a year), myoclonus, chorea, choreoathetosis, or ballismus. Tics may also occur.

White matter damage can occur with carbon monoxide poisoning (sometimes as a delayed, potentially devastating leukoencephalopathy involving the cerebral white matter) and may contribute to neurocognitive sequelae.

Psychiatric sequelae of carbon monoxide poisoning include anxiety and depression, and occasionally psychosis (Hopkins and Woon 2006). Secondary OCD has been described in patients with basal ganglia damage from carbon monoxide poisoning as well as other causes (Laplane et al. 1989). The exact mechanisms remain a matter of debate (Maia et al.

2008). One hypothesis draws on the observation that the OFC and medial thalamic nuclei are bidirectionally connected via excitatory glutamatergic projections. The GPi/SNpr inhibits thalamocortical transmission through a GABAergic projection. Thus, a lesion-related reduction in pallidal inhibitory activity could underlie well-described orbitofrontal hyperactivity in OCD by contributing to recurrent excitation in CSPTC circuits (Modell et al. 1988), as depicted in Figure 4–6. Since GPi may play a pivotal role in the termination of actions no longer contextually appropriate (Kropotov and Etlinger 1999), medial pallidal damage might explain why our patient was unable to interrupt his twirling compulsions once initiated. However, not all patients with medial pallidal damage develop OCD, and pallidotomy performed for Parkinson's disease is not associated with it, so the story is undoubtedly more complex.

Because of the pharmacological and anatomical complexity of the serotonergic system, mechanisms underlying treatment response in OCD to pro-serotonergic agents remain poorly understood. These mechanisms may include downregulation of hypersensitive 5-hydroxytryptamine receptors; inhibition of OFC and caudate hyperactivity via stimulation of GABAergic cortical interneurons; inhibition of glutamate release (Pittenger et al. 2011); and inhibition of dopamine release in the nucleus accumbens and ventral striatum.

In addition to severe OCD symptomatology attributable to bilateral pallidal damage, our patient developed apathy and dysexecutive deficits, including decreased reverse digit span, visuospatial planning, and problem solving; perseveration and concrete thinking; and memory impairment. A similar frontal-subcortical profile of deficits was observed by Laplane et al. (1989), likely reflecting the neurocognitive and behavioral importance of output channels in the GPi/SNpr to orbital, dorsolateral, and mesial frontal CSPTC circuits (Kropotov and Etlinger 1999). Preservation of recognition memory in the face of substantial encoding and uncued retrieval deficits is consistent with anoxic amnesia. Basal ganglia damage was reflected in parkinsonian signs (facial akinesia, resting tremor, cogwheel rigidity, bradykinesia, start hesitancy) and hyperkinetic manifestations (chorea and dystonia). The hyperkinetic manifestations emerged subacutely a few weeks after carbon monoxide poisoning, prior to neuroleptic treatment, thereby excluding tardive dyskinesia as the primary cause. Damage to the GPi/SNpr, which provides output channels for both the direct (excitatory) and indirect (inhibitory) CSPTC circuits (Figure 4–6), may explain why both hyperkinetic (chorea/choreoathetosis) and hypokinetic (parkinsonism) signs were present (Hallett 1993). Anoxic cerebellar hemispheric damage accounted for difficulties with finger-to-nose testing and rapid alternating movements despite normal tandem gait.

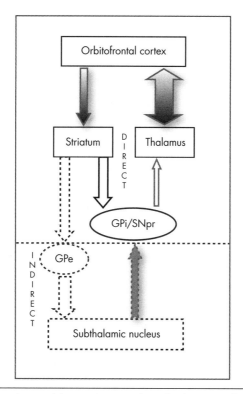

FIGURE 4–6. A possible mechanism by which internal pallidal damage could cause orbitofrontal overactivity in obsessive-compulsive disorder.
Excitatory (glutamatergic) connections are depicted with filled arrows; inhibitory (GABAergic) connections are indicated by open arrows. Specific elements of the indirect pathway are depicted with dashed borders.

The *direct* cortico-striato-pallido-thalamo-cortical loop begins with an excitatory projection to the striatum, which then inhibits the internal pallidum (GPi) and substantia nigra pars reticulata (SNpr). A second inhibitory connection runs from the GPi/SNpr to the thalamus. In normal functioning mode, the GPi/SNpr is inhibited by the striatum ("inhibition of inhibition"), leading to excitation in the thalamocortical portion of the loop. Thus, net activity in the *direct* pathway is *excitatory* at the cortical level.

The *indirect* pathway directs its inhibitory striatal projections to the *external* pallidum (GPe) and, from there, via an *additional* inhibitory connection to the subthalamic nucleus (STN). The STN in turn *excites* GPi, which inhibits the thalamus. Thus, the net effect of the indirect pathway is *inhibitory*. Note that in *both* the direct and indirect pathways, the GPi/SNpr inhibits the thalamus. Due to a reduction in pallidal inhibition (thin arrow), cortico-thalamo-cortical activity should increase (thick arrow).

While retaining heuristic utility from a clinical perspective, the classical model of basal ganglia functioning depicted above is highly simplified. For more elaborated contemporary models, see Montgomery (2007) and Mathai and Smith (2011).

In the management of this case, clomipramine was initially rejected because of its strong anticholinergic properties, given this patient's significant memory impairment. Considering the severity of the patient's OCD, high doses of SSRIs were needed to treat this condition, and buspirone was added as an anxiolytic as well as a possible augmenting agent. Benzodiazepines were avoided because of his prior history of alcohol dependence and prior failure to respond to clonazepam and alprazolam.

While SSRI treatment remains the mainstay of pharmacotherapy of OCD today, augmentation with low-dose atypical antipsychotics (Fineberg and Gale 2004), especially in patients with comorbid tic disorders, and/or a glutamatergic antagonist such as memantine (Pittenger et al. 2011) could be considered. Cognitive-behavioral therapy with exposure and response prevention procedures is frequently used adjunctively. Surgical treatments (Greenberg et al. 2010), including internal capsular deep brain stimulation, are reserved for severely refractory cases of primary OCD.

Key Clinical Points

- Carbon monoxide poisoning preferentially affects the hippocampus and globus pallidus.
- An anoxic amnestic syndrome and a frontal-subcortical profile of neurocognitive impairment and extrapyramidal signs may result from carbon monoxide poisoning.
- Cerebellar hemisphere involvement associated with carbon monoxide poisoning can produce limb ataxia with preserved tandem gait.
- Obsessive-compulsive symptomatology may result from lesions, degeneration, or dysfunction of basal ganglia structures.
- An "organic" etiology of obsessive-compulsive disorder does not preclude a response to a highly proserotonergic pharmacological approach.

Further Readings

Hopkins RO, Woon FL: Neuroimaging, cognitive, and neurobehavioral outcomes following carbon monoxide poisoning. Behav Cogn Neurosci Rev 5:141–155, 2006

Mathai A, Smith Y: The corticostriatal and corticosubthalamic pathways: two entries, one target—so what? Front Syst Neurosci 5:1–10, 2011

Montgomery EB Jr: Basal ganglia physiology and pathophysiology: a reappraisal. Parkinsonism Relat Disord 13:455–465, 2007

Stowe RM, Barnas DM, Diamond MS: OCD associated with pallidal lesions responds to serotonergic manipulation (abstract). Biol Psychiatry 29:312S, 1991

Zald DH, Kim SW: Anatomy and function of the orbital frontal cortex, II: function and relevance to obsessive-compulsive disorder. J Neuropsychiatry Clin Neurosci 8:249–261, 1996

References

Chacko RC, Corbin MA, Harper RG: Acquired obsessive-compulsive disorder associated with basal ganglia lesions. J Neuropsychiatry Clin Neurosci 12:269–272, 2000

Choi IS, Cheon HY: Delayed movement disorders after carbon monoxide poisoning. Eur Neurol 42:141–144, 1999

Fineberg NA, Gale TM: Evidence-based pharmacotherapy of obsessive-compulsive disorder. Int J Neuropsychopharmacol 8:107–129, 2004

Greenberg BD, Rauch SL, Haber SN: Invasive circuitry-based neurotherapeutics: stereotactic ablation and deep brain stimulation for OCD. Neuropsychopharmacology 35:317–336, 2010

Hallett M: Physiology of basal ganglia disorders: an overview. Can J Neurol Sci 20:177–183, 1993

Hopkins RO, Woon FL: Neuroimaging, cognitive, and neurobehavioral outcomes following carbon monoxide poisoning. Behav Cogn Neurosci Rev 5:141–155, 2006

Hopkins RO, Fearing MA, Weaver LK, et al: Basal ganglia lesions following carbon monoxide poisoning. Brain Inj 20:273–281, 2006

Kropotov JD, Etlinger SC: Selection of actions in the basal ganglia–thalamocortical circuits: review and model. Int J Psychophysiol 31:197–217, 1999

Laplane D, Levasseur M, Pillon B, et al: Obsessive-compulsive and other behavioural changes with bilateral basal ganglia lesions: a neuropsychological, magnetic resonance imaging and positron tomography study. Brain 112:699–725, 1989

Maia TV, Cooney RE, Peterson BS: The neural bases of obsessive-compulsive disorder in children and adults. Dev Psychopathol 20:1251–1283, 2008

Mathai A, Smith Y: The corticostriatal and corticosubthalamic pathways: two entries, one target—so what? Front Syst Neurosci 5:1–10, 2011

Modell JG, Mountz JM, Curtis GC, et al: Neurophysiologic dysfunction in basal ganglia/limbic striatal and thalamocortical circuits as a pathogenetic mechanism of obsessive-compulsive disorder. J Neuropsychiatry Clin Neurosci 1:27–36, 1988

Montgomery EB Jr: Basal ganglia physiology and pathophysiology: a reappraisal. Parkinsonism Relat Disord 13:455–465, 2007

Pittenger C, Bloch MH, Williams K: Glutamate abnormalities in obsessive compulsive disorder: neurobiology, pathophysiology, and treatment. Pharmacol Ther 132:314–332, 2011

PSYCHOSIS

Psychosis

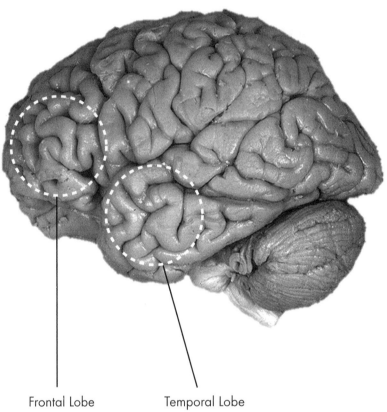

Frontal Lobe   Temporal Lobe

Introduction

Psychosis occurs comorbidly with a bewildering array of intrinsic structural brain diseases. These diseases are often multifocal, making it impossible to localize the crucial structures that must necessarily be compromised in order to produce psychosis. Epilepsy may be the one exception where psychosis is a well-established consequence of temporal lobe epilepsy and, to a lesser extent, frontal lobe epilepsy. This correlation is intuitively correct because these regions specialize in psychobehavioral functioning. The critical neuroanatomy remains unknown. The neurotransmitters involved include dopamine, given the beneficial effects of dopamine blockers on psychosis regardless of cause.

Dementia With Lewy Bodies

Marius Dimov, M.D., F.R.C.P.C.

A 65-year-old male, recently retired from working as a guard at a police station, was referred for an inpatient assessment because of confusion, gait disturbance, and visual hallucinations. His problems had started with mild difficulties with dexterity and especially with writing during the last few months of employment. He found himself to be "slower mentally" and "more forgetful." He also started making errors at work and, in general, was "easily tired" and "found it difficult to think." These problems had prompted his retirement earlier than planned.

Two months after retirement, he started experiencing visual disturbances, which he first described as "illusions." He saw small people in his yard, whereas in fact they were bushes or trees. At other times, he saw bugs crawling on him and the furniture. This happened during the day and at night, with no reported changes in his vision. Initially, he was able to realize that these were illusions and a misinterpretation of actual objects such as trees or bushes. However, as the visual experiences became more intense and vivid and occurred in different settings without triggers, he lost the ability to make this judgment and then failed to differentiate between reality and hallucinations. Thereafter, his behavior changed as he started shouting at the "strangers," using poles or sticks to chase them.

His mood also changed as he became more depressed and irritable. He started to experience sleep disturbances, waking up several times during the night disoriented, agitated, and with visual hallucinations of people in the house. His appetite was unchanged, as was his weight. He had difficulty with several household tasks that he had taken care of in the past, such as technical repairs. His performance and orientation fluctuated, showing some overall progressive decline. His gait became slower and his dexterity worsened. He had a few falls but without major injuries.

He was admitted to a local facility for management of these difficulties. Several antipsychotics were tried, including loxapine and ziprasidone. His perceptual disturbances settled, but his mobility worsened and he became more confused. A neuropsychiatric opinion was requested to assist in diagnosis and management. He was then transferred to a neuropsychiatric ward in a hospital for an assessment. The most probable diagnosis on transfer was dementia with Lewy bodies (DLB).

His previous medical history was positive for diabetes mellitus type 2, hypertension, and hyperlipidemia. His diabetes was well controlled. There was no history of angina or myocardial infarction and no previous neurological conditions, including stroke or seizures. He had a remote history of alcohol abuse but had been sober for more than 20 years. No previous psychiatric history was reported. His family history was positive for dementia in a distant relative. On admission he was taking loxapine 20 mg qd, ziprasidone 60 mg bid, metformin 1,000 mg bid, ramipril 10 mg bid, amlodipine 10 mg qd, and lansoprazole 30 mg qd.

Results of a complete blood count including differential, electrolytes, calcium, magnesium, phosphate, liver and renal chemistries, thyroid-stimulating hormone, C-reactive protein, and cerebrospinal fluid analysis and culture were within normal limits. He tested negative for HIV, syphilis, Lyme disease, and hepatitis A, B, and C. Brain imaging with computed tomography (CT) and magnetic resonance imaging (MRI) showed temporoparietal atrophy and a mild amount of nonspecific supratentorial white matter disease. Single-photon emission computed tomography (SPECT) showed decreased activity in the temporoparietal regions bilaterally. Electroencephalogram (EEG) showed widespread slowing and an absence of epileptiform discharges. Electrocardiogram and chest X ray had normal findings.

On mental status examination he was anxious and irritable. Speech was mildly dysarthric. His thoughts were scattered and tangential, with a preoccupation with the "people" and the "ghosts" that he was seeing.

On physical examination, blood pressure was 144/72 mm Hg, with a symptomatic systolic postural drop of 15, and heart rate was 88 beats/minute. He was overweight, but cardiovascular, respiratory, and abdominal examinations were unremarkable. On neurological examination he had a resting tremor with moderate-to-severe bilateral rigidity, right worse than left. He was bradykinetic, had difficulties with fine motor movements, and had moderate-to-severe postural instability.

After his delirium improved, focused neuropsychological testing revealed naming difficulties, problems with object recognition, and difficulties accessing semantic knowledge via pictures. He could not complete Trails B of the Trail Making Test. His memory was impaired. Nonverbal memory was worse than verbal memory. His overall total score on the Dementia Rating Scale–2 (DRS-2) was below the 1st percentile. A review of the DRS-2 subscales revealed mild impairment on Construction and Conceptualization, moderate impairment on Memory, and severe impairment on Initiation/Perseveration. An average score was obtained on the Attention subscale. His Montreal Cognitive Assessment (MoCA) score was 17/30 and the Mini-Mental State Examination score was 16/30, both indicating significant impairment.

During the hospitalization, the antipsychotics were tapered and discontinued. This led to a dramatic improvement in his parkinsonism, and he was eventually able to walk without a walker. His postural stability improved, and the rigidity and bradykinesia settled almost completely. His delirium slowly improved, but he continued to experience almost daily episodes of confusion. He had some reemergence of visual hallucinations, with a return of some insight that they were not real. Insomnia represented a significant challenge to treat. Eventually, he was able to report a relatively good night's sleep on a combination of trazodone (150 mg) and quetiapine (75 mg) at bedtime.

He was followed as an outpatient and continued to slowly deteriorate over the next year. His visual hallucinations became more intense and anxiety provoking. His memory, orientation, executive functioning, and judgment deteriorated (MoCA score of 11/30). He became progressively more aphasic. The confusional states became prolonged and frequent. His sleep dysfunction continued to represent a significant issue and, because of the emergence of depression, mirtazapine (30 mg) was added to trazodone (25 mg bid and 100 mg qhs). His parkinsonism remained mild, presenting mostly with mild rigidity, right worse than left. There was some noticeable worsening of his bradykinesia but no significant change in his postural stability. Quetiapine was replaced by clozapine (up to 25 mg/day) with some effect.

Discussion

The diagnosis of DLB is made clinically. The most recent revised consensus criteria (McKeith et al. 2005) include three features for diagnosis—central, core, and suggestive. The *central* features are dementia that results in severe and progressive cognitive-intellectual decline, with deficits in attention, memory, executive functioning, and visuospatial ability. Memory impairment may not occur initially but will eventually be evident as the disease progresses. The *core* features are problems with cognitive-intellectual abilities with pronounced variation in attention and alertness, recurrent well-formed visual hallucinations, and spontaneous features of parkinsonism. *Suggestive* features are REM (rapid eye movement) sleep behavior disorder (RBD), severe neuroleptic sensitivity, and low dopamine transporter uptake in the basal ganglia (viewed by SPECT or positron emission tomography [PET] imaging). Suggestive features combined with one core feature will support a diagnosis of probable DLB (Ferman and Boeve 2007; McKeith et al. 2005). In the absence of clearly established core features, the diagnosis of DLB can be difficult and the more prevalent Alzheimer's disease is usually considered. Patients with DLB may show greater deficits in attention and visual perception compared with patients with Alzheimer's disease, who show greater naming deficits (Ferman and Boeve 2007).

Parkinsonism in DLB must be clearly spontaneous and not secondary to antipsychotic use. In general, parkinsonism in DLB is less severe, at least initially, than in Parkinson's disease, but both Parkinson's disease dementia (PDD) and DLB show more bradykinesia and rigidity and less tremor. Furthermore, in DLB the parkinsonism is more symmetrical than in Parkinson's disease. Postural instability and gait difficulty are also reported more often in DLB and PDD than in Parkinson's disease (Ferman and Boeve 2007).

Visual hallucinations in DLB are detailed and well formed and could represent people, animals, or objects. The prevalence of visual hallucinations in autopsy-confirmed DLB is 59%–85%, versus 11%–28% for autopsy-confirmed Alzheimer's disease (Ferman and Boeve 2007). The etiology is thought to be a severe depletion of acetylcholine with involvement of the basal forebrain and ventral temporal lobe.

Fluctuations in cognitive-intellectual abilities, performance, attention, and arousal are similar to those in delirium without an identifiable acute medical etiology. The fluctuations are unpredictable, can occur suddenly at any time of the day, and are different from the "sundowning" typical for many delirious states and Alzheimer's disease. They have been described as variability in attention, incoherence of speech, sudden disorientation or somnolence, or an interruption of an activity with staring into space. Excessive daytime sleepiness, medication side effects, and the possibility of a sleep disorder (e.g., obstructive sleep apnea) need to be excluded.

REM sleep behavior disorder is defined as the loss of normal muscle atonia during the REM sleep stages. It presents with increased muscle tone and activity and might lead to complex movements and behaviors along with the presence of vivid dreams. A proposed mechanism of RBD is the involvement of the descending pontine-medullary reticular formation or sublaterodorsal nucleus (Ferman and Boeve 2007). RBD usually precedes the parkinsonism, visual hallucinations, and cognitive-intellectual decline as well as the diagnosis of DLB by many years.

The presence and density of Lewy bodies (intracytoplasmic alpha-synuclein-positive inclusions) correlate with the severity of the dementia in DLB. The cholinergic neuronal loss and depletion of choline acetyltransferase levels occur early in DLB and support the use of cholinesterase inhibitors in this condition. Patients with cortical Lewy bodies and numerous beta-amyloid plaques that may have neurofibrillary tangles characteristic of Alzheimer's disease are classified as having "Alzheimer's disease with DLB" or "Lewy body variant of Alzheimer's disease" (Ferman and Boeve 2007; Mesulam 2000).

As is the case for Alzheimer's disease patients, cholinesterase inhibitors are recommended for DLB patients. However, the evidence supporting this is weak. A Cochrane review concluded that there was only weak supportive evidence for the use of rivastigmine (Wild et al. 2003); patients' attention difficulties, hallucinations, and alertness, as well as the behavioral issues related to DLB, were shown to improve after administration of this class of drugs. Antipsychotics can be used short term in patients with DLB, but the recent literature points toward major morbidity and mortality associated with the use of this class of medications in dementia. Moreover, patients with DLB display a unique hypersensitivity to antipsychotics. Quetiapine (starting low with 12.5 mg/day) might be better tolerated than olanzapine. Olanzapine, with its anticholinergic effects, might worsen cognitive-intellectual abilities. As alternative symptomatic treatment, clozapine at low dosage (6.25–12.5 mg/day) can be used (Mollenhauer et al. 2010). Carbidopa-levodopa is better tolerated for parkinsonism than dopamine agonists and amantadine and can be used if mobility, balance, and bradykinesia become a significant issue (Ferman and Boeve 2007). For sleep, clonazepam and melatonin have been used in patients with DLB. Modafinil and methylphenidate have been used for daytime somnolence in selected patients (Ferman and Boeve 2007). Non-pharmacological approaches, as with other dementias, are helpful and include environmental and behavioral strategies.

In this patient the initial presentation was vague and atypical. The visual experiences were initially more consistent with illusions, and he showed relatively preserved insight and judgment. His parkinsonism was very subtle but became significantly worse with the use of antipsychotics. His cognitive-intellectual decline was also initially mild but progressed quickly within less than 6 months. Additionally, depression and sleep dysregulation, which could have represented a major depressive illness, were also prominent. His episodes of confusion and the worsening of his mental state, orientation, insight, and visual hallucinations could have been caused by delirium secondary to an acute medical condition rather than being symptoms of DLB. This presentation points to the importance of a complete workup to exclude major infectious and metabolic etiologies. SPECT showed decreased activity in the temporoparietal regions bilaterally, a finding that is typical of Alzheimer's disease but may also be found in DLB (Lobotesis et al. 2001).

His presentation also included an extrapyramidal movement disorder with bradykinesia, difficulties with fine motor skills and writing, and disturbed balance and gait. The differential diagnosis included an antipsychotic medication side effect and Parkinson's disease. His movement disorder, however, antedated the use of antipsychotics. The rapid and simultaneous onset of visual hallucinations, cognitive-intellectual decline, and fluctuations in cognitive-intellectual abilities leading to acute confusional states with partial resolution would be very atypical of idiopathic Parkinson's disease. Progressive supranuclear palsy should be considered, but there was no evidence of a vertical gaze palsy. Finally, multiple system atrophy, neurosyphilis, hypoparathyroidism, hydrocephalus, Creutzfeldt-Jakob disease, and Wilson's disease were also ruled out clinically and with the appropriate laboratory investigations and diagnostic studies.

Key Clinical Points

- The diagnosis of dementia with Lewy bodies can be challenging, and differentiating it from Alzheimer's disease is difficult. Mixed variants do exist. DLB is a clinical diagnosis, and a longitudinal history with follow-up is needed most of the time.

- The fluctuations in cognitive-intellectual abilities and awareness may be a sign of delirium secondary to an acute medical condition, and such delirium must be excluded by appropriate investigations and specialty consultations.

- Parkinsonism as a presenting feature has a wide differential diagnosis in the context of cognitive-intellectual decline, which in DLB may be mild. A referral to and assessment by a neurologist are often necessary.

- Once the diagnosis is established, treatment should focus on symptom management with trials of cholinesterase inhibitors and the well-considered and carefully monitored use of antipsychotics.

- Nonpharmacological strategies, with focus on safety and quality of life for the patient and family members, are integral to care.

Further Readings

David AS, Fleminger S, Kopelman MD, et al: Lishman's Organic Psychiatry: A Textbook of Neuropsychiatry, 4th Edition. Oxford, UK, Wiley-Blackwell, 2009

Ferman TJ, Boeve FB: Dementia with Lewy bodies. Neurol Clin 25:741–760, 2007

McKeith IG, Dickson DW, Lowe J, et al: Diagnosis and management of dementia with Lewy bodies: third report of the DLB Consortium. Neurology 65:1863–1872, 2005

References

Ferman TJ, Boeve FB: Dementia with Lewy bodies. Neurol Clin 25:741–760, 2007

Lobotesis K, Fenwick JD, Phipps A, et al: Occipital hypoperfusion on SPECT in dementia with Lewy bodies but not AD. Neurology 56:643–649, 2001

McKeith IG, Dickson DW, Lowe J, et al: Diagnosis and management of dementia with Lewy bodies: third report of the DLB Consortium. Neurology 65:1863–1872, 2005

Mesulam MM: Principles of Behavioral and Cognitive Neurology, 2nd Edition. New York, Oxford University Press, 2000, pp 498–500

Mollenhauer B, Forsti H, Gunther D, et al: Lewy body and parkinsonian dementia. Dtsch Arztebl Int 107:684–691, 2010

Wild R, Pettit TACL, Burns A: Cholinesterase inhibitors for dementia with Lewy bodies. Cochrane Database of Systematic Reviews. Issue 3, Art. No.: CD003672 2003 DOI: 10.1002/14651858.CD003672

Temporal Lobe Epilepsy Psychosis and Depression

Leon Berzen, M.B.B.Ch., F.F.Psych. (S.A.), F.R.C.P.C.
Eugene Wang, M.D., F.R.C.P.C.

A 26-year-old man was referred by his general practitioner for a neuropsychiatric consultation.

He was born in the Middle East. There were no complications during his prenatal or perinatal periods and no history of developmental delay.

There was no history of past sexual or physical abuse. His family history was noteworthy for paternal alcoholism and a vague report of epilepsy in some family members. Despite political turmoil in his homeland, he did not experience or witness any events of a severely traumatic nature.

He completed grade 12 in his birth country. Shortly afterward, he moved with his family to Canada for political reasons. He initially did manual labor and then obtained some college-level training in computers and design.

At the age of 18, he was diagnosed with epilepsy after a typical grand mal seizure. Prior to this, he had been having probable complex partial seizures, characterized by episodic word-finding difficulties or outright speech arrest; these seizures lasted approximately 1–2 minutes. He described his typical seizures as being sudden in onset and associated with experiences of déjà vu and recurrent emotional experiential phenomena. Sometimes his head turned to the right and he would see a bright light in his central vision. His eyes would fix on an object for a few seconds. He reported an associated involuntary clenching of both hands and the sensation that his arms were very loose. There was no other significant past medical or surgical history. He experimented with cannabis and alcohol in his late teenage years but without any negative effect on his social or educational functioning.

At the age of 21 years, he was admitted to an inpatient psychiatric unit for 4 weeks because of psychosis. He had become paranoid about the police, believing that they were going to charge him with rape and that he would go to jail. He also believed that social service agencies were following and monitoring him. His paranoia was not associated with any hallucinations. In addition to psychotic symptoms, he reported affective symptoms that included depressed mood, decreased sleep, poor appetite, decreased libido, suicidal ideation, low energy, and poor motivation. He had withdrawn from his friends and felt that he was not good enough to be around other people. His girlfriend was worried that he would commit suicide.

While in the hospital, he was started on olanzapine, which was titrated up to 20 mg/day. His psychotic symptoms diminished in intensity but did not resolve completely.

Over the next few years, he developed partial insight into his psychosis. He acknowledged that his paranoid ideas could be occurring in the context of a depression, but he still believed there was a reasonable basis for them. He experienced episodic depressed mood. His sleep was chronically poor. He experienced periods of improved socialization alternating with periods of social withdrawal, during which he had feelings of great inadequacy.

At the time of the initial neuropsychiatric consultation, he was living with his parents and had been unemployed for the preceding 3 years. His seizure control was excellent. His last grand mal seizure had occurred about

5 months prior to his neuropsychiatric assessment. However, since that last seizure he had been experiencing difficulty with concentration, short-term memory, and sustaining focus in his thinking. He also reported poor sleep, decreased energy, and decreased libido. He had become increasingly withdrawn from his friends and believed that he was not good enough to be around other people. His medications were carbamazepine 700 mg bid, topiramate 100 mg bid, and olanzapine 10 mg/day.

Initial mental status examination revealed a neatly groomed male of athletic build, fashionably dressed, and appearing his stated age. He came alone to the consultation. Good rapport was established from the start, and the self-report of his history was regarded as reliable. He spoke English with a Middle Eastern accent. He was hesitant in his responses. Even to routine questions, he mulled over responses with an air of excessive detail and deliberation. He frequently prefaced his remarks with "How can I say it?" He rated his subjective mood as 3/10. He endorsed suicidal ideation with no active plans. He endorsed the fixed belief that friends, strangers, and the police were monitoring him. When he was out in the streets, he believed that there were a greater than usual number of police cars driving about for the specific purpose of monitoring him. He reported experiencing flashes of light in his central visual field when he was having seizures. He had no other perceptual disturbances.

Initial neurological examination revealed normal cranial nerve findings. Testing of his motor system revealed normal tone and bulk. He had normal, grade 5 strength in all muscle groups. Sensory testing for light touch, pinprick, vibration, and proprioception was normal. His reflexes were grade 2+ bilaterally. Plantar reflexes were downgoing. His finger-to-nose and heel-to-shin tests were negative.

An initial MRI scan at age 19 had shown evidence of bilateral heterotopias. Unfortunately, this initial MRI scan could not be obtained from the radiology office where it was performed. A subsequent MRI scan, performed as part of an evaluation for possible epileptic surgery, revealed evidence of bilateral heterotopias in deep brain regions, at the trigone of the lateral ventricles, and cortically, in the left anterior temporal region. These lesions were considered to be inoperable.

His EEG revealed evidence of frequent epileptiform discharges, single or in brief trains, over the left midtemporal region, with occasional spread to the frontal region. The results of his laboratory studies (thyroid-stimulating hormone and others) were all negative.

The two diagnostic considerations were 1) a primary psychiatric disorder consisting of mood and psychotic components and 2) neuropsychiatric comorbidity arising from his seizure disorder. He was advised to continue olanzapine and was started on sertraline 100 mg/day to treat the depression.

Regular neuropsychiatric follow-up appointments were made for on-going medication management and for supportive and cognitive-behavioral therapy. Sertraline was increased to 200 mg/day. Over the next few years, the intensity of his psychotic and depressive symptoms fluctuated. Importantly, his psychotic symptoms appeared to be best controlled when he was experiencing intermittent breakthrough seizures. With improved anticonvulsant therapy, his subsequent EEGs revealed moderate dysrhythmia but no epileptiform discharges. During the times when his EEG "normalized" and he was seizure free, his psychotic symptoms worsened.

In follow-up and over time, he disclosed more about his own ideas around his psychotic symptoms. He believed that the reason he was being "monitored" was because he was a private person who did not give enough of himself in friendships. He believed that his friends were constantly taking offense from his social awkwardness and believed that he was a snob. He frequently attempted to make amends with his friends for these perceived transgressions, although he never told them that he believed he had wronged them. Cognitive-behavioral therapy approaches were adopted to target these symptoms. This led to periods of improved insight during which he reluctantly acknowledged that his delusional beliefs could be arising from his own mind. In addition to psychotherapy, his pharmacotherapy consisted of topiramate 200 mg bid, carbamazepine CR 700 mg bid, levetiracetam 500 mg bid, sertraline 200 mg/day, and olanzapine 20 mg/day. His social and occupational functioning gradually improved, and he was able to obtain employment in an art supply store.

Discussion

Patients with epilepsy have a high prevalence of psychopathology compared with the general population and those with other chronic medical conditions. This psychiatric comorbidity, which may represent an inhibitory response to the excessive excitatory state brought on by chronic seizures, includes depression, anxiety, psychotic disorders and cognitive-intellectual dysfunction. Psychiatric comorbidity may also arise from the use of anticonvulsants (antiepileptic drug–related neurobehavior disorders) (Blumer et al. 2004; Kerr et al. 2011).

Different classification schemes for the psychosis of epilepsy have been proposed in the literature. One classification scheme for psychosis in epilepsy defines symptoms by proximity to seizure occurrence (ictal or postictal psychosis), psychotic symptoms that are chronic and stable and occur independently of seizures (interictal psychosis), psychotic symptoms linked to seizure remission (alternative psychosis), and psychotic symptoms related to anticonvulsant medication (Kanner 2000).

The prevalence of psychosis in patients with epilepsy ranges from 4% in a neurological outpatient seizure clinic to 60% among inpatients in a psychiatric hospital (Blumer et al. 2004). Epileptic psychosis is most commonly seen in patients with temporal lobe epilepsy. Seizures are due to mesial temporal sclerosis in up to 70% of these cases. Temporal lobe seizures involving the limbic system structures (chiefly parahippocampus, hippocampus, and amygdala) manifest with autonomic effects, visceral sensations, altered perceptions, and hallucinations. Perceptual disturbances include hallucinations (most commonly auditory but also visual, gustatory, olfactory, and, even less often, tactile), derealization, and déjà vu (Berzen 2002).

The psychiatric comorbidity in patients with epilepsy, while sharing some commonalities with primary psychiatric disorders, has some distinct clinical features and treatment implications that must be considered by neurologists, psychiatrists, and other professionals working with this population. For example, antidepressant medication can be used in the treatment of both primary mood disorders and mood disorders related to epilepsy; however, in epileptic depression, antidepressants can become effective more rapidly and in lower doses (Blumer et al. 2004). In another example, it is possible to differentiate interictal psychosis from schizophrenic psychosis even though both involve a loss of reality testing. Interictal psychosis, in contrast to schizophrenic psychosis, demonstrates an increased frequency of visual hallucinations, better-preserved affect, a more benign prognosis with less personality and social deterioration, an absence of genetic loading for schizophrenia, and a low frequency of severe thought disorganization and negative symptoms (Salloway et al. 1997). The age at onset of interictal psychosis is usually early adolescence, which is earlier than the typical onset of schizophrenia.

In the 1960s, Landolt described the concept of *forced normalization*, in which psychiatric symptoms worsen when the EEG is normalized, often by anticonvulsant treatment (Lishman 1998; Salloway et al. 1997). Forced normalization has been observed in a subgroup of patients with interictal psychosis. Such patients may be considered as having *alternative psychosis*—that is, psychotic symptoms linked to seizure remission. This concept provides the rationale for using electroconvulsive therapy to provide controlled seizures when the psychosis proves resistant to all available antipsychotic medications.

Personality and behavioral changes have also been described in individuals with temporal lobe epilepsy. Norman Geschwind described an interictal syndrome of increased preoccupation with moral or religious issues, irritability, hyposexuality, and hypergraphia (Geschwind 1979; Waxman and Geschwind 1975). He attributed these changes to a spike focus in temporal limbic structures. Terms such as *viscosity* and *stickiness* have been used to describe the heightened attention to detail and order displayed by patients with epilepsy. When the viscosity is severe, excessive detail will dominate the patient's thinking and communication style. Interactions become frustratingly slow, creating distress and constituting a significant barrier to the provision of treatment.

The clinical workup of patients with epilepsy presenting with psychotic symptoms should include a detailed seizure and psychiatric history, electroencephalography, and neuroimaging. When routine electroencephalographic studies are negative, a sleep-deprived EEG may be helpful. Prolonged video-electroencephalographic monitoring is also an option when further diagnostic clarification is sought. MRI is essential, in particular to identify the presence of mesial temporal sclerosis. The clinical challenge is then to understand the relationship of the psychosis to the seizures, which may only become apparent over time.

This case exemplifies some of the common neuropsychiatric issues that occur in patients with epilepsy, specifically symptoms related to mood disturbances, psychosis, and personality changes. The enduring nature of the patient's psychotic symptoms and their reemergence in times of optimal seizure control are consistent with interictal psychosis and alternative psychosis, respectively. He also exhibited personality features seen in individuals with chronic seizure disorders.

Key Clinical Points

- Seizure disorders, especially temporal lobe epilepsy, are frequently associated with interictal (chronic) mood and psychotic disorders and personality changes.

- Treatment providers for individuals with seizure disorders must be familiar with the unique features and challenges of neuropsychiatric issues in this population.

- International consensus practice guidelines now exist for the treatment of neuropsychiatric conditions associated with epilepsy.

- Interictal psychosis involves a spectrum of schizophrenia-like symptoms, and the possibility of alternative psychosis and forced normalization should be considered.

Further Readings

Blumer D, Montouris G, Davies K: The interictal dysphoric disorder: recognition, pathogenesis, and treatment of the major psychiatric disorder of epilepsy. Epilepsy Behav 5:826–840, 2004

Kerr MP, Mensah S, Besag F, et al: International consensus clinical practice statements for the treatment of neuropsychiatric conditions associated with epilepsy. Epilepsia 52:2133–2138, 2011

References

Berzen L: Epilepsy and psychosis. Canadian Psychiatric Association Bulletin, February 2002. Available at: http://ww1.cpa-apc.org:8080/publications/archives/bulletin/2002/february/specialfeatureberzen.asp. Accessed August 11, 2012.
Blumer D, Montouris G, Davies K: The interictal dysphoric disorder: recognition, pathogenesis, and treatment of the major psychiatric disorder of epilepsy. Epilepsy Behav 5:826–840, 2004
Geschwind N: Behavioural changes in temporal lobe epilepsy. Psychol Med 9:217–219, 1979
Kanner AM: Psychosis of epilepsy: a neurologist's perspective. Epilepsy Behav 1:219–227, 2000
Kerr MP, Mensah S, Besag F, et al: International consensus clinical practice statements for the treatment of neuropsychiatric conditions associated with epilepsy. Epilepsia 52:2133–2138, 2011
Lishman WL: Organic Psychiatry, 3rd Edition. Oxford, UK, Blackwell Science, 1998
Salloway S, Malloy P, Cummings JL: The Neuropsychiatry of Limbic and Subcortical Disorders. Washington, DC, American Psychiatric Press, 1997
Waxman SG, Geschwind N: The interictal behavior syndrome of temporal lobe epilepsy. Arch Gen Psychiatry 32:1580–1586, 1975

Frontal Lobe Epilepsy and Its Neuropsychiatric Manifestations

Vinod H. Srihari, M.D.
Warren T. Lee, M.D., Ph.D.

A 23-year-old right-handed pizza deliveryman was referred for assessment of new-onset psychosis. He had a history of auditory hallucinations lasting for 2 days associated with violent outbursts that were out of character with his usual self, and he had been admitted to an early psychosis treatment unit. His family reported that he also had social withdrawal and anhedonia for a few weeks prior to the episode. There was no psychiatric, substance abuse, or medical history of note. Family history was also negative. Six months prior to the onset of his symptoms, he had sustained a head injury in the course of his work. He reported that prior to this admission, he had not lost consciousness or experienced other postconcussive symptoms and had gone back to work.

In the mental status examination, he appeared disheveled and bewildered, exhibiting poor eye contact. Although he denied feeling depressed, his affect was markedly constricted. He was oriented to person, place, and time. He reported command auditory hallucinations and persecutory delusions, and his insight was impaired. Results of a physical examination and laboratory testing, including a noncontrast CT scan of the brain, were within normal limits. The provisional diagnosis was brief psychotic disorder.

Per protocol he was started on risperidone, but he experienced no amelioration in his symptoms even when the dosage was titrated up to 6 mg/ day. Two weeks into his hospitalization, he experienced five episodes of nocturnal seizures. These seizures occurred in clusters while he was asleep and were observed by the nursing staff. They reported that he would suddenly become agitated, appear to be terrified, and then start screaming. He exhibited asymmetric tonic posturing of his right leg and also grabbed at the bedsheets with his hands. There was rapid secondary generalization followed by a short period of postictal confusion. He was amnestic for these episodes.

An interictal EEG showed high-amplitude, rhythmic, high-frequency waves with postictal slowing in left-sided frontal leads (Figure 5–1). A brain MRI scan showed normal findings. He was started on valproate and his psychotic symptoms improved significantly. His seizures did not recur.

An EEG done 1 month after starting valproate showed normal findings (Figure 5–2). He had no more hallucinations or delusions, and risperidone was slowly tapered and discontinued, with no reemergence of psychotic symptoms. At 6-month and 1-year follow-up, he remained seizure free and was functioning closer to his premorbid state, when he was on valproate monotherapy. However, he was not able to continue working as a pizza deliveryman.

Discussion

This patient's initial presentation was classically that of brief psychotic disorder or first-episode psychosis, which is often a prelude to an eventual diagnosis of schizophrenia. The workup was standard practice to exclude an organic basis to his symptoms. However, he did not respond to

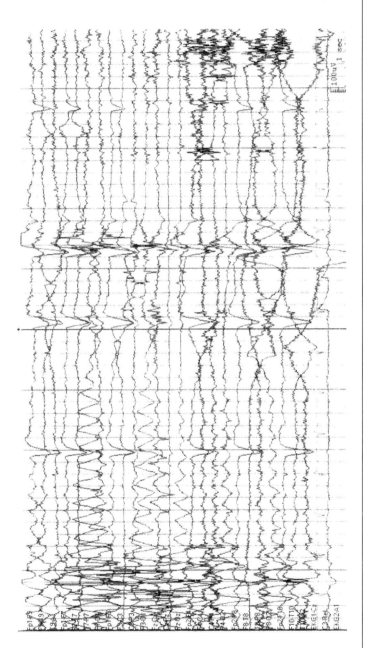

FIGURE 5–1. Interictal electroencephalogram from a 23-year-old male done after the seizures, showing high-amplitude, rhythmic, high-frequency waves with postictal slowing in the left-sided frontal leads.

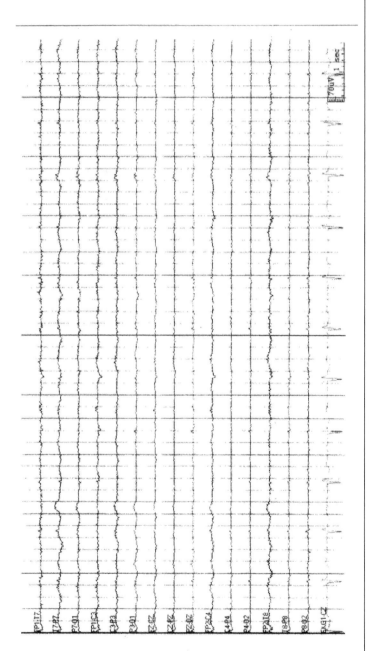

FIGURE 5–2. Electroencephalogram (EEG) from same patient whose EEG is shown in Figure 5–1 after 1 month of antiepileptic medication.

antipsychotic medications. Following a series of witnessed seizures and a subsequent interictal EEG, frontal lobe epilepsy with postictal psychosis was diagnosed.

Epilepsy is a well-known cause of psychosis and has been described for both temporal and much less commonly frontal lobe epilepsy (Adachi et al. 2000; García-Morales et al. 2008). The relationship of the seizures to psychosis varies (Sachdev 1998). Psychosis may be the presenting feature of nonconvulsive status epilepticus—an *ictal psychosis* (Takaya et al. 2005). Psychosis may follow a seizure as in this case—a *postictal psychosis*. In postictal psychosis there is typically a lucid interval of a few days before the psychosis surfaces; during this lucid interval, the patient appears to be back to normal. Psychosis may occur years after the onset of epilepsy, typically 10–14 years later—a chronic *interictal psychosis*. Lastly, psychotic symptoms may surface when the seizure disorder goes into remission—an *alternative psychosis*.

Frontal lobe epilepsy can be identified by the ictal psychobehavioral manifestations, which include terrifying fear (La Vega-Talbot et al. 2006; Takaya et al. 2005), agitation, irritability, complex automatisms, and ictal laughing and singing (Enatsu et al. 2011). Some of the symptoms can provide localizing clues. For example, prominent speech disturbance may suggest dominant hemisphere involvement. Unilateral or bilateral tonic posturing, facial grimacing, vocalization, speech arrest, and complex automatisms including kicking may point toward supplementary motor area involvement. A unique feature of supplementary motor area seizures results from the fact that each supplementary cortex area controls bilateral musculature, which may lead to bilateral tonic posturing without loss of awareness or consciousness. Simple partial motor seizures with clonic movements may implicate the primary motor cortex. Tonic and clonic movements usually (but not always) point to a contralateral lesion in the frontal lobe. Complex behaviors like motor agitation, viscerosensory symptoms, strong emotions, and repetitive motor activity are more likely associated with the medial frontal, frontopolar region or cingulate gyrus (Kellinghaus and Luders 2004; Kotagal and Arunkumar 1998; O'Brien et al. 2008). Moreover, compared with temporal lobe seizures, frontal lobe seizures tend to begin and end abruptly, are brief (<1 minute in duration), are often frequent, and show a tendency to occur at night and in clusters.

Frontal lobe epilepsy is attributable to several causes, including cortical dysgenesis, gliosis, vascular malformations, neoplasms, head trauma, infections, and anoxia. As a result of advances in genetics, an expanded number of genetically inherited syndromes have been described. Autosomal dominant nocturnal frontal lobe epilepsy is typified by brief, stereotypical seizures, ranging from simple arousals from sleep to dramatic, bizarre behaviors, with retained awareness during the episode (Kurahashi and Hirose 2010). The etiology of the patient's frontal lobe epilepsy in this case remains unresolved; the role of his preceding head trauma is uncertain since it was reportedly mild and his MRI scan had normal findings.

Should outpatient EEG be done routinely for first presentation of psychosis? It is uncommon to see frontal lobe epilepsy presenting as psychosis in regular psychiatric practice. The American Psychiatric Association practice guideline for schizophrenia recommends EEGs only when clinically indicated, such as in patients with atypical presentations, including head injury, poor response to antipsychotic medications, and a family history of epilepsy (American Psychiatric Association 2004). Clinical judgment remains important in pursuing a suspected diagnosis of epilepsy, because a single EEG is a relatively insensitive test for an underlying seizure disorder. Even for those with an established epileptic disorder, an initial outpatient interictal standard EEG shows abnormalities in only 29%–55% of patients (Goodin et al.1990). Furthermore, much of the frontal lobe is inaccessible for scalp EEGs.

For the psychiatrist, there are some clinical clues that suggest that the bizarre behavior in question may be the ictal phenomena of frontally originating seizures. Ictal behavioral episodes are stereotypic and typically brief (less than 60 seconds). Motor behavior is repetitive and may include finger tapping, kicking, rubbing, pelvic thrusting, thrashing, picking, genital manipulations, scratching, rearranging clothes, speech arrest or disturbance, moaning, grunting, and vocal repetitions. Given some of the bizarre complex movements, distinguishing nonepileptic events (psychogenic nonepileptic seizures, also called "pseudoseizures") from epileptic seizures can prove challenging. The preservation of awareness during bilateral manual activity and the explosive onset and abrupt termination with minimal postictal features may add to diagnostic confusion.

When in doubt, video-electroencephalographic monitoring is indicated. All patients should undergo high-resolution gadolinium-enhanced brain MRI. However, a distinct lesion may not be visible in a sizable percentage of patients with frontal lobe epilepsy. There may also be a role for functional neuroimaging like PET and SPECT (Kotagal and Arunkumar 1998).

Key Clinical Points

- Patients with frontal lobe epilepsy may exhibit bizarre behaviors and thus may be seen by a psychiatrist before being seen by a neurologist.

- Although epilepsy is a well-known cause of psychosis, pychotic symptoms per se are rarely due to frontal lobe epilepsy.
- Routine electroencephalograms are not recommended for first presentation of psychosis unless there is an indication such as history of head trauma, family history of epilepsy, or poor response to treatment.

Further Readings

Beleza P, Pinho J: Frontal lobe epilepsy. J Clin Neurosci 18:593–600, 2011

Haut S: Frontal lobe epilepsy, 1994–2002. Available at: http://emedicine.medscape.com/article/1184076. Accessed August 11, 2012.

Kim HF, Yudofsky SC, Hales RE, et al: Neuropsychiatric aspects of seizure disorders, in The American Psychiatric Publishing Textbook of Neuropsychiatry and Behavioral Neurosciences, 5th Edition. Edited by Yudofsky SC, Hales RE. Washington, DC, American Psychiatric Publishing, 2008, pp 649–675

References

Adachi N, Onuma T, Nishiwaki S, et al: Inter-ictal and post-ictal psychoses in frontal lobe epilepsy: a retrospective comparison with psychoses in temporal lobe epilepsy. Seizure 9:328–335, 2000

American Psychiatric Association: Practice Guideline for the Treatment of Patients With Schizophrenia, 2nd Edition. Arlington, VA, American Psychiatric Association, 2004

Enatsu R, Hantus S, Gonzalez-Martinez J, et al: Ictal singing due to left frontal lobe epilepsy: a case report and review of the literature. Epilepsy Behav 22:404–406, 2011

García-Morales I, de la Peña Mayor P, Kanner AM: Psychiatric comorbidities in epilepsy: identification and treatment. Neurologist 14:S15–S25, 2008

Goodin DS, Aminoff MJ, Laxer KD: Detection of epileptiform activity by different noninvasive EEG methods in complex partial epilepsy. Ann Neurol 27(3):330–334, 1990

Kellinghaus C, Luders HO: Frontal lobe epilepsy. Epileptic Disord 6:223–239, 2004

Kotagal P, Arunkumar GS: Lateral frontal lobe seizures. Epilepsia 39:S62–S68, 1998

Kurahashi H, Hirose S: Autosomal dominant nocturnal frontal lobe epilepsy. Gene Reviews Available at: http://www.ncbi.nlm.nih.gov/books/NBK1169/. Accessed August 11, 2012.

La Vega-Talbot M, Duchowny M, Jayakar P: Orbitofrontal seizures presenting with ictal visual hallucinations and interictal psychosis. Pediatr Neurol 35:78–81, 2006

O'Brien TJ, Mosewich RK, Britton JW, et al: History and seizure semiology in distinguishing frontal lobe seizures and temporal lobe seizures. Epilepsy Res 82:177–182, 2008

Sachdev P: Schizophrenia-like psychosis and epilepsy: the status of the association. Am J Psychiatry 155:325–336, 1998
Takaya S, Matsumoto R, Namiki C, et al: Frontal nonconvulsive status epilepticus
   manifesting somatic hallucinations. J Neurol Sci 234:25–29, 2005

Atypical Psychosis in Mitochondrial Disease

Magdalena Ilcewicz-Klimek, M.D., F.R.C.P.C.

A 35-year-old woman was admitted for psychosis. Her health problems had started in late childhood. She developed frequent headaches, which were predominantly right-sided and accompanied by nausea and vomiting. She experienced visual auras of scintillations and scotomata. Around the same time, she had to deal with increased stress at school related to bullying by her peers due to her short stature. Her grades were average during most of the school years, but she failed grade 10 because she was severely affected by the bullying. At that time she developed her first episode of depression. She quit school in grade 11. Her depressive symptoms improved spontaneously, and she got a job as a store clerk. She had a few brief romantic relationships but was never married and had no children.

Her family history was positive for migraines in both of her siblings, mother, and maternal grandmother. Her mother went through periods when she was very withdrawn, but no psychiatric or medical diagnosis was ever made.

Over time, her migraines became more frequent and severe, and in her early 20s she noticed episodes of poor balance and exercise intolerance. At age 28 she experienced a severe migraine that lasted for a week. She was treated with intravenous dihydroergotamine in the emergency room. While she was still in the hospital, she suffered a stroke in the right occipital area and presented with a left homonymous hemianopia. The stroke was attributed to vasospasm as a result of a migraine and ergotamine. A few months later she started to experience left-sided twitching and was successfully treated with phenytoin for seizures. A year later she presented with left-sided hemiparesis, and an X-ray computed tomography (CT) head scan showed a new right temporoparietal infarct.

Investigations into rare causes of the strokes had negative findings. On physical examination there was limb ataxia and action myoclonus. Based on the clinical presentation, a provisional diagnosis of mitochondrial disorder was made. She soon suffered several more strokes, with some localized in the left occipital area, resulting in cortical blindness. Eventually, the seizures worsened to the point of status epilepticus, and she was treated in an intensive care unit (ICU) with intravenous antiepileptic agents for a week. She eventually improved and was discharged.

At age 35, she was found unconscious in her apartment; she had taken an overdose of valproic acid, which had been prescribed for her seizures. She was admitted to an ICU with severe metabolic acidosis, hyperammonemia, and encephalopathy. She required hemodialysis, and her recovery was prolonged.

She later reported that she had suffered from severe depression for a few months prior to the suicide attempt, which had been precipitated by significant losses that had occurred within a short period of time: her mother and her best friend had died from cancer. Her medical history also revealed that she had experienced recurrent episodes of depression over the years but had never been treated for them.

After the ICU stay, the patient was transferred to a psychiatric ward for management of psychotic depression. She continued to have severe depressive symptoms with prominent psychomotor retardation, anhedonia, and ongoing thoughts that life was not worth living. She experienced auditory hallucinations, such as the nurses making derogatory comments, causing her to believe that the nurses were plotting against her. An EEG did not show encephalopathy. She was prescribed venlafaxine XR 150 mg/day and risperidone 2 mg/day. However, her mobility started to deteriorate, to the point that she had problems with ambulating independently despite only minimal rigidity noted on examination. Once her psychiatric symptoms improved, she was able to go home with assistance. Shortly after discharge, she decided to stop risperidone, and her mobility improved significantly.

A few months later, she was brought to the emergency room again with an acute onset of visual and tactile hallucinations accompanied by bizarre delusions. She was seeing monsters and enormous insects and felt them biting her skin. She had become severely agitated, barricading herself in a bathroom while holding a big kitchen knife and stabbing at her hallucinations, which she believed were going to kill her. She denied any use of alcohol or illegal substances. Further inquiry revealed that she had experienced at least one seizure a few days before the onset of psychosis.

On examination she was found to have a complete left homonymous hemianopia and right upper quadrantanopia to finger motion, and far visual acuity was 20/200 in the left eye and 20/300 in the right eye. She had no ptosis or external ophthalmoplegia. Her head was drooped because of neck weakness. She had flattening of the left nasolabial fold. Her hearing was decreased bilaterally, with slow and mildly dysarthric speech. She had proximal muscle and neck flexor weakness, pyramidal weakness in the left upper extremity, and increased deep tendon reflexes and tone on the left side. She was unable to walk without assistance because of cerebellar ataxia, action tremor, and myoclonus.

Investigations were ordered to clarify the diagnosis. An EEG showed generalized epileptiform discharges with a left temporal lobe focus. Magnetic resonance imaging (MRI) of the brain confirmed the presence of old infarcts, which did not follow vascular territories (Figure 5–3). MRI also demonstrated global atrophy. Atrophy was greater in the cerebellum compared with the cerebrum. MRI spectroscopy revealed a reduction in the NAA (N-acetylaspartate) peak and an increased lactate peak over the lateral ventricles. Audiology testing confirmed bilateral sensorineural hearing loss. Her echocardiogram and electrocardiogram showed normal findings.

With the exception of elevated postprandial lactate and serum ammonia, her extensive blood work and urine tests had normal results. Valproic acid level was within the therapeutic range. Electromyography results were inconclusive, and nerve conduction studies had normal findings. A muscle biopsy confirmed mitochondrial myopathy with abnormal mitochondria and ragged red fibers.

The results of these investigations and the clinical picture confirmed the diagnosis of a mitochondrial disorder, most likely MELAS (mitochondrial myopathy, encephalopathy, lactic acidosis and stroke-like episodes) syndrome. When the patient was switched from valproic acid to lamotrigine, her myoclonus became much worse. This was followed by a trial of clonazepam, which caused sedation and only minimal improvement in myoclonus. Olanzapine was prescribed for psychosis and her psychiatric symptoms resolved within a few days, which may not have been attributable to this recently introduced neuroleptic. On the other hand, her mobility deteriorated; she became wheelchair-bound and required assistance with the basic activities of daily living. After the dose of olanzapine was lowered to 2.5 mg/day, her mobility improved slightly.

As her acute psychiatric symptoms resolved, cognitive-intellectual problems became apparent. She displayed short-term memory and executive function deficits. Her behavior was childlike, with impulsive reactions, concrete thinking, poor attention, and limited insight into her deficits. Only a limited neuropsychological assessment was possible because of her severe visual and physical limitations. Overall, global cognitive-intellectual impairment was confirmed, with more specific deficits

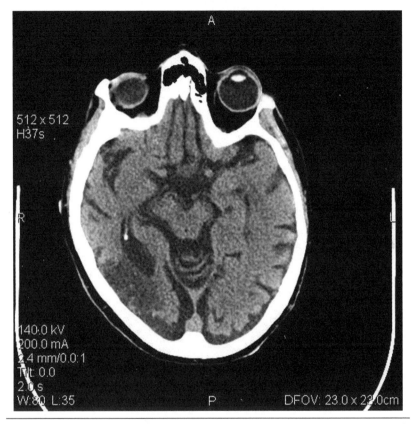

FIGURE 5–3. Axial computed tomography scan from the patient with mitochondrial disorder showing stroke-like changes in a nonvascular distribution in the right posterior temporal lobe.

in verbal and prospective memory. Her recognition memory was relatively good, suggesting a problem with retrieval rather than encoding. Her verbal IQ was in the extremely low range, with verbal fluency in less than the 4th percentile and category fluency at the 1st percentile. Her processing speed was slow, with right-left confusion, apraxia, poor performance on mental arithmetic tasks, and a kindergarten-level spelling ability. Digit span was 3 forward and 2 backward.

She was discharged to a nursing home because she required assistance with most activities of daily living. After discharge, valproic acid was retried several times at low doses to suppress her myoclonus but had to be stopped. Although myoclonus improved dramatically with this medication, she developed psychosis with prominent visual hallucinations each time. She continued to have recurrent depression, which was treated successfully with various antidepressants. She was also prescribed a mito-chondrial cocktail of supplements, including coenzyme Q_{10}, arginine, and vitamins, but her physical condition continued to gradually deteriorate.

Discussion

MELAS syndrome is due to a mitochondrial cytopathy that occurs spo-radically or through maternal inheritance. Multiple different mitochon-drial mutations have been associated with MELAS. The most prevalent of these mutations is an A-to-G transition mutation at nucleotide 3243 (m.3243A>G) of the tRNALeu(UUR) gene. The diagnosis is based on the presence of stroke-like episodes, typically before age 40; encephalop-athy; and evidence of a mitochondrial myopathy with lactic acidosis, ragged red fibers, or both. Other possible features include short stature, hearing loss, exercise intolerance, elevated cerebrospinal fluid protein, migraine-like headaches, seizures, cognitive-intellectual impairment, cerebellar ataxia, myoclonus, cardiomyopathy, cardiac conduction defects, diabetes mellitus, gastrointestinal dysmotility, and nephropathy. The hallmark of the strokes in MELAS syndrome is that they do not conform to the terri-tories supplied by major cerebral arteries. The mechanism whereby de-fects in mitochondrial DNA cause the histological and clinical features of MELAS syndrome is not known (Sproule and Kaufmann 2008).

The common neuropsychiatric manifestations of mitochondrial disor-ders are depression, psychosis, delirium, and cognitive-intellectual impair-ment. Prevalence data are, however, limited (Fattal et al. 2006; Finsterer 2009, 2010; Koene et al. 2009; Mancuso et al. 2011). Rates of depression have been reported to be as high as 42% in MELAS syndrome. Depression can occur early in the disease process, sometimes preceding other physical symptoms (DiMauro and Schon 2008; Fattal et al. 2006). For instance, in this case, depressive symptoms were already present in late childhood. Be-cause psychiatric presentations can be an early sign of mitochondrial disease, psychiatrists may be among the first physicians involved in providing care and responsible for initiating investigations and making the correct diagnosis.

Global cognitive-intellectual impairment or mitochondrial dementia, as seen in this case, has been observed in up to 60%–70% of patients with various mitochondrial disorders. Cognitive-intellectual deficits can also be focal if they are directly related to the underlying stroke-like lesions (Finsterer 2009).

In this patient's case, several factors may have played a role in her psy-chosis. First, the psychosis may have been directly related to the mito-chondrial dysfunction. Based on the current literature, atypical psychosis appears to be especially common in MELAS syndrome. Only one of this patient's episodes of psychosis could be accounted for on the basis of a depression (Finsterer 2010).

The acute onset of predominantly visual hallucinations in one decompensation suggests possible encephalopathy or delirium. This is an unlikely explanation because there was no decreased or fluctuating level of consciousness, there was no confusion, and the EEG did not show typical diffuse slowing. Based on her EEG, the patient's presentation also could not have been due to partial status epilepticus, which has been described in patients with mitochondrial disorders who have presented with acute behavioral and mental status changes. Her report of a seizure a few days prior to the onset of psychosis, as well as the rapid resolution of her symptoms, is suggestive of a postictal psychosis.

Sensory deprivation may have contributed to her hallucinations and psychosis. Her significant visual impairment raises the possibility of Charles Bonnet syndrome, at least to account for her visual hallucinations or illusions. However, in this syndrome, visual hallucinations are not typically associated with delusions and hallucinations in other modalities, and insight is usually well preserved.

The final factor that played an important part in this patient's psychosis was her medication. Psychotic symptoms were consistently triggered by the use of valproic acid, settling when stopped. The potential negative effect of certain medications on mitochondrial disorders is well known. Indeed, one of the most important issues in management of patients with these conditions is the avoidance of mitochondrion-toxic medications. Examples include antiepileptic agents like valproic acid and barbiturates (Finsterer 2010). Neuroleptic medications, especially typical antipsychotics and risperidone, have been shown to inhibit mitochondrial oxidative phosphorylation and may trigger psychiatric and physical symptoms; therefore, these medications must be used with great caution in patients with mitochondrial disorders (Ahn et al. 2005; Finsterer 2010; Modica-Napolitano et al. 2003). In this case, mobility deteriorated dramatically when she was treated with risperidone. The patient was also sensitive to the side effects of olanzapine, but to a lesser degree.

There are no available guidelines for the management of psychiatric symptoms in mitochondrial disorders. In the event of depression, serotonin reuptake inhibitors are generally considered effective and well tolerated. Therapeutic options for cognitive-intellectual impairment in patients with mitochondrial disorder are still experimental. Supplements and various vitamin cocktails may offer some benefits for the physical and neuropsychiatric manifestations. For instance, there are several reports of a positive response of psychotic and cognitive-intellectual symptoms to coenzyme Q_{10} (Ahn et al. 2005; Fattal et al. 2006; Finsterer 2009, 2010).

The role of mitochondrial dysfunction in many primary psychiatric disorders, including unipolar depression, bipolar disorder, schizophrenia, autism, and neurodegenerative disorders, has become an area of interest. However, no clear conclusions can be made at this point and further studies are needed (Clay et al. 2011; Finsterer 2010; Kato 2001).

Key Clinical Points

- Mitochondrial disorders should be considered in patients with multiorgan symptoms and signs that include exercise intolerance, migraines, seizures, stroke-like episodes, hearing loss, diabetes, and short stature.

- Psychosis, cognitive-intellectual impairment, delirium, and depression are common neuropsychiatric symptoms of mitochondrial disorders.

- Mitochondrion-toxic medications like valproic acid should be avoided in patients with mitochondrial disorders because of the risk of worsening their underlying illness.

- Many neuroleptics have been shown to inhibit mitochondrial function and need to be used with caution in these patients.

- There is no established treatment for mitochondrial disorders. Supplements like coenzyme Q_{10} and vitamins may be helpful.

Further Readings

Finsterer J: Central nervous system manifestations of mitochondrial disorders. Acta Neurol Scand 114:217–238, 2006
Finsterer J: Treatment of central nervous manifestations in mitochondrial disorders. Eur J Neurol 18:28–38, 2011

References

Ahn MS, Sims KB, Frazier JA: Risperidone-induced psychosis and depression in a child with a mitochondrial disorder. J Child Adolesc Psychopharmacol 15:520–525, 2005
Clay HB, Sillivan S, Konradi C: Mitochondrial dysfunction and pathology in bipolar disorder and schizophrenia. Int J Dev Neurosci 29:311–324, 2011
DiMauro S, Schon EA: Mitochondrial disorders in the nervous system. Annu Rev Neurosci 31:91–123, 2008
Fattal O, Budur K, Vaughan AJ, et al: Review of the literature on major mental disorders in adult patients with mitochondrial diseases. Psychosomatics 47:1–7, 2006

Finsterer J: Mitochondrial disorders, cognitive impairment and dementia. J Neurol Sci 283:143–148, 2009

Finsterer J: Psychosis as a manifestation of cerebral involvement in mitochondrial disorders, in Recent Advances in Clinical Medicine: Proceedings of the International Conference on Medical Pharmacology. WSEAS Press, 2010, pp 90–96

Kato T: The other, forgotten genome: mitochondrial DNA and mental disorders. Mol Psychiatry 6:625–633, 2001

Koene S, Kozicz TL, Rodenburg RJ, et al: Major depression in adolescent children consecutively diagnosed with mitochondrial disorder. J Affect Disord 114:327–332, 2009

Mancuso M, Orsucci D, Ienco EC, et al: Psychiatric involvement in adult patients with mitochondrial disease. Neurol Sci December 23, 2011 [Epub ahead of print]

Modica-Napolitano JS, Lagace CJ, Brennan WA, et al: Differential effects of typical and atypical neuroleptics on mitochondrial function in vitro. Arch Pharm Res 26:951–959, 2003

Sproule DM, Kaufmann P: Mitochondrial encephalopathy, lactic acidosis, and strokelike episodes: basic concepts, clinical phenotype, and therapeutic management of MELAS syndrome. Ann N Y Acad Sci 1142:133–158, 2008

HYPERKINETIC STATES

Hyperkinetic States

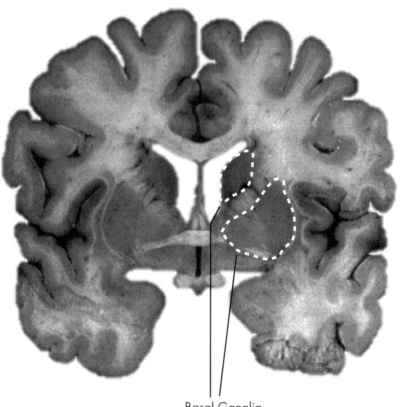

Basal Ganglia

Introduction

There is a well-known comorbidity of psychopathology and movement disorders. The psychopathological manifestations of movement disorders include anxiety, depression, obsessions and compulsions, and psychosis. A disturbance of the basal ganglia is the cause of the movement disorders, and disruption in their limbic connectivities is presumably responsible for the co-occurring psychiatric presentations. The crucial connectivities and critical neurotransmitter systems are, however, unknown.

Tourette's Disorder in Adults

Anton Scamvougeras, M.B.Ch.B., F.R.C.P.C.

A 29-year-old male pharmacist was referred for assessment and optimal management of tics that had bothered him since childhood.

He was the second born of a pair of identical twins. His mother had an uneventful pregnancy, with a normal vaginal delivery. He had suffered a very brief period of hypoxia perinatally but did not need to be in the intensive care unit. Milestones were all normal. He had always been slightly shorter than his twin brother.

When he was 6, a teacher noted that he was blinking excessively in class and occasionally "making faces." He was referred to an allergy specialist, found to have allergies to pollen and dust mites, and treated with eyedrops. The eyedrops appeared to be unhelpful, so their use was discontinued after a few months. His parents noticed that he had begun to make "rolling" shoulder movements while watching television and would sniff, grunt, and grimace repeatedly while playing with his brother, who made no such movements. His mother thought he might have Tourette's disorder after reading an article in a popular magazine, and when he was 7, his general practitioner referred him to the neuropsychiatry unit at the local children's hospital, where the diagnosis of Tourette's disorder was confirmed. Treatment with a low-dose dopamine blocker was recommended, but his parents declined.

Tic severity fluctuated throughout his childhood and teens. Despite this, he progressed well both academically and socially. At age 15, tics interfered with his quality of life enough for him to attempt a trial of haloperidol, but he stopped after a few days because he complained that the medication made him feel "like a zombie." The lifetime intensity of his tics was greatest when he was 19 and studying at a university, and they continued to fluctuate in intensity through his 20s.

At age 29, at the time of commencing a new job, his tics were again prominent and he was referred by his family doctor to an adult neuropsychiatry clinic.

Assessment revealed that he was in physically good health, and he initially denied symptoms of any comorbid psychiatric conditions. He demonstrated motor tics, including blinking, grimacing, head rotation, and shoulder movements. Some of the tics had a dystonic quality, with brief sustained posturing at the conclusion of the tic. One such tic was very forceful, involving hyperextension of the neck in conjunction with tonic tensing of arm and shoulder musculature. This tic was the most problematic symptom, causing neck pain and having been present for 4 years.

Neurological examination was otherwise normal. Blood investigations ruled out rare secondary causes of tics. The diagnosis of Tourette's disorder was again confirmed. Magnetic resonance imaging (MRI) brain scan was normal but for a small subarachnoid cyst in the vicinity of the anterior pole of the left temporal lobe.

Even though his tics seemed objectively intrusive and painful, he only rated them 6/10 on an informal lifetime severity scale, in contrast with the 10/10 severity that had occurred during his years at the university. Nonetheless, on being educated thoroughly about the nature of his condition and available management, he elected to attempt a trial of medication. He commenced a trial of risperidone, starting at the very low dose of 0.25 mg hs, with the intention of slowly titrating the dose upward. At 0.5 mg hs, he noted an uncomfortable sense of physical and mental slowness during the day, and this became unbearable at 1 mg. His tics remained unchanged and he elected to stop the medication trial.

A year passed before his return. Tics had again increased to the point of intrusiveness; he now rated them 7/10 in severity. His partner of 1 year was expecting a child, and although he welcomed this development, he was anxious with regard to the prospect of being a father. He asked about another trial of medication. Various agents were discussed, and a follow-up appointment was booked to answer further questions and allow time for him to consider his options.

When he returned for that appointment 1 month later, it was remarkable that his tics had in the interim spontaneously settled to the point that he found them far less intrusive. Both he and his clinician were struck by the fact that if they had indeed started a new medication at the previous appointment, they would both have attributed his improvement to that intervention. He rated the tic severity at only 4/10, and there was clearly no need to consider commencing any medications.

He returned for another appointment 2 months later to say his tics remained well controlled, but he revealed that he suffered significant ego-dystonic intrusive thoughts, often with violent content, that he found somewhat embarrassing to discuss. These thoughts met criteria for obsessions and were intrusive and pervasive enough to merit a diagnosis of obsessive-compulsive disorder (OCD). They had been present since his teens, and he admitted to having downplayed this symptom during prior assessments. He had never acted on any of these violent thoughts, nor was he assessed to be at risk of doing so. The obsessions benefited from the introduction of a selective serotonin reuptake inhibitor (SSRI) medication, with their degree of intrusiveness decreasing by an estimated 50% over the first 3 months of treatment.

His tic involving forceful hyperextension of his neck increased in frequency and intensity again, causing significant neck pain and now with the added symptoms of paresthesia in both hands. Cervical imaging revealed degenerative arthritic change far out of proportion to his age, but there was no evidence of cord injury. Electrophysiological testing showed no objective evidence of significant radiculopathy. This tic was obviously a cause for concern, and he again elected to attempt a trial of medication. On this attempt he managed to tolerate low-dose haloperidol starting at 0.5 mg nightly and building to a dose of 1.5 mg nightly. Tic intensity decreased from 7/10 to 4/10 and initial side effects of a sense of slowness and heaviness settled substantially, but not completely, over the first 6 weeks of treatment.

This was the beginning of his beneficial but somewhat ambivalent relationship with medications. Over the next 8 years, he went through periods of attempting to withdraw completely from haloperidol, but he always chose to return because he found it offered significant overall benefit to his quality of life. He bemoaned the fact that at times he felt that it "took the edge off" his enjoyment of life, but at the same time he acknowledged that the severe symptoms that surfaced when he attempted to go without medications intruded more. He was also pleased to note that his obsessions and compulsions were even more thoroughly controlled when he used haloperidol in combination with the SSRI. His quality of life was better overall when he was taking these medications. He is aware that both tics and obsessions may spontaneously decrease over time, and his management plan will include careful trials of medication reduction in years to come.

Discussion

Tourette's disorder is a neurodevelopmental condition with genetic and environmental causes that has as its central symptoms motor and vocal tics

(Jankovic 2001). By virtue of association at the genetic and pathophysiological level, individuals with Tourette's disorder have an increased chance of having comorbid conditions, in particular attention-deficit/hyperactivity disorder, mood disorders, OCD, pathological grooming disorders, and pervasive developmental disorders. Birth trauma increases the probability that the syndrome will manifest in genetically susceptible individuals.

The onset of Tourette's disorder usually occurs before the age of 10 years, and the condition most commonly peaks in intensity in the late teens. Most individuals with Tourette's disorder experience a significant decrease in their tic severity as they grow into adulthood. For a minority, however, the tics continue to interfere significantly with their quality of life. In addition, there is a group of individuals who suffer Tourette's disorder–like syndromes of late onset (Chouinard and Ford 2000).

A thorough assessment or reassessment in adulthood is prudent, even in those patients who have had a classic course since childhood. Psychiatric assessment will include careful review of the current status of comorbid conditions, which often prove to interfere more with quality of life than the tics themselves. Neurological assessment confirms the nature of the tics and screens for any signs of atypical neurodevelopment or other neurological conditions. Rare causes of "secondary" tics, such as Wilson's disease, acanthocytosis, Huntington's disease, and basal ganglia injury, should be excluded. MRI brain scan serves to screen for rare structural causes of tics and to exclude chance comorbidities. Such scans rarely indicate causative pathology, but they will demonstrate evidence of atypical neurodevelopment, such as subarachnoid cysts and heterotopias, at a higher rate than in the general population.

Once diagnosis is confirmed, education about tics should be revisited; adults will be capable of a more detailed understanding of the causes and mechanisms of their condition than they were in childhood. Tics should be explained as being strongly genetically determined and the result of overactivity of circuits responsible for important motor subprograms that are evolutionarily beneficial.

Tics show the classically described "waxing and waning" intensity over any time frame. This baseline variation appears to be the result of normal physiological fluctuation in the activity of dopamine-mediated neural circuitry, and it would occur even if all other variables could be held steady. Tic intensity will also vary with factors such as anxiety from psychosocial stressors, attention-demanding tasks, and fatigue. Baseline fluctuation in tic intensity makes interpretation of the outcome of treatment trials particularly challenging. Clinicians and patients are at risk of making false-positive or false-negative attributions, misinterpreting natural tic fluctuation as being the result of changes in treatment. The only way to avoid this pitfall is to assess response to treatment over longer time frames, rather than responding too rapidly and too frequently to short-term changes. Use of some form of measure of tic severity, such as an informal 0–10 lifetime tic intensity scale or an instrument such as the Yale Global Tic Severity Scale, is recommended (Storch et al. 2005).

There is a great deal of interpersonal variation in the degree to which individuals find tics intrusive, and this should be carefully assessed when judging the need for intervention. Some individuals may be able to adapt well and live happy and productive lives despite severe tics, whereas others may be distracted or even devastated by what appear objectively to be the most subtle of tics. Education of the patient, along with family members when it is appropriate to do so, will often be the only intervention necessary.

When it is clear that the tics are affecting quality of life to a more significant degree, more active therapies may be necessary. Behavioral therapies have met with some success, and some clinicians would recommend a trial of techniques such as habit reversal training before entertaining use of medications (Franklin et al. 2010). That said, there are patients who choose to go directly to trials of medications.

All medications used to treat tics aim to decrease activity of dopaminergic neurons, and the three main groupings of agents are 1) dopamine blockers such as haloperidol and risperidone, 2) alpha$_2$-agonists such as clonidine, and 3) the amine-depleting agent tetrabenazine.

There are no universally accepted algorithms for choice of medications. Neurologists often prefer to start treatment with tetrabenazine, probably because they are all too familiar with the severe tardive dyskinesia that can result from use of dopamine-blocking agents in other contexts. In contrast, psychiatrists are aware of the catastrophic dysphoria and severe depressions that can be a side effect of tetrabenazine, and are thus more comfortable commencing treatment with medication such as risperidone.

It should be remembered that when neuroleptics are used to treat tics in this population, we are actually seeking the slowing of motor circuitry, the very effects that we consider side effects when using the identical agents to treat psychosis. Thus it should not be surprising that older and "dirtier" agents such as haloperidol may be more effective than newer atypical antipsychotics in some patients.

Use of tetrabenazine carries a very clear risk of depressed mood (Kenney et al. 2006); less well known is that use of dopamine-blocking agents also carries a significant risk of depression and dysphoria in this population (Margolese et al. 2002). Equally important is the fact that individuals with Tourette's disorder are at risk of tardive dyskinesia, but they are probably less vulnerable to this side effect than those receiving neuroleptics for mood disorder or psychosis (Silva et al. 1993).

There is a great deal of interpersonal variation in the response to medications, with no known reliable methods for identifying in advance who will respond to which agents. Thus two individuals, each with moderately severe motor and vocal tics, may appear identical in almost every way, and yet one ends up responding extremely well to very low-dose haloperidol whereas the other's tics remain completely treatment resistant even on trials of high-dose combination therapies. The most prudent approach is, therefore, an empirical one, with systematic trials of medications, and careful record keeping over time regarding response to treatment.

Comorbid syndromes are often more disabling than tics, and it is not unusual for management to focus more on symptoms such as intrusive obsessions, depressed mood, or sleep disturbance than on the tics themselves (Eddy et al. 2011). Intriguingly, OCD associated with Tourette's disorder is different from OCD that occurs unrelated to Tourette's disorder (Nestadt et al. 2009). Those in the former group have more obsessions with violent and sexual content, more touching compulsions, more preoccupation with symmetry, and fewer concerns regarding contamination and cleaning than those in the latter group.

It is common for patients to have questions about deep brain stimulation for Tourette's disorder, given that some anecdotal cases have been widely publicized. The procedure is a promising alternative for severe treatment-resistant Tourette's disorder but is still in the experimental stage, with multidisciplinary centers around the world developing protocols and investigating optimal neuroanatomical targets.

The aim of all Tourette's disorder therapies is improvement of quality of life rather than eradication of a specific tic. Education in this regard can often redirect a patient's efforts and expectations in a very productive fashion.

The majority of individuals experience a decrease in tic intensity with aging, as dopaminergic systems mature and overactivity of related circuits wanes. Patients can almost all be reassured that they likely have time on their side in this regard.

Key Clinical Points

- Tics fluctuate at baseline, and care must be taken to keep that fluctuation in mind when assessing the effects of changes in management.

- Symptoms of comorbid conditions such as obsessive-compulsive disorder or a mood disorder may interfere more with quality of life than the tics themselves and oftentimes will be the main focus of management.
- Education of the patient and family regarding the nature of Tourette's disorder may be all the management required in some cases.
- All medications that directly decrease tics appear to do so by decreasing dopaminergic activity, by receptor blockade (haloperidol, risperidone), alpha$_2$-receptor agonism (clonidine), or amine depletion (tetrabenazine).
- There is a significant risk of emergence of depressed mood when tetrabenazine or dopamine blockers are used for treatment of tics.

Further Readings

Jankovic J: Tourette's syndrome. N Engl J Med 345:1184–1192, 2001

Scahill L, Erenberg G, Berlin CM Jr, et al: Contemporary assessment and pharmacotherapy of Tourette syndrome. NeuroRx 3:192–206, 2006

Swain JE, Scahill L, Lombroso P, et al: Tourette syndrome and tic disorders: a decade of progress. J Am Acad Child Adolesc Psychiatry 46:947–968, 2007

References

Chouinard S, Ford B: Adult onset tic disorder. J Neurol Neurosurg Psychiatry 68:738–743, 2000

Eddy CM, Cavanna AE, Gulisano M, et al: Clinical correlates of quality of life in Tourette syndrome. Mov Disord 26:735–738, 2011

Franklin SA, Walther MR, Woods DW: Behavioral interventions for tic disorders. Psychiatr Clin North Am 33:641–655, 2010

Jankovic J: Tourette's syndrome. N Engl J Med 345:1184–1192, 2001

Kenney C, Hunter C, Mejia N, et al: Is history of depression a contraindication to treatment with tetrabenazine? Clin Neuropharmacol 29:259–264, 2006

Margolese HC, Annable L, Dion Y: Depression and dysphoria in adult and adolescent patients with Tourette's disorder treated with risperidone. J Clin Psychiatry 63:1040–1044, 2002

Nestadt G, Riddle MA, Grados MA, et al: Obsessive-compulsive disorder: subclassification based on co-morbidity. Psychol Med 39:1491–1501, 2009

Silva RR, Magee HJ, Friedhoff AJ: Persistent tardive dyskinesia and other neuroleptic-related dyskinesias in Tourette's disorder. J Child Adolesc Psychopharmacol 3:137–144, 1993

Storch EA, Murphy TK, Geffken GR, et al: Reliability and validity of the Yale Global Tic Severity Scale. Psychol Assess 17:486–491, 2005

Psychosis Associated With Huntington's Disease

Anthony Feinstein, M.B.B.Ch., M.Phil., Ph.D., F.R.C.P.C.

A 38-year-old married woman, the mother of three young children, was brought to the emergency room by her husband. She had been speaking of hearing voices for approximately 6 months, but only when she began wearing her son's football helmet to keep out the voices did her husband decide to act. She had initially resisted her family's pleas for her to seek help for her troubling symptoms, fearing she would be kept in the hospital against her will once she had been assessed. She frequently reminded her husband that such an outcome had been the fate of her father, now deceased, who suffered from Huntington's disease. In keeping with her reluctance to seek psychiatric help for the "voices," she had refused repeated requests from her general practitioner to undergo testing for the Huntington gene.

On further psychiatric inquiry, the woman readily admitted to hearing voices with mixed positive and negative content. There were multiple voices identified, and they would comment on her appearance and behavior. At times, these voices would also address her directly by commanding her to do things, such as buying a new hair product or contacting her vicar about obtaining a divorce. She had since started to act on some of these instructions, resulting in further distress to her husband. The third-person comments were, however, initially complimentary, with the voices praising her beauty and predicting she was destined for better things in life than marriage to her farmer husband. She began wearing the football helmet only when the voices began denigrating her, the praise interspersed with derogatory comments laced with profanities.

She spoke openly of her plans for a different future. She claimed a well-known local neurosurgeon was in love with her and that she would soon divorce her husband to marry him. This, she was convinced, would be followed by the acquisition of great wealth. Mood, sleep, and memory were reported to be unaffected, and anxiety was not endorsed. Libido was poor, which she attributed to having "cooled" toward her husband.

This emergency room visit was the first time that she had made contact with psychiatric services. Past medical history was unremarkable.

A family history, obtained from her husband, was notable for documented Huntington's disease going back at least two generations. Her father and paternal grandfather were thought to have had the disease, as did other relatives on the paternal side. Of note was the fact that both her father and grandfather had been treated by psychiatrists and had spent years in psychiatric hospitals. Neither had displayed abnormal, involuntary movements until well after the onset of psychosis. In both relatives, significant mental state changes characterized by a mix of grandiose and persecutory beliefs had signaled the onset of the illness. Both had committed suicide, the father in his late 40s and the grandfather in his mid-50s. Neither reportedly suffered from dementia.

She grew up in the shadow of her troubled family history. She was one of two children, and her younger sister was reportedly well. Birth, milestones, and schooling passed without note despite frequent visits to the local psychiatric institution to visit her father and his brother. She was able to recall when she first had become aware of the family's genetic history: she was 18 years old at the time, and with this knowledge also came a determination to live life to the fullest notwithstanding the risk of inheriting the gene. This resolve was accompanied by a consistent refusal to undergo genetic testing. She married at age 21 to a man who had been apprised of her risk for developing Huntington's disease. Her husband confirmed this fact but also divulged that the true extent of his in-laws' psychiatric disturbance had been withheld from him.

The mental status examination on admission revealed an unkempt appearance. Only with some coaxing did she agree to remove the football helmet. For the remainder of the assessment, she was cooperative. Subtle choreoathetoid movements involving the upper limbs were present. Speech was mildly dysarthric. Mood was reported to be "very good." Affect was incongruent with mood and appeared blunted. Thought form was characterized by tangential thinking, while thought content was notable for grandiose and persecutory delusions. There were no thoughts of self-harm or plans to harm others. Prominent auditory hallucinations, including command hallucinations, dominated the mental state assessment; at times she would respond to them by either complimenting or admonishing the source of these voices. She disaffirmed visual, gustatory, and olfactory hallucinations. Cognitive-intellectual functions were impaired, with a Mini-Mental State Examination (MMSE) score of 25/30. One point was lost for disorientation, another 2 for short-term memory deficits, 1 for impaired sequencing, and 1 for poor constructional ability. Insight into the psychosis was absent, but awareness was partially intact for the cognitive deficits. Her lack of empathy toward her spouse and three children was striking.

Brain MRI revealed mild generalized atrophy with evidence of more selective atrophy involving the caudate nuclei bilaterally, as shown by the loss of convexity of the margins of the anterior horns of the lateral ventricles. A single-photon emission computed tomography (SPECT) brain scan revealed hypoperfusion in both caudate nuclei. A reduction in alpha rhythm was present on the electroencephalogram.

Given her lack of insight and her determination to contact and pursue the neurosurgeon she was planning on marrying, she was detained in the hospital involuntarily. Treatment began with quetiapine as a first-choice antipsychotic agent, the rationale being that the drug has a relatively innocuous side-effect profile with respect to involuntary movements. The dosage was titrated up to 1,200 mg/day without any benefit. A trial of risperidone at a dosage of 6 mg/day was equally ineffective. Treatment was therefore switched to olanzapine, with the dosage increased to 40 mg/day. The only noticeable change was a marked increase in her appetite. Treatment was changed to clozapine, but at a dosage of 600 mg/day, this medication had to be discontinued because it caused excessive sialorrhea and sedation. A small improvement in the auditory hallucinations was, however, noted, when she stopped wearing her son's football helmet.

Six months had elapsed by now without any progression in her abnormal movements. Her cognitive-intellectual functioning, on the other hand, had declined. An MMSE of 22 was obtained, and concerns were expressed that the high doses of clozapine were contributing to this result. The medication was therefore stopped, the MMSE returned to 25, but the hallucinations again became florid. At that point, a trial of haloperidol was begun. Haloperidol at a dosage of 4 mg/day partially relieved the auditory hallucinations, did not further impair cognitive-intellectual ability, had no effect on the delusions, and produced some mild psychomotor slowing that in fact diminished the choreoathetoid movements. Of note was that throughout this period, she consistently refused genetic testing, which had been proposed repeatedly to confirm the clinical diagnosis of Huntington's disease. Her husband, who had been appointed responsible for making medical decisions for her after she was deemed incapable, also declined confirmatory testing on her behalf. The husband had also refused to consent to a trial of electroconvulsive therapy, despite being given reassurances as to the safety of the procedure. At that point, she was transferred to a long-term mental health facility.

Discussion

This case history demonstrates a number of interesting features about patients with Huntington's disease, an autosomal dominant inherited neurodegenerative disorder that arises as a result of expansion of the trinucleotide (CAG) repeat in the short arm of chromosome 4. Before describing these features, it is important to note that the diagnosis in this case was made clinically in the absence of a confirmatory genetic test. The first observation pertains to the patient's age at onset of the disorder, which was younger than her father's age at onset, which in turn was younger than his father's symptom onset. Such a phenomenon is termed *anticipation*, which results from the increasing length of the expansion of the triplet (CAG) repeat in the offspring of those with Huntington's disease. Given that the age at onset of the disorder is related to the size of the repeat, children may become symptomatic at an earlier age than their parents. There is also evidence that the triplet instability is more marked in male gametes, which translates into anticipation appearing more prominently in the children of males with the disease (Nance 1997). In addition, an association between the size of the expansion and the severity of the disease as demonstrated clinically and measured by neuroimaging has been reported (Roth et al. 2005). In the patient described here, the loss of convexity in the frontal horns of the lateral ventricles observed on MRI, indicative of atrophy of the head of the caudate nuclei (Malekpour and Esfandbod 2010), and the bilateral caudate hypoperfusion noted on SPECT (Gemmell et al. 1989) were present at symptom onset. The characteristic electroencephalographic abnormality was likewise present early in the disease.

The most striking aspect of this patient's presentation was her florid psychosis accompanied by minimal abnormal, involuntary movements, an identical clinical picture to that of the previous two generations in her family. Huntington's disease presenting primarily with an alteration in mental state is well described. Changes in personality, including apathy or increased argumentativeness, may be a harbinger of the neurological difficulties to come. Anxiety and depression are much more common than in the general population, as is psychosis, most typically that of a paranoid delusional state. A more florid schizophrenia-like picture characterized by auditory hallucinations and various types of delusional thinking may also occur.

Some Huntington pedigrees have been described in which the psychotic features have defined the phenotype in all or most affected members across generations, with these changes long predating the emergence of the choreoathetoid movements or dementia (Corrêa et al. 2006). Such a clinical picture fits with the familial phenotype described in this case report. In a study that compared two groups of Huntington patients with and without psychosis ($n=22$ in each group), the psychotic patients were more likely to have a first-degree relative with psychosis (Tsuang et al. 2000). Significantly, the age at onset of psychosis was lower in patients with a higher number of trinucleotide repeats. Moreover, in all but one of nine families with a psychotic Huntington's disease subject who had a first-degree relative with psychosis, the relative's psychosis was also linked to Huntington's disease. The observations led the authors to suggest that the CAG expansion in some families may enhance the ability of other, nonspecified genetic factors to determine the clinical presentation in Huntington's disease.

One final aspect of family history, germane to this case report, deserves emphasis: the suicides of the patient's father and grandfather. Huntington's disease is one of a handful of neurological conditions, which also include multiple sclerosis, traumatic brain injury, stroke, and epilepsy, in which the suicide rate relative to the general population is increased (Arciniegas and Anderson 2002).

Treating psychosis in a patient with Huntington's disease can present a challenge, as this case report illustrates. Trials of quetiapine, risperidone, olanzapine, and clozapine all proved ineffective. The absence of published treatment guidelines meant that the approach adopted was that of trial and error. Quetiapine was used initially, the rationale being that the drug had a low likelihood of causing additional extrapyramidal side effects. When it proved ineffective, risperidone was tried. A literature review provided some evidence for treatment efficacy here (Cankurtaran et al. 2006), but the patient failed to respond as hoped. Clozapine was abandoned because of side effects. Haloperidol, a fifth choice, was marginally more helpful and, not surprisingly, reduced the subtle signs of involuntary movement given the side effect of bradykinesia. Aripiprazole was not tried, for funding reasons, notwithstanding a single case report describing its effectiveness in a psychotic patient with Huntington's disease who had not responded to olanzapine.

The reasons for this patient's lack of response to antipsychotic medication are unclear. Certainly, the small published treatment literature, often limited to single case reports, does indicate therapeutic benefits with most antipsychotic agents. Electroconvulsive therapy was considered after the failure of five antipsychotic drugs. Electroconvulsive therapy has been used safely and effectively, albeit rarely, in patients with Huntington's disease, the majority of whom had severe depression. There is also, however, a single case report of its efficacy in a primary, nonaffective psychosis associated with Huntington's disease.

Patients with Huntington's disease have a life expectancy of 10–15 years from the time of diagnosis. In the case described here, the onset of such a florid psychotic illness early in the disease added significantly to the patient's morbidity, more so given her poor response to psychiatric treatment. Given the difficult clinical and family situation, efforts were made to boost the involvement of other disciplines, including social work and occupational therapy, in the patient's management. This included providing appropriate services to the patient's husband and children.

Key Clinical Points

- Huntington's disease is an autosomal dominant neurodegenerative disorder that arises as a result of expansion of the trinucleotide (CAG) repeat in the short arm of chromosome 4.
- Psychosis may be the presenting clinical feature of Huntington's disease.
- In some families with Huntington's disease, psychosis may be the predominant phenotype across generations, long predating the development of the characteristic choreoathetoid movements.
- The onset of Huntington's disease may be earlier in the offspring of male patients, reflecting an increasing length of the trinucleotide repeat—a phenomenon termed *anticipation.*
- The characteristic neuroimaging findings, not always present, include dilatation of the anterior horns of the lateral ventricles on magnetic resonance imaging and hypoperfusion of the caudate nuclei on single-photon emission computed tomography/positron emission tomography.
- A small published literature suggests that the newer antipsychotic drugs are the treatment of choice for psychosis associated with Huntington's disease, but as this case report indicates, not all patients respond adequately. Electroconvulsive therapy may prove effective in patients whose psychosis has not responded adequately to antipsychotic medication.

Further Readings

David AS, Fleminger S, Kopelman MD, et al: Lishman's Organic Psychiatry, 4th Edition. Chichester, UK, Wiley-Blackwell, 2009

Guttman M, Alpay M, Chouinard S, et al: Clinical management of psychosis and mood disorders in Huntington's disease, in Mental Dysfunction in Movement Disorders. Edited by Bedard MA, Agid Y, Chouinard S, et al. Totowa, NJ, Humana Press, 2002, pp 409–426

References

Arciniegas DB, Anderson CA: Suicide in neurologic disease. Curr Treat Options Neurol 4:457–468, 2002

Cankurtaran ES, Ozalp E, Soygur H, et al: Clinical experience with risperidone and memantine in the treatment of Huntington's disease. J Natl Med Assoc 98:1353–1355, 2006

Corrêa BB, Xavier M, Guimarães J: Association of Huntington's disease and schizophrenia-like psychosis in a Huntington's disease pedigree. Clin Pract Epidemiol Ment Health 2:1, 2006

Gemmell HG, Sharp PF, Smith FW, et al: Cerebral blood flow measured by SPECT as a diagnostic tool in the study of dementia. Psychiatry Res 29:327–329, 1989

Malekpour M, Esfandbod M: Images in clinical medicine: Huntington's chorea. N Engl J Med 363:e24, 2010

Nance MA: Clinical aspects of CAG repeats. Brain Pathol 7:881–900, 1997

Roth J, Klempíi J, Jech R, et al: Caudate nucleus atrophy in Huntington's disease and its relationship with clinical and genetic parameters. Funct Neurol 20:127–130, 2005

Tsuang D, Almqvist EW, Lipe H, et al: Familial aggregation of psychotic symptoms in Huntington's disease. Am J Psychiatry 157:1955–1959, 2000

Tardive Dyskinesia

Silke Appel-Cresswell, M.D.
David Sherman, M.Sc., M.D.

A 37-year-old zookeeper was seen for assessment of involuntary movements. He had been diagnosed with bipolar I disorder at the age of 29 and had required seven involuntary hospitalizations for mania. The manic episodes were severe. On one occasion, he had stood on the runway of a major airport trying to stop a large passenger plane. The depressive phase of his illness had led to suicidal ideation, but there had not been any suicide attempts. Over the years he had been treated with numerous typical and atypical neuroleptics, including flupenthixol, loxapine, aripiprazole, risperidone, and olanzapine. In addition, he received long-term treatment with lithium for mood stabilization, intermittent antidepressants (SSRIs), and phenytoin and levetiracetam for a seizure disorder. Clozapine had been tried briefly in a severe manic phase with what he described as "disastrous effects": it made him feel "evil" and "caused me to throw a chair out of a window."

He developed involuntary movements around the age of 35 and was treated with loxapine 25–50 mg/day po, in addition to lithium, phenytoin, and levetiracetam. When he was seen at age 37, the involuntary dyskinetic movements had become more severe and enduring and were very distressing for him. They involved the perioral, jaw, and tongue muscles, resulting in jaw clenching, teeth grinding, blowing of the cheeks, tongue protrusion, and grimacing. He was frequently biting the inside of his cheeks. The dyskinesias affected the respiratory muscles, resulting in problems with breathing and occasionally choking while eating. Subsequently the movements also began to involve the shoulders. He denied any tic-like urge or relief when the movements occurred. They stopped during sleep. However, if he awoke during the night, he would have difficulty resuming sleep because of the recurrence of the movements.

Intense exercise alleviated the dyskinesias, and he would spend at least 2 hours each day exercising and training for long-distance running events. His occupation was also an important physical outlet for him. However, in the previous 3 months the movements had progressed to being constant. He could not continue with his work as a zookeeper because the abnormal movements were antagonizing the animals and he had been bitten twice. Not being able to work and having to give up running led to a further deterioration in both mood and movements. He described his movements as painful and embarrassing, and he had become severely depressed and socially withdrawn as a result of them.

His past medical history included a focal seizure disorder due to a cavernous angioma in the right occipitoparietal region; this angioma had been resected. He required seizure prophylaxis consisting of phenytoin 300 mg/day. Levetiracetam had been stopped a few months prior. His psychiatric symptoms were independent of his seizures or seizure medications. He had tried cocaine, ecstasy, and LSD a decade previously and currently smoked marijuana regularly. There were no involuntary movements associated with his substance use in the past, nor did he have a movement disorder such as tics in childhood. He had a family history of mental health disorders in his grandparents' generation and probably even in the generations before, but no other movement disorders were known.

At his first appointment at the movement disorder clinic, he presented as a casually dressed athletic young man who was adequately kempt. His eye contact was limited and he was constantly moving around. His mood was low, with intense feelings of sadness. He endorsed hopelessness and feelings of being punished, but there were no true psychotic symptoms. He denied suicidal ideation. Both he and his parents blamed the incessant involuntary movements for his low mood. On the Beck Depression Inventory he scored 35, indicating severe depression.

Physical examination demonstrated marked and continuous dyskinetic stereotypies and dystonic movements. The movements affected respiratory muscles, leading to sniffing sounds and poorly coordinated breathing at times. He had tongue protrusion, jaw closure, teeth grinding, shoulder shrugging, and elbow flexion. Some movements appeared more choreiform and stereotypical, whereas others led to more sustained dystonic postures. He could stop most of his movements for a few seconds when asked, and they improved slightly with voluntary movements. He did not have any marks suggesting chewing of his lips or tongue, a behavior often seen in neuroacanthocytosis. Cranial nerve examination, apart from the involuntary movements, was unremarkable. Voluntary tongue protrusion was reasonably sustained, and there was no delay in initiating either saccades or slow saccades (both of which can be seen in Huntington's disease). There was no bradykinesia, rigidity, tremor, or significant ataxia. The remainder of the neurological examination was normal.

Computed tomography scans of the brain revealed no changes beyond what was expected after his neurosurgical procedure. In particular, the heads of caudate were unremarkable, arguing against Huntington's disease. Laboratory investigations to rule out competing causes of the movements, particularly those that could lead to mental health problems such as Wilson's disease, neuroacanthocytosis, lupus erythematosus, or Huntington's disease, were negative. A dedicated ophthalmological examination did not find evidence for sunflower cataracts or Kayser-Fleischer rings, which could indicate Wilson's disease.

Shortly before he was seen at the movement disorder clinic, loxapine, then at 50 mg/day, was replaced with olanzapine 5 mg qhs. A past attempt to control his depression with fluoxetine 20 mg/day po had led to a worsening of his movements, and the fluoxetine was stopped. Benztropine, an anticholinergic, had not led to an improvement of the involuntary movements in the past. Hence when first seen in the clinic, he was taking olanzapine 5 mg qhs, phenytoin 300 mg/day, and lithium 1,200 mg/day.

Given the severity of the symptoms, it was decided to give tetrabenazine a cautious trial. He was apprised of the risk of depression, akathisia, and parkinsonism associated with a dopamine depleter. An electrocardiogram was ordered to rule out a prolonged QTc interval when on both tetrabenazine and olanzapine. He took only two doses of tetrabenazine 12.5 mg and then stopped it because he felt his depression worsen.

He was started on clonazepam 0.5 mg tid with a warning that clonazepam can be addictive, particularly given his previous history of drug abuse. Olanzapine was decreased to 2.5 mg qhs, and over the next few months, the dyskinesias seemed to improve. Unfortunately, he decided to take loxapine again for a few days, which led to a deterioration of his involuntary movements. Increasing the clonazepam to 1.5 mg tid did not lead to a significant improvement in the following months.

Botulinum toxin injections into the very severely involved jaw and perioral muscles were tried once. However, he did not find them useful. Vitamin E was used as an adjunct but did not lead to a clear benefit.

Given his severe disability, tetrabenazine was given another trial. This time he slowly increased the dose to 25 mg tid. However, the medication was tapered off again because he did not feel that it had any effect on his dyskinesias and he had significant akathisia and mild parkinsonism. He complained that "tardive has completely ruined my life." At that time, the movements were mostly dystonic, and so he was given another trial of benztropine. He was referred to neurosurgery for evaluation of his suitability for deep brain stimulation to treat his tardive dyskinesia (TD).

However, over the next few months, his TD improved and was manageable when he was emotionally calm; the TD worsened during emotional arousal. Unfortunately, he was not compliant with his psychotropic medication and experienced further manic episodes with grandiose, spiritual, and paranoid delusions. He had two further involuntary hospitalizations lasting several months. Care was taken not to reexpose him to typical neuroleptics during his admissions.

Plans for the future included changing his antiseizure medication to valproate, which would have a mood-stabilizing effect and might be able to replace lithium. Both phenytoin and lithium can induce choreiform movements, and lithium is associated with an increased risk for the development of TD.

The possible use of clozapine was discussed with him, but he was not willing to give this another try after his past experience. In addition, clozapine decreases the seizure threshold, which was of concern given his previous history of seizures.

Discussion

Tardive dyskinesia refers to abnormal, involuntary movements induced by dopamine receptor blocking agents (DRBAs), usually after at least 1 month of exposure and lasting at least 1 month after the offending drug is discontinued. Definitions vary, and in rare cases TD has been described after only a few exposures. *Tardive* means "late," which reflects the distinction from the acute drug-induced movement disorders that occur early in the course of treatment and are usually reversible.

Classically, *tardive dyskinesia* described orofacial-lingual-masticatory stereotypies with pursing and smacking of lips, chewing movements, and tongue protrusion, but the term is now often used as a synonym for any abnormal, involuntary movement induced by DRBAs. These movements can include stereotypies, dystonia, akathisia, myoclonus, tics, or tremor. In contrast to the random and unpredictable choreiform movements occurring in Huntington's disease and other movement disorders, the hyperkinetic movements in TD tend to be more stereotypical, predictable, and repetitive in nature (Soares-Weiser and Fernandez 2007). Tardive dyskinesia can also affect respiratory muscles as in this case, leading to irregular respiration. Tardive dystonia typically affects axial muscles, which may manifest as opisthotonos and retrocollis. Arms and legs might be flexed and extended in a repetitive fashion. There is a broad range of severity of TD. The patient in this case represents the severe end of the spectrum. Many patients, particularly if they only have orolingual TD, are not aware of their movements.

This patient had several risk factors associated with the development of TD: high total drug exposure, affective rather than psychotic disorders, use of lithium, and preexisting brain damage. Other risk factors for TD include older age, dementia in the elderly, previous drug-induced parkinsonism, alcoholism, diabetes mellitus, HIV-positive status, and smoking. Older female patients appear to be at higher risk of developing stereotypical TD, especially orolingual dyskinesias, whereas younger patients might be more prone to developing tardive dystonia. As seen in this case, many patients will have a combination of movements.

Tardive dyskinesia is a clinical diagnosis, and additional investigations are only performed to exclude competing diagnoses. The differential diagnosis for TD includes diseases that lead to both hyperkinetic movements and psychiatric symptoms, such as Huntington's disease, Wilson's disease, and neuroacanthocytosis. Additional findings on the neurological or general medical examination or abnormal imaging and laboratory test results should raise red flags. Even in drug-naive patients with schizophrenia, an increased rate of involuntary movements is well documented. If movements are predominantly craniofacial, primary dystonic disorders such as blepharospasm, Meige syndrome, and cervical dystonia are a consideration; edentulous perioral dyskinesias are considered in the elderly.

Prevalence rates vary widely in the literature. More recent data suggest that about 10%–20% of patients on long-term atypical neuroleptics and about 30% on typical neuroleptics develop TD. In 5%–10% of cases, TD interferes significantly with function (Aia et al. 2011; Bakker et al. 2011; Correll and Schenk 2008). The development of TD in patients with schizophrenia might be associated with higher mortality rates (Chong et al. 2009; Dean and Thuras 2009).

Among the atypical neuroleptics, the likelihood of TD is least with clozapine (if TD can be triggered by clozapine at all), followed by quetiapine, risperidone at low dosages, olanzapine, ziprasidone, and risperidone at high dosages (Tarsy et al. 2002). Aripiprazole has also been reported to cause TD. Spontaneous remission rates are low if treatment with DRBAs continues, which is often a necessity. Stopping the offending agent significantly increases chances for remission. Remissions usually occur in the first year and rarely up to 5 years after stopping the offending agent.

Another very important agent causing TD is metoclopramide, a dopamine blocker used to treat nausea and other gastrointestinal symptoms. Obtaining a thorough drug history, including from collateral sources such as prescription records, is paramount. Other medications such as antidepressants or lithium might rarely lead to tardive movement disorders as well.

The dopamine receptor hypersensitivity hypothesis proposes that TD results from increased sensitivity to dopamine of nigrostriatal system dopamine receptors as a consequence of chronic antipsychotic-induced dopamine receptor blockade. The pathophysiology is still surprisingly unclear, but several theories have been proposed. Tardive dyskinesia is most commonly associated with typical neuroleptics, which are potent D_2 dopamine receptor blockers. Both imaging and animal studies suggest that D_2 blockade leads to D_2 upregulation and increased receptor sensitivity, which are important etiological factors for TD. The relatively stronger serotonergic versus dopaminergic blockade of atypical compared with typical DRBAs is thought to be protective against TD. Other potential factors suggested include individual susceptibility, oxidative stress, and degeneration of GABAergic and cholinergic interneurons in the basal ganglia. Amine depleters such as tetrabenazine do not cause TD, although they can cause an acute dystonic reaction.

Prevention is key because once TD manifests it is often treatment resistant and, as seen in this case, can become as disturbing as the psychiatric condition itself. DRBAs should only be used when necessary. Schizophrenia and other psychotic disorders will usually require DRBAs, but insomnia, depression, and anxiety can be treated with alternative medications. Atypical neuroleptics should be favored over typical ones.

Once TD has developed and particularly if it is clinically significant, the first line of treatment should be the removal or replacement of the offending agent if possible. Switching to an antipsychotic medication with a lower risk of TD, such as clozapine or quetiapine, should be considered. Clozapine is associated with a 1%–2% incidence of agranulocytosis and requires monitoring. Dopamine-depleting agents such as tetrabenazine or reserpine can be quite effective but frequently induce treatment-limiting parkinsonism, depression, and akathisia, as seen in this patient.

The antioxidant vitamin E (1,200–1,600 IU/day) might improve TD or prevent further worsening of TD, but study outcomes have been variable (Soares-Weiser and Fernandez 2007). Smaller studies have reported some benefit with the use of branched-chain amino acids (isoleucine, leucine, and valine), propranolol, benzodiazepines (clonazepam), amantadine, and levetiracetam. Levetiracetam carries a U.S. Food and Drug Administration warning concerning the infrequent side effects of psychosis, suicidality, and other behavioral symptoms. Injections with botulinum toxin can be very useful in focal TD, especially in perioral, tongue, and jaw movements, and are generally well tolerated.

Anticholinergic medications such as benztropine and trihexyphenidyl can be useful for acute dystonic reactions and possibly tardive dystonia but can worsen stereotypical TD. Increasing the offending DRBA can lead to a temporary improvement of TD but is associated with an increased risk of persistence and possible worsening of TD in the long term and should be avoided if possible. Deep brain stimulation can be considered in the most severe cases (Welter et al. 2010).

Key Clinical Points

- Tardive dyskinesia emerges after prolonged exposure to a dopamine receptor blocking agent and can also occur when an offending drug is reduced in dosage or discontinued.

- TD is iatrogenic, and prevention is key. Atypical antipsychotics should be favored over typical ones and used only where irreplaceable and at the lowest effective dose. If possible, they should be tapered off slowly once the first signs of TD occur.

- Metoclopramide is an important agent causing TD. Obtaining a thorough drug history, including from pharmacy and physician records, is paramount.

- Risk factors for TD include previous brain damage, previous drug-induced parkinsonism, female sex, and older age, as well as higher drug dosage and longer exposure.

- TD persists in a significant proportion of patients. Treatment strategies are diverse, but there is no established gold standard.

Further Readings

Aia PG, Revuelta GJ, Cloud LJ, et al: Tardive dyskinesia. Curr Treat Options Neurol 13:231–241, 2011

Soares-Weiser K, Fernandez HH: Tardive dyskinesia. Semin Neurol 27:159–169, 2007

References

Aia PG, Revuelta GJ, Cloud LJ, et al: Tardive dyskinesia. Curr Treat Options Neurol 13:231–241, 2011

Bakker PR, de Groot IW, van Os J, et al: Long-stay psychiatric patients: a prospective study revealing persistent antipsychotic-induced movement disorder. PLoS One 6:e25588, 2011

Chong SA, Tay JA, Subramaniam M, et al: Mortality rates among patients with schizophrenia and tardive dyskinesia. J Clin Psychopharmacol 29:5–8, 2009

Correll CU, Schenk EM: Tardive dyskinesia and new antipsychotics. Curr Opin Psychiatry 21:151–156, 2008

Dean CE, Thuras PD: Mortality and tardive dyskinesia: long-term study using the US National Death Index. Br J Psychiatry 194:360–364, 2009

Soares-Weiser K, Fernandez HH: Tardive dyskinesia. Semin Neurol 27:159–169, 2007

Tarsy D, Baldessarini RJ, Tarazi FI: Effects of newer antipsychotics on extrapyramidal function. CNS Drugs 16:23–45, 2002

Welter ML, Grabli D, Vidailhet M: Deep brain stimulation for hyperkinetics disorders: dystonia, tardive dyskinesia, and tics. Curr Opin Neurol 23:420–425, 2010

SOMATOFORM AND SOMATOFORM-LIKE DISORDERS

Somatoform and Somatoform-Like Disorders

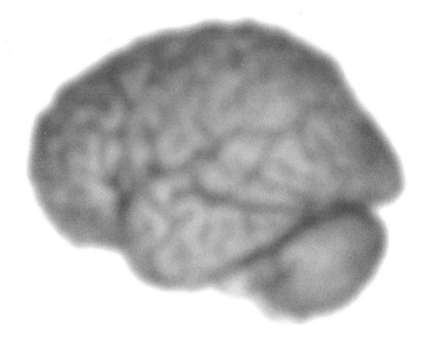

INTRODUCTION

Patients who present with physical complaints in the absence of an explanatory organic pathology are a diagnostic and management challenge. Most commonly, such patients are unconsciously converting psychological distress into somatic symptoms. Emergent motor-sensory symptoms involve only those aspects of neurological functioning over which there is voluntary control. Where the presentation is neurologically unexplained cognitive-intellectual symptoms, the newly coined term *cogniform disorder* is applied. Less commonly, typical disease initially presents atypically or accurate diagnosis is delayed. The error here is to mislabel such presentations as somatoform, which is to the detriment of both patient and physician.

Multiple Physical Symptoms That Remain Undiagnosed

Marius Dimov, M.D., F.R.C.P.C.

A 52-year-old woman in an assisted living setting was referred for assessment and management as an inpatient following a progressive decline in her mobility and self-care. She required mechanical lifts for her transfers. She was previously a healthy nurse, whose problems started 5 years before admission while she was working as a supervisor in a nursing home. The only health issue reported at the time was mild asthma, which started to worsen after exposure to dust during construction work at her workplace. Her breathing problems sharply escalated to the point of her requiring a painter's mask on top of two other masks when exposed to normal, "nonpurified" environments. Without the mask she would immediately start suffocating and experience an acute sensation of "squeezing and burning" in her throat. She started having episodes of "passing out" and collapsing, with loss of voluntary muscle control, on any exposure to air without a protective mask. At times she would become lethargic, fatigued, and "spaced out," with poor cognitive-intellectual and physical functioning for days thereafter. She also started to have muscle twitches and erratic choreiform movements in the upper and lower extremities, to the point of completely losing balance and falling. These movements would be triggered by simple movements, stress, or exposure to scents, exhaust, or dust. Other physical symptoms included tingling sensations in her extremities, difficulty swallowing, diplopia, constipation for several days, and vague arthralgias.

Over time her mobility progressively declined; at first she needed a cane, then a walker, and finally a motorized wheelchair. She was forced to sell her apartment and move to an assisted living facility, where she required total care. Any body movement would trigger acute suffocation (even with the mask). She would collapse and become unresponsive for a few minutes to hours, experiencing residual post-event fatigue that lasted for days. She also had episodes of unprovoked sudden collapse, described as "the sleeping thing," in which she would remain slouched over for 2–6 hours while continuing to maintain awareness of her surroundings. These episodes would resolve with no apparent residual confusion. Her symptoms fluctuated in severity over time, but her overall disability was progressive, especially during the year before admission, leading to her referral for inpatient assessment on a neuropsychiatric ward.

On examination she was in a motorized wheelchair. She wore a painter's mask with two large filters on both sides. She was neither in pain nor in distress, but rather was calm and jovial. There was no psychomotor agitation or retardation. Her affect was bright. Speech demonstrated normal speed and prosody. Her thought form was goal directed. Her thought content showed a striking satisfaction with her life despite her current state.

She had been reluctant to proceed with the hospital admission and firmly believed that despite no definitive diagnosis, she had a very severe and progressive neurological condition that had worsened during the past year. There was no appetite loss or sleep disturbance, and energy level was only affected by the frequency and severity of her episodes, with residual fatigue postevent. No suicidal ideation or gestures or perceptual disturbances were reported. She had no language deficits. She complained of problems with attention and memory but showed no such difficulties on formal testing.

Her vital signs were stable, and cardiovascular, respiratory, and abdominal exams were unremarkable. She started suffocating instantly when asked to take off the mask, becoming unresponsive and shaking and slumping down into her chair. Oxygen saturation (SaO_2), measured via pulse oximetry, remained unchanged at 99%.

On neurological examination, she was alert and fully oriented. Recent and remote memory were intact, and visuospatial and executive functioning were adequate. Cranial nerves were normal. There was no spasticity or rigidity. Attempts to test any voluntary movement resulted in uncontrollable shaking of her whole body, slumping and almost falling off the chair, and becoming unresponsive for a few seconds, head down. Coordination, gait, and balance were not tested because of her uncontrollable shaking. Her presentation was not consistent with any known neurological disorder as reviewed by a neurologist. Multiple sclerosis and myoclonus had been considered and excluded.

Laboratory testing included a complete blood count and differential, electrolytes, fasting blood sugar, renal function, thyroid function, liver enzymes, calcium, magnesium, phosphate, albumin, erythrocyte sedimentation rate, C-reactive protein, C3, C4, and vasculitis screen; all results were normal or negative. Spine computed tomography (CT) and magnetic resonance imaging (MRI) brain scans showed no abnormality. Electroencephalographic findings were normal, with no epileptiform discharges or slowing. Electrocardiographic, echocardiographic, and chest X ray findings were normal.

There was no family history of movement disorders or Huntington's disease. Her previous medical history was significant only for asthma, which she developed as a child when exposed to horses. She had been treated for asthma over the years, but it was at its worst 5 years prior to admission; at that time she used prednisone as needed and multiple inhalers. She gave a history of multiple allergies, even though allergy testing was inconclusive. No allergies to medications were reported.

She was the oldest of three children, with two younger sisters. She described sexual abuse perpetrated by her father toward her and her sisters. Despite this she described normal milestones and did well in school. She graduated as a nurse and worked in different settings throughout her life. Her relationships were overall unsatisfactory. She recalled having been engaged several times, but she never married and never had a child. She feared intimacy, and although she did have sexual experiences, she described hiding in a closet afterward (to her partner's dismay). At one point she had confronted her father with the sexual abuse, but he had dismissed her and it remained a family secret. The worsening of her health had coincided with her working as a nurse with disabled adults. She was also going through perimenopausal changes. As her health declined and she became more and more physically dependent, her father became more involved with her care. She had to sell her apartment, and the money went into a joint account with her father.

The working diagnosis was a somatoform disorder presumed to be due to an underlying major depressive disorder with an associated somatic psychosis. There was also evidence of alexithymia (difficulty in describing or being aware of emotions or mood), with a pervasive belief that "good girls don't cry." A formulation was offered to her explaining that her illness was caused by an underlying neurochemical depression but was surfacing as severe disabling physical symptoms.

She showed some superficial understanding initially, embracing the psychiatric concepts provided to her by an authority figure (doctor). She agreed to start taking a combination of fluoxetine and risperidone. She was also seen by an occupational therapist and physiotherapist, and a progressive rehabilitation program was initiated. Psychotherapy was started and continued on a daily basis in the hospital. The emphasis was on dealing with difficult and conflicting emotions, including her attitude and feelings toward her father.

With therapy she became more aware of her underlying depression and began to display appropriate affect, including sadness, anxiety, and anger. She experienced a peculiar left temporal discomfort when dealing with strong emotions. She became more assertive and was better able to establish her boundaries. She demonstrated a simultaneous improvement in her physical symptoms. She began to regain control of her movements, and the episodes of slumping and unresponsiveness decreased in frequency. She started to get up from a chair on her own and assisted with her transfers with less jerkiness and better postural stability. By the time of discharge, she was walking with the assistance of a walker and was able to independently perform all her activities of daily living. She remained hypersensitive to ambient air and continued to have laryngospasms when her mask was off; therefore, she continued to use a mask, but a lighter one with less protection.

She was discharged to her assisted living facility with a walker and arrangements for follow-up with a physiotherapist and psychiatrist. She remained independent with a walker. Attempts to transition her to a cane were unsuccessful even though she was able to walk perfectly well when asked to push the walker with her index fingers, thus not using it as support. Moreover, if she tried to use two canes or just stand without touching anything, she would instantly start jerking, remaining on her feet with very complex choreiform-like movements that disappeared once she touched any stable ambient object.

Although more comfortable with strong emotions, she continued to present with an avoidance of emotionally laden issues. She appeared to take comfort in the sick role and remained enmeshed with her father, who continued to be overinvolved with her care. She also continued to avoid same-age contacts and was more comfortable with the older residents in her care facility. Despite these issues she achieved a level of stability, and no further deterioration was noted 2 years after discharge from the hospital. She continued to take fluoxetine 50 mg/day and risperidone 2 mg/day.

Discussion

Patients with multiple physical symptoms that remain undiagnosed represent a major diagnostic and treatment challenge. The initial workup is often prolonged, as various specialists attempt to uncover organic disease. Patients may travel to various doctors and centers worldwide in search of a cure. Treatments with unproven benefits and sometimes significant risks are offered. Despite these challenges, no patient should be diagnosed with a somatoform disorder without a full and comprehensive search for organic etiologies. These investigations need to be reviewed by the treating psychiatrist to ensure that due diligence has been done to exclude disease.

Somatization is a process whereby psychological distress is expressed by way of physical symptoms. The hallmark of somatization is the presence of physical symptoms that do not match the known organic damage patterns, supported by a negative diagnostic workup that confirms the absence of underlying disease that would account for the presenting symptoms (Hurwitz 2003; Thomas and Jancovic 2004). The patient in this case met these criteria. Although she was previously diagnosed with asthma, her breathing problems did not fit the typical asthma presentation. The striking feature of laryngospasm was also not related to a structural deficit or dystonia but represented a severe anxiety response, with air hunger in reaction to any exposure to "nonpurified" air. Her extremely dramatic reaction of suddenly slumping over and becoming unresponsive when subjected to a mild stress in the form of odors, car exhaust, or dust or when asked to perform simple tasks (even when a mask was present) is outside the range of known allergic reactions.

Somatization is driven by underlying psychological distress. The source of this distress in patients with chronic somatization is uncertain. Major depressive disorder has been identified as the most common underlying psychiatric illness in patients with chronic conversion disorders (Hurwitz 2003). The possibility of other diagnoses should, however, be considered; other diagnoses may include psychosis, posttraumatic stress disorder, and anxiety disorders. The mechanism of symptom production is also unknown. Patients' symptoms may arise from fixed beliefs of somatic dysfunction (somatic delusions) that control neurological pathways to produce patterns of loss or gain of function that do not match the known organic damage patterns (Hurwitz and Prichard 2006).

Somatoform patients may also often demonstrate alexithymia. Unexpressed emotions may then surface in the form of organically unexplained physical symptoms. These symptoms may be shaped by the patient's knowledge and beliefs about how disease should present—a process known as *symptom modeling* (Hurwitz 2003). Symptom modeling was likely in this case because the patient was a nurse who had worked with severely physically disabled patients.

The pharmacological treatment is chosen depending on the presumed underlying psychological disturbance. Because in most cases the proposed mechanism is a major depressive illness with a somatic psychosis, an antidepressant and an atypical antipsychotic may be used. Electroconvulsive therapy (ECT) should be considered in severely disabled patients who remain unresponsive to medications (Hurwitz 2003). Patients will also benefit from physical rehabilitation, which is needed both for activation and to deal with secondary deconditioning. Psychotherapy, including expressive-supportive therapy and cognitive-behavioral therapy, is essential to explore conflicts and stressors, uncover emotions, and help patients accept that they have a psychiatric illness (Beutel et al. 2008; Rosebush and Mazurek 2011). Finally, narcoanalysis may sometimes be used to help patients recover lost neurological functions, gain insight, and accept the psychogenic origin of their symptoms (Beutel et al. 2008; Poole et al. 2010).

In caring for patients with somatoform disorders, clinicians must at all times remain vigilant for newly occurring signs and symptoms and the potential of an unrelated and independent organic illness to manifest itself in the future (Aybek et al. 2008; Stone et al. 2009). New investigations or referral to appropriate specialists should be pursued to avoid misdiagnosis, which is now less common given the availability of increasingly sophisticated diagnostic tools.

Key Clinical Points

- Comprehensive investigation and exclusion of possible organic diagnoses is necessary before making a diagnosis of somatoform disorder.
- Major depressive disorder is the most common underlying primary psychiatric disturbance, with alexithymia as an emotional communication style. The differential diagnosis is wide, and periodic reassessment is needed to identify emergent psychopathology.
- Treatment strategies often include an antidepressant augmented by an atypical antipsychotic and psychotherapy.
- A multidisciplinary approach is often beneficial.
- Changes in the physical symptoms or the emergence of new ones should prompt additional investigations or consultations with the appropriate specialists to rule out the occurrence of a new organic condition.

Further Readings

BC Neuropsychiatry Program: Somatoform disorders brochure, February 2008. Available at: http://psychiatry.vch.ca/docs/pdf/somatoform_disorders.pdf. Accessed August 12, 2012.

Hurwitz T: Somatization and conversion disorder. Can J Psychiatry 49:172–178, 2003

Rosebush P, Mazurek M: Treatment of conversion disorder in the 21st century: have we moved beyond the couch? Curr Treat Options Neurol 13:255–266, 2011

Stone J, Carson A, Duncan R: Symptoms "unexplained by organic disease" in 1144 new neurology out-patients: how often does the diagnosis change at follow-up? Brain 132:2878–2888, 2009

References

Aybek S, Kanaan RA, David AS: The neuropsychiatry of conversion disorder. Curr Opin Psychiatry 21:275–280, 2008

Beutel ME, Michal M, Subic-Wrana C: Psychoanalytically oriented inpatient psychotherapy of somatoform disorders. J Am Acad Psychoanal Dyn Psychiatry 36:125–142, 2008

Hurwitz T: Somatization and conversion disorder. Can J Psychiatry 49:172–178, 2003

Hurwitz TA, Prichard JW: Conversion disorder and fMRI. Neurology 12:1914–1915, 2006

Poole N, Wuerz A, Agrawal N: Abreaction for conversion disorder: systematic review with meta-analysis. Br J Psychiatry 197:91–95, 2010

Rosebush P, Mazurek M: Treatment of conversion disorder in the 21st century: have we moved beyond the couch? Curr Treat Options Neurol 13:255–266, 2011

Stone J, Carson A, Duncan R: Symptoms "unexplained by organic disease" in 1144 new neurology out-patients: how often does the diagnosis change at follow-up? Brain 132:2878–2888, 2009

Thomas M, Jancovic J: Psychogenic movement disorders: diagnosis and management. CNS Drugs 18:437–452, 2004

Complex Illness After a Fall

Anton Scamvougeras, M.B.Ch.B., F.R.C.P.C.

A 46-year-old woman working as a nursing aide in a hospital on the Canadian prairies had a fall while descending the stairs at work, slipping and landing on her lower back and buttocks. Immediately after the fall she complained of pain in the lower back, coccyx, and buttocks, with numbness radiating into her right leg. Her family doctor ordered an X ray of her lumbar spine and pelvis, which revealed no bone injuries.

Her pain persisted and then worsened. She was unable to work. Six weeks postinjury she was again assessed; she was found to have no specific neurological deficits, and a diagnosis of sciatica was entertained. Disability insurance agencies became involved, and she was enrolled in a rehabilitation program.

Pain symptoms persisted. Five months postinjury she was noted to appear "slow" and, for the first time in an interview, tearful. Three months later, "inconsistent strength" was noted on assessment of lower-limb power and was thought to represent psychogenic amplification of symptoms. A myelogram showed slight posterior disk protrusion at L4–L5, with mild degenerative changes in the lumbar spine.

Over the next 10 years, the woman was serially reassessed and treated by rehabilitation specialists and three psychiatrists. After 2 years of illness, all involved agreed that she was suffering from major depression. Concurrently, she suffered a gait disturbance described as "bizarre" by various clinicians, judged to be psychogenic, and diagnosed as conversion disorder. There was some debate between her treating physicians and disability agencies as to whether she was consciously inducing her physical symptoms. Computed tomography and MRI of her thoracolumbar spine did not demonstrate any significant pathology. She received physical rehabilitation. Trials of medications, including analgesics, selective serotonin reuptake inhibitors, and tricyclic antidepressants, were either unsuccessful or aborted because of side effects. There was no change in her level of function, and she remained very severely disabled by her illness.

Twelve years postinjury, at age 58, she was admitted to a neuropsychiatry unit for assessment. She described constant "tight and burning" pain of "excruciating" severity in her neck, back, legs, feet, arms, upper chest, and abdominal wall, with intermittent "spasms" of pain in various parts of the body. Pain was worsened by heat, movement, and any effort, without any relieving factors. She dated the onset of the pain to the time of her fall, with steady worsening since; it was now "as bad as ever."

She complained of associated weakness in her legs and was unable to walk without the assistance of a cane or walker. For 8 years prior to admission to the neuropsychiatry unit, she had required a wheelchair for all excursions from home.

Her mood was depressed and frustrated. Anhedonia was complete, even to the point that spending time with her grandchild was of no enjoyment. Sleep was disturbed, with initial insomnia and reduced duration.

Fatigue was constant, and her appetite was poor. Despite the poor appetite, her weight had increased by 30 pounds since illness onset. Libido was absent, and all sexual activity had discontinued. She complained she "used to have a brain like a computer" but now her memory was poor. There was no suicidal ideation, and no overt psychotic symptoms.

The resultant overall disability was severe. She required help with her personal care and with cooking and cleaning. For an average of 4 days a week she would be largely confined to bed. She had a "medical" bed at home and various physical adaptations to the house to accommodate her needs.

On examination, she looked older than 58. She made poor eye contact, staring at the floor in front of her. Her speech was droning and monotonous. Affect was flat and depressed, with no spontaneity. She wept periodically during the interview, her nose often running profusely without her making any move to wipe it. Her husband was in the habit of rising and wiping her face as she wept. Thought form was very circumstantial, and she was preoccupied with her physical symptoms.

Cognitive-intellectual testing was noteworthy for slowness, reduced attention, normal naming, reduced short-term verbal memory, normal nonverbal memory, bizarrely poor calculation ability (she claimed she was unable to multiply 2 by 2), concrete thinking, and incessant pessimistic self-commentary concerning her performance.

Physical examination revealed that her entire body was tender to the very slightest touch. Muscles of the back and shoulders were held tonically contracted. She demonstrated idiosyncratic variable responses to numerous examination tasks. When asked to follow a target with her eyes, she would at times perform the task in a normal fashion but at other times close her eyes or look away. There were no objective cranial nerve deficits. Tests of power revealed variable muscle effort. She was unable to perform some movements to specific request, yet at other times she was able to demonstrate power in relevant muscles when distracted. There was no muscle atrophy, reflexes were normal, and she was able to walk with a cane held in her right hand, with an unstable gait that fluctuated inconsistently.

There was, thus, very clear evidence of psychogenic overlay. There was nothing to suggest conscious amplification of symptoms: she genuinely appeared to believe that she was ill in this fashion.

She had been born in a small town. Her mother died when she was a child, and she had been raised by her grandparents in modest circumstances. Upon completing grade 10, she trained as a nursing aide and found a job in the hospital in a medium-size town nearby. She had held this job for more than 20 years at the time of her injury. At 18 she had met her husband, who was then 25 and who worked as a custodian in the same hospital. Their marriage was a happy one, with three children and one grandchild. She was known to be hardworking, energetic, independent, and family oriented. Before her fall she was mildly overweight but otherwise healthy.

Past psychiatric history revealed premorbid mild obsessional personality traits, no prior psychiatric illness, and no substance use or abuse. Past medical history was noteworthy for absence of neurological symptoms. She had three pregnancies with three normal deliveries.

Her mother had died in her 40s of a presumed ruptured brain aneurysm, and her maternal grandmother had died in her 60s, also apparently the result of an intracranial bleed. An aunt had died of myocardial infarction at the age of 42. There was no family history of psychiatric illness.

A provisional diagnostic formulation was made.

Severe somatoform disorder with:

> Chronic complex somatoform pain
> Conversion disorder (presenting as leg weakness; gait disturbance)
> Cogniform features (psychogenic cognitive-intellectual deficits)
> Major depression

Special investigations were performed to screen for possible medical causes for the physical and psychiatric symptoms. Results of blood investigations, electrocardiogram, and chest X ray were normal.

MRI head scan revealed a large region of encephalomalacia in the deep left frontal lobe; the encephalomalacia was seen adjacent, superior, and lateral to the anterior horn of the lateral ventricle, with some extension to superior aspects of the left basal ganglia. The lesion measured 4 cm×2 cm× 2 cm and was most consistent with an old infarct (see Figure 7–1).

A magnetic resonance angiogram showed that intracranial vascular structures were within normal limits, with no evidence of stenosis, occlusions, or aneurysms. Carotid ultrasound showed no significant plaque formation or stenosis. Echocardiographic findings were normal.

Investigations had now, for the first time, established that the patient had sustained a stroke or cerebrovascular accident affecting her left frontal lobe. With her family history, it was hypothesized to have possibly been caused by a ruptured berry aneurysm, although the site is not classic for an intracerebral hemorrhage resulting from such a rupture. It was impossible to date the stroke; perhaps it had actually caused her fall. She had in fact presented with right leg symptoms, which correlates with the visualized left-sided stroke. There was a very high likelihood that this lesion had caused or was contributing to her depression. Further, the fron-

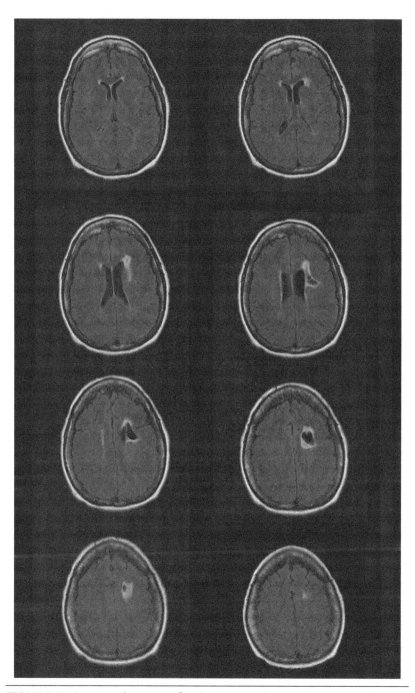

FIGURE 7–1. Axial FLAIR (fluid-attenuated inversion recovery) magnetic resonance brain images demonstrating a large region of encephalomalacia deep in the left frontal lobe.

tal lobe injury likely explained the incessant perseverative quality of her complaints.

An understanding of her disorder was shared with her and her husband. Her comprehension of body physiology was rudimentary, and the illness was thus described in a straightforward fashion. It was explained that the stroke was likely causing her depression, and that most of the physical symptoms were the result of the depression being indirectly expressed as pain and weakness. It was emphasized that this was a very real illness and not imagined.

Management options were discussed, with recommended use of physiotherapy and medications. In view of chronicity, severity, and the number of prior trials of medications, the patient was also offered the choice of ECT. The patient elected to attempt a trial of medications and was started on sertraline, nortriptyline, and risperidone. They were well tolerated and were increased to therapeutic range.

Her sleep improved for the first time in years, but mood, pain, and other physical symptoms were unchanged. Guided by her family, she requested a course of ECT and received 11 right unilateral treatments. Sleep improved further, and preoccupation with physical symptoms decreased. Pain "spasms" were much improved and were described as "less than half the size." Her mood began to improve.

Physiotherapy assisted gait and mobility, and an occupational therapist encouraged activities of interest. Daily psychotherapy consisted largely of support and basic educational and cognitive techniques regarding the nature of her illness and a path to recovery.

At discharge after a 4-month admission, her pain and "spasms" were still present but rated to be at least 30% improved. Sleep was good and mood had improved to 6/10, compared with 2/10 at admission. She was walking with a cane but still used a wheelchair for excursions. She was far less preoccupied with her physical symptoms, and the perseverative quality of her complaints was greatly reduced. Family noted that she was less agitated and "less emotional." Medications at the time of discharge were sertraline 200 mg/day, nortriptyline 20 mg qhs, and risperidone 2 mg qhs.

Her course over the years since that admission has essentially been that of someone with a large left frontal region stroke and a partly treatment-responsive depressive disorder. Treatment has included trials of different antidepressant regimens as well as stimulants and antiparkinsonian medications. At 20 years postinjury, now 66 years old, she is followed and treated by a psychiatrist in a mental health team close to home. This patient's sleep remains good, but her depressed mood, pain syndrome, and gait disturbance all remain moderately problematic. She walks more and no longer uses a wheelchair, but her insight into her illness remains partial. Her overall function is, therefore, only modestly improved, and she has never regained her premorbid level of function.

Discussion

This is the story of a physical illness masquerading as a psychiatric illness masquerading as a physical illness.

A left frontal stroke likely caused this woman's initial fall, and the immediate musculoskeletal consequences of the fall likely masked any neurological signs of the relatively silent stroke. The neuropsychiatric effects of the brain lesion then caused the development of a major depression in the months thereafter, which manifested with mood and neurovegetative changes, but more obviously through somatization as a "pancorporeal" pain syndrome and a psychogenic gait disturbance.

The most important lesson from the case is that whenever a psychiatric disorder is diagnosed, the clinician should take steps to screen for general medical conditions that may cause those psychiatric signs and symptoms. This patient had been ill with depression for many years, and the depression had been relatively resistant to treatment, without at any point being investigated with a head scan. Brain imaging is recommended as part of the workup for any individual with severe major depression, especially when there are atypical features such as late onset, treatment resistance, or prominent comorbid physical symptoms.

It is interesting to speculate about why this patient had not received a brain scan. She had, over the first 12 years of illness, received at least four scans of her lower back. Clearly the clinicians working with her were distracted by the site of her injury and by her complaints of pain. Furthermore, when depression is diagnosed in the face of prominent pain, it may be consciously or unconsciously assumed by the clinicians to be "secondary" to the pain, and thus a possible gross organic cause for the depression may not be pursued. There is also the possibility that chronicity itself tends to adversely affect new assessments, with the risk that "follow-up" assessments may be biased by earlier opinions and less complete than those conducted when a patient first comes into contact with a discipline.

Identifying a general medical condition as the cause of or a contributor to major depression is of varying importance in subsequent management. In the case described, discovering the stroke, and making the highly probable link to the presenting complaints and overall decrease in function, was of only limited value. Subsequent management would have been similar without this finding. The patient would have continued to receive treatment for major depression and a somatoform syndrome. Discovery of the stroke did, however, give the patient, family, and clinicians clarity regarding diagnosis. Hence it was easier for the patient and family to see the whole disabling syndrome as a "real" illness, something that, of course, would have been reinforced regardless of whether a stroke was demonstrated or not. The concrete finding probably allowed for more tenacious subsequent treatment, with positive effects.

Frontal lobe strokes can cause major depressive illness. Initial work suggested that left-sided lesions were considerably more likely to cause depressive symptoms, with proximity of the lesion to the left frontal pole believed to put the individual at higher risk (Robinson 1986). Cumulative evidence now shows that the relationship is less straightforward, with correlation between frontal lobe stroke laterality and depressed mood varying by time since stroke and by whether the individual is in an inpatient or community setting (Bhogal et al. 2004).

Aspects of this patient's illness, considered with the benefit of hindsight, did show frontal lobe lesion features. She demonstrated scanning speech and a perseverative quality to her somatic concerns. There had also been evidence on cognitive-intellectual testing that she had more limitations in left hemisphere function than in right hemisphere function. Short-term verbal memory was more impaired than short-term nonverbal memory, and there were problems with language tasks such as animal naming and story recall. However, the meaning of these correlations was enhanced by post hoc understanding; we had not had a high index of suspicion for a possible left-sided lesion based on clinical findings alone.

The local musculoskeletal pain in the weeks and initial months after the fall was not unexpected, but the severity, chronicity, and anatomical distribution of the subsequent pain were all highly suggestive of a somatoform pain syndrome. Certain brain lesions may cause specific pain syndromes, "thalamic pain" being the most described form (Hong et al. 2010; Kumar and Soni 2009). The demonstrated lesion is not, however, at an anatomical site classically associated with such a syndrome (Kalita et al. 2011).

Atypical and inconsistent patterns of weakness in all four limbs, and of gait disturbance, were not consistent with symptoms of any known general medical condition. A medical condition, the stroke, was assessed to be the most likely cause of the patient's depression, but no medical condition was found to be directly causing her weakness or gait disturbance. Thus it was concluded that she had a psychogenic illness. She was judged over a series of clinical assessments to fully believe that she was ill in the fashion in which she presented, and was thus judged to have a somatoform condition as opposed to either a factitious disorder or a form of malingering.

The focus of treatment was on education and support regarding the nature of the combination of stroke, depression, and somatoform symptoms; on physical therapies for the psychogenic gait disturbance; and on biological treatments for the underlying major depression.

The prognosis of a somatoform disorder is more closely linked to the prognosis of the underlying cause of the emotional distress than it is to the nature of the somatized physical symptoms (Hurwitz 2003). This patient's overall course followed that of an individual with a poststroke, partly treatment-responsive depressive disorder.

Key Clinical Points

- Whenever a psychiatric disorder is diagnosed, care must be taken to screen for general medical conditions that may be causing the psychiatric syndrome.
- Brain imaging is recommended in the workup of severe major depression, especially in the face of treatment resistance or any atypical features.
- Discovering a probable general medical cause for a psychiatric syndrome such as major depression will not necessarily alter treatment, but it will add to the clinician's and the patient's understanding of the condition.
- The relationship between laterality of the neuroanatomical site of stroke and the onset of major depression is more complex than previously thought, with factors such as time since stroke being important.
- Physical symptoms and signs that do not follow the known damage patterns of general medical conditions are judged by the clinician to be psychogenic. If they are not consciously produced, they are judged to be somatoform in nature.

Further Readings

Hurwitz TA: Somatization and conversion disorder. Can J Psychiatry 49:172–178, 2003

References

Bhogal SK, Teasell R, Foley N, et al: Lesion location and poststroke depression: systematic review of the methodological limitations in the literature. Stroke 35:794–802, 2004

Hong JH, Bai DS, Jeong JY, et al: Injury of the spino-thalamo-cortical pathway is necessary for central post-stroke pain. Eur Neurol 64:163–168, 2010

Hurwitz TA: Somatization and conversion disorder. Can J Psychiatry 49:172–178, 2003

Kalita J, Kumar B, Misra UK: Central post stroke pain: clinical, MRI, and SPECT correlation. Pain Med 12:282–288, 2011
Kumar G, Soni CR: Central post-stroke pain: current evidence. J Neurol Sci 15:10–17, 2009
Robinson RG: Post-stroke mood disorder. Hosp Pract 21:83–89, 1986

Lyme Disease

Catherine Chiles, M.D., D.F.A.P.A., F.A.P.M.

A 65-year-old woman, who was a retired litigation attorney, presented to her primary care physician with complaints of fatigue, decreased concentration, memory deficits, depressed mood, and chronically disturbed sleep. Since retirement in the preceding year, she had moved from her urban condominium to a home in the Connecticut countryside. Her property abutted a wildlife sanctuary, a haven for white-tailed deer and songbirds. After a legal career that was spent primarily indoors, she was enjoying spending time outdoors and had become an avid gardener. Her backyard garden was quite overgrown, so she had been spending many hours doing a spring season cleanup. At the end of one long day working in the garden, she noted excessive fatigue, muscle aches, and a mild headache; she attributed these symptoms to her gardening labors in the sun. She went to sleep early but found her sleep disturbed.

Over the ensuing weeks, symptoms of depression set in, and she decided to call her physician. Her symptoms were a mystery to her, because she had long anticipated this transition in life in a positive, planned way. During the evaluation, family history revealed thyroid disease. Her mother had a history of chronic major depression after her husband passed away. Medical history included hypothyroidism, which had been treated successfully with thyroxine replacement since age 50. She was postmenopausal, with no residual symptoms. Social history included an upbringing in Brooklyn, New York, as the only child of a first-generation immigrant family. Her parents had sacrificed their own ambitions to provide her an education. She had moved to Connecticut after law school when her husband sought a teaching position there. She was married for 35 years, until the death of her husband 4 years earlier due to pancreatic cancer.

Psychiatric history included symptoms of depression during her bereavement that had responded to treatment with a support group therapy and a selective serotonin reuptake inhibitor for 1 year. She had been close to her son, a schoolteacher in California, and daughter, a research scientist in North Carolina, but they visited less frequently now. She had become more socially isolated after her husband died and consequently less involved in her community. During the review of systems, the physician elicited a history of a skin rash in the late spring, approximately 8 or 9 weeks prior to the visit, that had appeared on her leg as erythematous and circular; this information raised his concern for Lyme disease. Because the rash had disappeared, she had not sought care for it or thought about it since.

Laboratory tests included thyroid indices, a complete blood count, electrolytes, vitamin B_{12}, folate, liver and renal function tests, urinalysis, and a urine toxicology screen, as well as serology for Lyme antibody, syphilis, and HIV. An electrocardiogram during the office visit was unremarkable. On mental status examination, the physician detected short-term memory loss and deficits in attention that were new since the patient's last office visit. She was referred for a computed tomography brain scan, neuropsychological testing, and psychiatric follow-up; recurrent mood disorder remained in the differential diagnosis. She was given a 10-day course of doxycycline for possible Lyme disease. She was educated that a bite from a deer tick was a known vector for this illness in the area, and that May and June were the months in which transmission by tick bite was likely (Bacon et al. 2008).

She completed the antibiotic course. Test results had not revealed any medical causes for her symptoms. She was euthyroid, and her Lyme titer was negative. Because her symptoms had persisted unchanged, she was referred to a psychiatrist for depression and possible early dementia. The psychiatrist reviewed available results of laboratory investigations and neuropsychological tests, which were consistent with early-onset dementia. She had become frustrated by her condition and was dysphoric about her lapses in memory. She had no family history of dementia, and her premorbid cognitive functioning had been high. The psychiatrist ordered a brain MRI scan, lumbar puncture, and electroencephalogram (EEG), all with negative results. She accepted additional sessions for diagnostic evaluation. She was thereafter evaluated by an infectious disease specialist, who repeated many of the initial tests.

Meanwhile, she had searched the Internet to find answers and learned that Lyme disease is common in New England and the Mid-Atlantic states and may go undetected with standard screening tests. She sought the advice of several prominent specialists who focused on the rheumatological, immunological, neurological, and infectious aspects of Lyme disease. She implored the psychiatrist at a follow-up visit to refer her for a single-photon emission computed tomography (SPECT) scan, a test she had read about as having an ability, albeit equivocal at times, to detect neurological evidence of Lyme disease. Pursuit of this test was much debated in the on-line chat rooms for chronic Lyme disease sufferers that she had joined.

The psychiatrist coordinated a meeting of the primary care physician, the neurologist, the patient, and herself to develop a treatment plan in or-der to limit "doctor shopping" and to advocate for the patient to receive more specific tests for Lyme disease. She was considered for long-term an-tibiotic treatment by the local Lyme disease specialist after the results of a SPECT scan and the two-stage immunoassays (ELISA [enzyme-linked im-munosorbent assay] followed by Western blot) were found to be consistent with Lyme disease.

Discussion

Lyme disease (borreliosis) is an infection caused by the spirochete *Borrelia burgdorferi* and is the most commonly reported vector-borne disease in the United States. Annually, 15,000–20,000 new cases are diagnosed in the United States, but this may represent only 10% of actual cases (Bacon et al. 2008). Borreliosis is diagnosed predominantly in northeastern states but occurs across the United States and in Europe.

Historically, the clinical manifestations (rash, multisystem illness) of a bite by the tick *Ixodes* were recognized in Europe in 1909, well before the elucidation in the United States that the tick is an infective vector of *Borrelia* (Fallon and Nields 1994). In 1975, Yale researcher Dr. Allen C. Steere and colleagues studied an unusual cohort of arthritis cases centered in Lyme, Connecticut. Later, they linked many of the cases to tick bites. Based on these cases, medical entomologist Dr. Willy Burgdorfer and his colleagues isolated the infectious agent *Borrelia* from the vector tick in 1982. Thereafter the illness became known as Lyme disease and the in-fectious agent was named *Borrelia burgdorferi*. Neuropsychiatric sequelae of tick bites had been identified as early as the 1920s, and today these se-quelae are often early clinical findings in Lyme disease (Burgdorfer et al. 1982; Fallon and Nields 1994).

B. burgdorferi occurs naturally in reservoir hosts such as mice and squir-rels. Transmission to humans occurs after the bite and blood feeding of the carnivorous tick species *I. scapularis* and *I. pacificus*. The tick requires mam-malian blood to molt and to evolve from a larva to a nymph, and then from a nymph to an adult—three blood meals over its 2-year life cycle. After *Ixo-des* feeds on a reservoir host, at a subsequent blood meal (either as a nymph or as an adult female tick), infection is transmitted to another host or to humans. Infection is most commonly transmitted by the nymph, which is barely if at all detectable at 2 mm in size and often falls off after feeding. Lyme disease peaks clinically in the summer in relation to the nymphal tick's increased activity in May and June. *I. scapularis* (deer tick) is the vector in most U.S. cases of Lyme disease. The white-tailed deer is not a reservoir host nor is it infected with *B. burgdorferi;* however, just like waterfowl and songbirds, it is integrally involved as a transporter for the tick and thus its survival. *I. pacificus* (black-legged tick) is the vector in many midwestern or southern regions of the United States; *I. ricinus* is the predominant vector in Europe. *Ixodes* ticks can transmit other infections as well, causing co-infection with *Babesia microti* (babesiosis), *Anaplasma phagocytophilum* (anaplasmosis), human granulocytic or monocytic ehrlichiosis, or less commonly *Francisella tularensis* (tularemia). Whereas borreliosis most commonly affects fixed tissues, babesiosis occurs solely in red blood cells (Bacon et al. 2008; Hildenbrand et al. 2009; Krause et al 1996; Wormser et al. 2006).

Lyme disease occurs in several stages, similar to other spirochetal infections such as syphilis. The tick must stay attached to the skin for 24–48 hours (Hildenbrand et al. 2009). In some reported cases, transmission occurs as quickly as 12 hours (Bacon et al. 2008). Borreliosis in Europe is caused by the genospecies *B. garinii* and has more neurological symptoms relative to U.S. cases (Hildenbrand et al. 2009).

The early stage or incubation occurs within days to weeks after the infectious tick bite. Erythema migrans, or a "target" lesion, develops as an enlarging, reddened, pruritic, raised rash (≥ 5 cm in diameter) with or without a central clearing zone. The rash may be followed by a flulike syndrome (headache, fever, myalgia, mild stiff neck, malaise). For most patients, the rash or target lesion of stage 1 is recalled only later. However, early clinical evidence of erythema migrans remains the hallmark of illness onset and is critical for a confirmed diagnosis (Bacon et al. 2008; Fallon and Nields 1994; Hildenbrand et al. 2009).

Subsequent stages may be the initial presentation if the first stage is mild. Within days to weeks the infection spreads hematogenously if untreated, and may enter the central nervous system (CNS) and cause a variety of neuropsychiatric presentations that range from mild confusional states to (rarely) encephalitis, which can occur weeks to months later. Disseminated infection may present as multiple target lesions or with neurological (meningitis, radiculopathy, facial palsy) or cardiac (carditis, atrioventricular block) symptoms. Months to years after the initial infection, peripheral neuropathy and chronic mono- or oligo-articular arthritis of large joints, especially the knee, may develop (Bacon et al. 2008; Fallon and Nields 1994; Hildenbrand et al. 2009).

Since many of the presenting symptoms of Lyme disease involve the CNS, the psychiatrist may be consulted before the diagnosis of Lyme disease is confirmed. A wide range of psychiatric disorders have been reported as manifestations of Lyme disease, including depression, paranoia, dementia, panic attacks, anorexia nervosa, and obsessive-compulsive disorder. Symptoms of neuroborreliosis may include fatigue, low mood, insomnia, and difficulty in concentration; these symptoms may be mistaken for major depression, as seen in the patient in this case. In addition, profound cognitive changes can occur, as seen in depression or dementia (Fallon and Nields 1994). As demonstrated in this case, the differential diagnosis includes recurrent depression and new-onset dementia, as well as mood or cognitive disorder due to a general medical condition, such as relapsed hypothyroidism. The patient's history of exposure (working outdoors with sleeves rolled up, in a rural setting in a state where Lyme disease is common) and new onset of cognitive and mood symptoms increase the chances of Lyme disease.

The very nature of the spirochete, in its ability to metamorphose into undetectable forms, challenges the search for laboratory proof of *Borrelia* infection. Most suspected patients are tested for titers of antibodies against the infection, but there is a high false-negative rate early in the course of the illness. In later stages, the evidence of immune response may be detected by a two-step process: ELISA or indirect fluorescent antibody assay (first step), and then, if the assay results are positive or equivocal, immunoblot or Western blot test (second step) (Hildenbrand et al. 2009). Along with physician-diagnosed evidence of erythema migrans, these tests confirm the diagnosis of Lyme disease according to standards of research and disease surveillance set by the Centers for Disease Control and Prevention (Bacon et al. 2008). Clinical evidence of neuroborreliosis may be corroborated by a SPECT scan that provides evidence of antibiotic-reversible frontal lobe hypoperfusion. MRI brain scan may demonstrate frontal cortex white matter changes in half of patients with neuroborreliosis that may persist despite successful antibiotic treatment (Hildenbrand et al. 2009).

Preventive measures against tick bites are strongly recommended; these measures include wearing light-colored protective clothing, using tick repellents, checking the body daily for ticks, and prompt removal of attached ticks. Treatment with antibiotics against a proven infection of Lyme disease or Lyme neuroborreliosis remains the standard of care. The best evidence for the utility of antibiotics is seen when the attached, engorged tick can be identified as *I. scapularis* in the nymph or adult female stage and treatment is given within 72 hours of exposure to the tick (Wormser et al. 2006). In areas in which infected ticks are endemic (e.g., 25%–40% of ticks in northeastern states carry the infectious agent for Lyme disease) and evidence for exposure is high, the threshold to treat with antibiotics is lowered. Parenteral antibiotics may be used in cases of CNS involvement or in chronic, refractory cases of Lyme disease. In this case, the use of a course of oral doxycycline was ineffective. Consideration of parenteral and longer courses of antibiotics is made when there is evidence by clinical examination and diagnostic tests of neuroborreliosis. For many patients with Lyme disease, chronic symptoms may persist or migrate to a new site, despite adequate treatment (Wormser et al. 2006).

Key Clinical Points

- Lyme disease, a tick-borne spirochetal infection, is the most common, and still rapidly emerging, vector-borne illness in the United States. Only 10% of cases are reliably detected.
- *B. burgdorferi* enters the CNS early in the infection process; thus, patients with Lyme disease may present first to a psychiatrist.
- Early-stage tests for Lyme antibody titers have high false-negative rates. The two-step tests (ELISA or indirect fluorescent antibody assay, followed by immunoblot or Western blot) have increased sensitivity at later stages.
- Preventive measures against tick bites remain critical to combat the spread of Lyme disease.
- Parenteral antibiotics may be required for severe CNS disease.

Further Readings

Hajek T, Paskova B, Janovska D, et al: Higher prevalence of antibodies to Borrelia burgdorferi in psychiatric patients than in healthy subjects. Am J Psychiatry 159:297–301, 2002

Halperin JJ, Shapiro ED, Logigian E, et al: Practice parameter for the treatment of nervous system Lyme disease (an evidence-based review): report of the Quality Standards Subcommittee of the American Academy of Neurology. Neurology 69:91–102, 2007

Hildenbrand P, Craven DE, Jones R, et al: Lyme neuroborreliosis: manifestations of a rapidly emerging zoonosis. AJNR Am J Neuroradiol 30:1079–1087, 2009

References

Bacon RM, Kugeler KJ, Mead PS; Centers for Disease Control and Prevention: Surveillance for Lyme disease—United States, 1992–2006. MMWR Surveill Summ 57:1–9, 2008

Burgdorfer W, Barbour AG, Hayes SF, et al: Lyme disease—a tick-borne spiro-
chetosis? Science 216:1317–1319, 1982

Fallon BA, Nields JA: Lyme disease: a neuropsychiatric illness. Am J Psychiatry
151:1571–1583, 1994

Hildenbrand P, Craven DE, Jones R, et al: Lyme neuroborreliosis: manifestations
of a rapidly emerging zoonosis. AJNR Am J Neuroradiol 30:1079–1087,
2009

Krause PJ, Telford SR, Spielman A, et al: Concurrent Lyme disease and babesiosis: evidence for increased duration and severity of illness. JAMA 275:1657–
1660, 1996

Wormser GP, Dattwyler RJ, Shapiro ED, et al: The clinical assessment, treatment,
and prevention of Lyme disease, human granulocytic anaplasmosis, and babesiosis: clinical practice guidelines by the Infectious Diseases Society of
America. Clin Infect Dis 43:1089–1134, 2006

Epilepsia Partialis Continua and Pseudoseizures

Warren T. Lee, M.D., Ph.D.

A 27-year-old right-handed, married white woman, who worked as a secretary, came to the emergency room, at the insistence of her husband, for twitching movements of her left hand and forearm that had begun suddenly 4 weeks before. The episodes were stereotypic: beginning with numbness and tingling sensation of the right hand and progressing to the arm, and followed by a shift to the left hand, which then began to twitch. At times, these episodes would be preceded by an aura of "feeling off" and "listlessness" for an hour or more. The episodes lasted from minutes to as long as 4 hours and occurred one to three times a week. She denied that the episodes were precipitated by heightened emotion or sleep deprivation. During the episodes, she remained awake and cognizant of her surroundings. Her postseizure symptoms were limited to fatigue, without weakness of the limbs or clouded sensorium. She was not particularly worried about this new problem and did not feel it was important enough to have kept a seizure journal.

She did not have a past history of febrile seizures, encephalitis, meningitis, tics, or myoclonic jerks. She denied any past or current medical or psychiatric problems or use of substances. The results of her physical examination and detailed neurological examination were all within normal limits. Two interictal EEGs did not reveal any epileptiform discharges. The findings from initial routine laboratory investigations, an MRI scan, and cerebrospinal fluid analysis from a lumbar puncture were also within normal limits.

A diagnosis of possible epilepsia partialis continua (EPC) was considered based on her seizure semiology. A major workup for EPC was undertaken, including additional toxic, endocrine, metabolic, autoimmune, and paraneoplastic investigations and extensive body scanning.

Once a bed was available, the patient was transferred to a continuous video-electroencephalographic unit and monitored for 72 hours. She was aware of the purpose of the investigation and was cooperative. She had two recorded episodes during the period of telemetry. The episodes began with subjective numbness of the right hand and face followed by left hand and arm flexion-extension movements. These mostly involved the entire hand, with arrhythmic flexion-extension movements at the metacarpophalangeal joints. Each episode lasted for 15–20 minutes. The episodes would arrest briefly when the patient was distracted by verbal interventions or instructions to perform mental tasks or physical tasks with the contralateral hand. From the video, she appeared unconcerned about the episodes. The EEG showed electromyographical artifact but no epileptiform activity or other abnormalities. Furthermore, an ictal SPECT scan did not reveal perfusion abnormalities.

She was told that her witnessed episodes were most likely nonepileptic in origin, and she was referred to the consultation-liaison psychiatrist for further assessment and joint management.

At the first psychiatric interview, she expressed reservations and reluctance about being seen by a psychiatrist. She was persuaded to participate in the assessment by her husband. She was generally pleasant and able to maintain eye contact, but at times she appeared distant and uninterested, with an air of *la belle indifférence*. She explicitly denied current and past anxiety and depressive symptoms, and this was borne out by scores in the "mild" range on the Beck Anxiety Inventory and Beck Depression Inventory. Her Montreal Cognitive Assessment score was 30/30. There was no evidence of psychosis, mania, or other psychiatric symptoms. She denied any past or recent trauma, childhood problems, or substance use. Family history was negative for psychiatric and neurological disorders. She rejected the feedback that her "seizures" were psychogenic in origin and believed that epilepsy would still be eventually confirmed. She reported, with some reticence, tremendous stress in the year prior to the onset of her symptoms. The stress arose in the context of her work and adjusting to newly married life. However, she declined to discuss any marital discord further. She also declined further psychiatric assessment or treatment and psychological interventions that were offered. At a neurology outpatient follow-up 4 months after discharge, she reported that there had been no more seizures. She had separated from her husband and had taken up another job.

Discussion

EPC is a rare focal motor epilepsy and is defined as spontaneous clonic activity (usually 0.1–6 Hz) of cortical origin that affects a limited part of the body (usually on one side) and continues for a prolonged period (usually defined as longer than 1 hour). If captured during an electroencephalographic recording, epileptiform features with a fixed temporal coupling to the muscle jerks are confirmatory (Bien and Elger 2008). Routine EEGs may not, however, always show epileptiform correlates because cortical neurons over a large area need to fire synchronously for the electroencephalographic activity to be reflected on the scalp electrodes. In adults, the most common causes of EPC are neoplastic, paraneoplastic, infectious, inflammatory, and vascular. In children, the most common cause is Rasmussen encephalitis. Less common causes include cortical dysplasia and neurotoxins.

Other possible neurological diagnoses that were considered in this patient included motor tics, myoclonic jerks, and other movement disorders, but none were consistent with her clinical presentation. A diagnosis of psychogenic nonepileptic seizures (PNES) was made after an extensive negative workup and in particular the absence of any electrographic correlates during prolonged video-electroencephalographic monitoring, which captured two of her stereotypic events. Moreover, the evolution of side-switching symptoms without loss of consciousness, starting on one side and moving to the other, follows no known epileptic pattern. The hallmark of psychogenic neurological disorders is that they do not follow the known organic damage patterns.

Psychogenic nonepileptic seizures is now the commonly used term to describe this problem, replacing *pseudoseizures;* the former is considered less pejorative. PNES and other conversion disorders often evoke the ire of physicians because these disorders are viewed as not being "real" neurological problems. This negative countertransference is made worse by the fact that similar nonorganic presentations can be seen in patients with factitious disorders or who are malingering.

Since the time of Jean-Martin Charcot, physicians have wrestled with the etiological basis of conversion disorders (Figure 7–2). Charcot used the term *functional* to describe conversion disorders because, in spite of the absence of demonstrable neuropathology, neurological function was clearly disturbed (Sackellares and Kalogjera-Sackellares 2002). Pierre Janet, a student of Charcot, proposed that "dissociation" could explain the symptoms, especially in the context of a traumatic experience. Freud, on the other hand, countered that such difficult experiences were "repressed into the unconscious" and "converted" into physical symptoms. However, the notion of PNES being wholly psychological is untenable in an era where the brain-mind dichotomy is eroding rapidly.

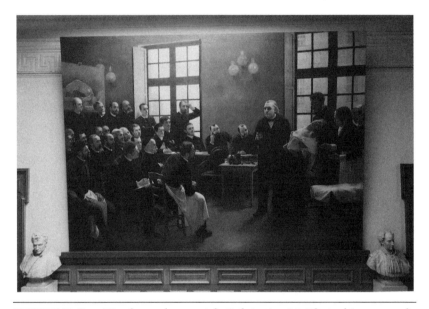

FIGURE 7–2.   *Une leçon clinique à la Salpêtrière* (*A Clinical Lesson at the Salpêtrière*), a painting by Pierre-André Brouillet, in Université Paris Descartes (1887).

This painting depicts a female patient fainting during a clinical demonstration of hysteria. Jean-Martin Charcot was a pioneer in investigating hysterical seizures. His students, Joseph Babinski (supporting the patient), and Gilles de la Tourette, and others can be seen in the painting. *Photo credit:* W. Lee, 2012.

The development of advanced neuroimaging techniques has provided the means to study the neural basis of conversion disorders. Werring and colleagues (2004) compared five patients with medically unexplained visual loss whose symptoms met the criteria for conversion disorder with normal control subjects and found that during visual stimulation, these patients had reduced activation in their visual cortex but increased activation in their left inferior frontal cortex, insula, posterior cingulate cortex, and limbic structures and bilateral thalami and striatum. Using SPECT scanning in seven patients with conversion disorder who presented with unilateral sensorimotor impairment, Vuilleumier and colleagues (2001) found reduced blood flow in the thalamus and basal ganglia contralateral to the deficit, which resolved after recovery from the sensorimotor symptoms.

These and other studies have demonstrated that there are anatomical changes in the brains of patients who have psychogenic deficits and that these changes involve neural structures that normally control the affected, symptomatic body parts. Yet the neurological symptoms do not reflect the known damage pattern when such structures are organically injured. This points to the role of the mind in conversion disorder and the likelihood that idiosyncratic somatic beliefs have assumed control over the symptomatic neural structures but are disrupting neurobehavioral expression in such a way so as to produce the bizarre somatic symptoms seen clinically (Hurwitz and Prichard 2006).

PNES is the most common nonepileptic condition seen in major epilepsy centers, where PNES cases make up 20%–30% of referrals. However, it has been estimated that 5%–15% of PNES patients have concurrent epileptic seizures (Benbadis and Allen Hauser 2000; Martin et al. 2003). Neurologists have identified positive signs to differentiate PNES from epileptic seizures based on clinical semiology. Some of the major features of a nonepileptic seizure are listed in Table 7–1, but these are only suggestive of a PNES diagnosis rather than definitive.

Routine EEGs are not useful for diagnosing PNES because of their low sensitivity. Even in bona fide epilepsy, routine EEGs may not reveal epileptiform activity in the interictal phases because most routine EEGs only sample about 15 minutes of brain electrical activity. However, repeated normal routine EEGs in the context of frequent attacks and lack of response to antiepileptic medications may suggest PNES.

The accepted gold standard for diagnosis of PNES is video-electroencephalography (Ghougassian et al. 2004). As long as the seizure episode is recorded during the monitoring period, the combination of the video semiology in the absence of a correlating electroencephalographic epileptic discharge allows for a definitive diagnosis. Hyperventilation, photic stimulation, and suggestion may be employed to increase the yield during video-electroencephalographic monitoring.

Video-electroencephalography does have limitations. The EEG may be difficult to interpret because of excessive movement artifact, and scalp EEG may not detect epileptic seizure activity if the ictal cortical region is small (Tao et al. 2007). Moreover, cortical ictal activity in areas remote from electrode positions such as mesial or basal cortex may not be cap-

TABLE 7–1. General features of a nonepileptic seizure

Setting

Environmental gain (e.g., audience present)

Seldom sleep related and does not occur in sleep

Often triggered (e.g., by stress)

Attack

Atypical movements, often bizarre or purposeful

Seldom results in injury

Often starts and ends gradually

Out-of-phase movements of extremities

Side-to-side movements

Examination

Restraint accentuates the seizure

Flexor plantar response

Reflexes intact (corneal, pupillary, and blink)

Consciousness preserved

Autonomically intact

After attack

No postictal features (lethargy, tiredness, abnormal electroencephalographic findings)

Prolactin normal (after 30 minutes)

No or little amnesia

Source. Adapted from Kim et al. 2008, p. 657.

tured by scalp electrodes. Although an episode may be correctly identified during video-EEG as PNES, it is important to bear in mind that in such cases PNES may coexist with an underlying epileptic disorder.

Included in the differential diagnosis of nonepileptic seizures are 1) factitious disorder, in which the patient consciously and deliberately feigns seizures but the deception is a pathological need for a sick role; and 2) malingering, in which the reasons for the conscious and deliberate deception are tangible and rational and are either to obtain some interpersonal benefit or to avoid some noxious social consequence. Proving feigning or the absence of feigning is difficult and places the physician in an invidious adversarial role in his or her interactions with the patient. PNES is predicated on the assumption that the actions are generated outside of conscious awareness and intention, which is simple and clear in theory but often very difficult for the physician to determine in practice.

In addition, there are physiological conditions that can lead to episodic seizure-like events but are not epilepsy per se; examples include transient ischemic attack, convulsive syncope, dysautonomia, complicated migraine, and substance intoxication or withdrawal. The term *pseudopseudoseizures* has been used to describe symptoms that have the appearance of PNES but are eventually found to be due to an underlying organic cause, such as paraneoplastic encephalitis (Caplan et al. 2011). Hence, a detailed medical and neurological assessment should always be completed before a diagnosis of PNES is made.

A diagnosis, once made, should be communicated to the patient in an empathic, nonjudgmental, and yet unambiguous way. The patient and family may react with denial, disbelief, indignation, and even hostility. Written information in addition to verbal explanation may be helpful. Psychological and emotional issues have to be addressed with sensitivity and discretion. Treatment includes psychotherapy and the use of adjunctive medications to treat coexisting anxiety and depression if appropriate. Cognitive-behavioral therapy, in particular, has been reported to be helpful (Goldstein et al. 2010).

Key Clinical Points

- Epilepsia partialis continua is a rare motor epilepsy that can persist for hours and may have the appearance of psychogenic nonepileptic seizures.
- PNES can often be differentiated from epileptic seizures based on semiology, but the gold standard for diagnosis is video-electroencephalographic monitoring.
- Other causes of nonepileptic seizure-like events include physiological causes such as transient ischemic attack, convulsive syncope, cardiac arrhythmia, autonomic dysfunction, complicated migraines, and substance intoxication or withdrawal.
- An extensive medical workup is indicated for all suspected PNES.
- Treatment of PNES is directed at the underlying psychological distress, which needs to be identified, and includes the use of psychotherapy and medications for depression and anxiety.

Further Readings

Benbadis SR: Psychogenic nonepileptic seizures, October 6, 2011. Available at: http://emedicine.medscape.com/article/1184694. Accessed August 12, 2012.

Bien C, Elger C: Epilepsia partialis continua: semiology and differential diagnoses. Epileptic Disord 10:3–7, 2008

Syed T, LaFrance W: Nonepileptic seizures, in The Neuropsychiatry of Epilepsy, 2nd Edition. Edited by Trimble M, Schmitz B. Cambridge, UK, Cambridge University Press, 2011, pp 124–132

References

Benbadis SR, Allen Hauser W: An estimate of the prevalence of psychogenic non-epileptic seizures. Seizure 9:280–281, 2000

Bien C, Elger C: Epilepsia partialis continua: semiology and differential diagnoses. Epileptic Disord 10:3–7, 2008

Caplan JP, Binius T, Lennon VA: Pseudopseudoseizures: conditions that may mimic psychogenic non-epileptic seizures. Psychosomatics 52:501–506, 2011

Ghougassian DF, d'Souza W, Cook MJ: Evaluating the utility of inpatient video-EEG monitoring. Epilepsia 45:928–932, 2004

Goldstein LH, Chalder T, Chigwedere C: Cognitive-behavioral therapy for psychogenic nonepileptic seizures: a pilot RCT. Neurology 74:1986–1994, 2010

Hurwitz TA, Prichard JW: Conversion disorder and fMRI. Neurology 12:1914–1915, 2006

Kim HF, Yudofsky SC, Hales RE, et al: Neuropsychiatric aspects of seizure disorders, in The American Psychiatric Publishing Textbook of Neuropsychiatry and Behavioral Neurosciences, 5th Edition. Edited by Yudofsky SC, Hales RE. Washington, DC, American Psychiatric Publishing, 2008, pp 649–675

Martin P, Burneo JG, Prasad A: Frequency of epilepsy in patients with psychogenic seizures monitored by video-EEG. Neurology 61:1791–1792, 2003

Sackellares JC, Kalogjera-Sackellares D: Psychobiology of psychogenic pseudoseizures, in The Neuropsychiatry of Epilepsy. Edited by Trimble M, Schmitz B. Cambridge, UK, Cambridge University Press, 2002, pp 210–225

Tao JX, Baldwin M, Hawes-Ebersole S: Cortical substrates of scalp EEG epileptiform discharges. J Clin Neurophysiol 24:96–100, 2007

Vuilleumier P, Chicherio C, Assal F: Functional neuroanatomical correlates of hysterical sensorimotor loss. Brain 124:1077–1090, 2001

Werring DJ, Weston L, Bullmore ET: Functional magnetic resonance imaging of the cerebral response to visual stimulation in medically unexplained visual loss. Psychol Med 34:583–589, 2004

Cogniform Disorder

Brenda Kosaka, Ph.D., R.Psych.

A 43-year-old man was referred for neuropsychological assessment because of cognitive difficulties, including failing memory. His other problems were atypical posttraumatic headaches and depression. He had been involved in a motor vehicle accident 15 months previously; he had apparently run a red light, had struck two cars, and may have had a loss of consciousness (although the loss of consciousness never was clearly established). At the time of his assessment, he could still not recall any details of the motor vehicle accident, but there were no medicolegal implications because all litigation had been settled. He had been unable to return to work in the software industry since his accident.

He was highly concerned about his cognitive difficulties, which had undermined his self-esteem, and provided many details about these difficulties. He had been very proud of his premorbid abilities and had been tested by Mensa (the society for people with high IQs) in his late 20s and was a member. Premorbidly his spelling was "terrifically phenomenal." He could read upside down and backward, and he did not suffer fools gladly. Now he felt that he was not as smart as he was before the accident. He said that he had a "sieve" for a brain—information floated away, and he could not remember what his boss or wife told him. To compensate he carried a notebook, but he would forget to use it. He felt there was a difference in his "lexicon." He was still able to play chess but said that it physically hurt. He read a lot, and he could sustain reading for up to 3–4 hours if the book was a Tom Clancy novel or science fiction.

On direct inquiry he endorsed verbal, spatial, and prospective memory problems. He also noted problems with calculation. By contrast, remote memory and skill-based learning were unaffected. He reported that he could improve his memory if he drank caffeinated diet cola. His wife confirmed his "progressive memory problems."

He wondered if his memory difficulties had in fact started 22 years earlier when a hydraulic jack fell off a cabinet and clipped his head. He may have had a brief loss of consciousness. Following that accident he went to the hospital, where he was extremely emotionally labile and complained of severe headache. Skull X ray findings were negative, and the diagnosis at the time was concussion. That night, he was found to be gritting his teeth, hanging onto his head, and trembling for 5–10 minutes. The results of seizure investigations at that time were negative. This event was followed by subjective memory difficulties and difficulties with complex calculations in his 20s and 30s. Despite such concerns, he had still passed the Mensa testing.

His headaches were intense, like "a nuke" exploding in his head, and associated with light and sound sensitivity, but he did not have vomiting or visual disturbance. His headache pain was rated as a 7 to 8 out of 10. Headaches were associated with occasional vertigo and were improved by sleep and sex. He had no history of migraines. He was taking ibuprofen and acetaminophen for pain relief on an as-needed basis.

He rated his mood as a 3 to 4 out of 10. His low mood was coupled with low self-esteem, limited energy, decreased interest, and intermittent suicidal thoughts when he missed a day of his antidepressant, bupropion. Marital tension added to his depression. His wife had quit her job because of the "stress" of his difficulties.

He was the eldest of three siblings from a Mennonite family. He described himself as socially introverted and avoidant, a "bookworm immersed in science fiction." There was no history of physical abuse, but his father was a strict disciplinarian. The patient had completed 2 years of college but did not obtain a diploma. He had no real career or life goals. He had worked for 20 years as a graphic artist and had been employed in a software business. He had loved this job but was laid off when the software industry slowed down. He did part-time software work for a catalog business but did not find it rewarding. He had a talent for designing and drafting plans of fictional spaceships. He had done this for over 20 years and had sold over 1,000 of the plans commercially. Each plan displayed a deck, compartments, and subsystems, and visual details of the interior and exterior of the imagined vessel.

He was heterosexual and in his second marriage. His first had ended after 9 years when his wife had an affair with his best friend. This first marriage had produced one child, a son who lived with the mother in another Canadian province.

He described himself as being compulsive in nature and said that he would take risks at work and in his personal life. He had been overinvolved with pornography for 20 years, although he had made three or four attempts to stop this activity. His stepson from his current wife's previous marriage and who lived with them, had discovered several of his pornographic computer files. A recent referral had been made to a sexual medicine clinic to address the pornography issue. His libido was reduced since the motor vehicle accident, but he noted with some pride that he was "infamous" in this particular area of functioning.

His previous medical history was significant for glucose intolerance, managed by diet, and irritable bowel syndrome. Five years prior to the current assessment, he had had another unexplained episode where he had grabbed the sides of a hot tub and had burst into tears. A seizure disorder was once more suspected and investigated but again not confirmed.

Previous psychiatric history included marital counseling at age 30. Following his divorce, he attempted suicide by an overdose of medications; this attempt prompted a brief admission to the hospital, followed by outpatient monitoring, and he was on stress leave for 2 years. He had had a "head injury" 3 years previously when his head struck the rear door of his vehicle. His wife had found him on the ground seconds later and had observed a brief period of amnesia. This "head injury" had precipitated daily headaches and escalating depression. He was treated for this depression with paroxetine for approximately 1 year and was free of headache and depression until his motor vehicle accident.

Family medical and psychiatric history was positive for diabetes mellitus in his grandmother, systemic lupus erythematosus in his mother, and alcohol problems in his father and brother.

He was taking bupropion 75 mg bid but no other regular medications. His neurological examination was normal. His EEG showed no evidence of epileptiform activity, and brain CT and MRI showed normal intracranial anatomy.

His treating psychiatrist had diagnosed major depression, posttraumatic headaches, and cognitive problems in the context of depression. He had been offered a trial of treatment with nortriptyline and dextroamphetamine, but he had declined because of a fear of medications and concerns that the proposed new medications could reduce his libido.

There had been no previous neuropsychological assessments associated with any of his prior difficulties. Rapport during testing was fair. On the first day of testing he was very energized, but he calmed down by the second day. His responses were at times slow and consistently correlated with his attempts to be accurate and precise in his approach.

His Full Scale IQ (from the Wechsler Adult Intelligence Scale—Third Edition) was at the 93rd percentile (Superior range). There was a nonsignificant 4-point difference between his Performance IQ, which was at the 93rd percentile (Superior range), and his Verbal IQ, which was at the 88th percentile (High Average range). Working Memory Index and Processing Speed Index scores were in the average range. He was penalized for slowness on a task of mazes but made no errors. Yet on a more demanding timed task of verbal abstraction he was at the 88th percentile.

Comprehensive testing (Figure 7–3) showed very little significant cognitive impairment. Variability was seen within some cognitive domains. For example, he was found to do better on the more difficult paired-associates memory test. His effort was poor on a list-learning task; he appeared to give up when he did not recall all 15 words on the first trial. Recognition testing for either verbal or nonverbal memory was excellent, suggesting no difficulties with encoding.

Emotionally, his trait anxiety was at the 93rd percentile, whereas his state anxiety was only at the 67th percentile. He was alexithymic on the Toronto Alexithymia Scale (TAS-20). He had a moderate degree of depression on the Multiscore Depression Inventory. Depressive symptoms on this inventory included a moderate degree of low energy, low self-esteem, social introversion, pessimism, sad mood, and learned helplessness.

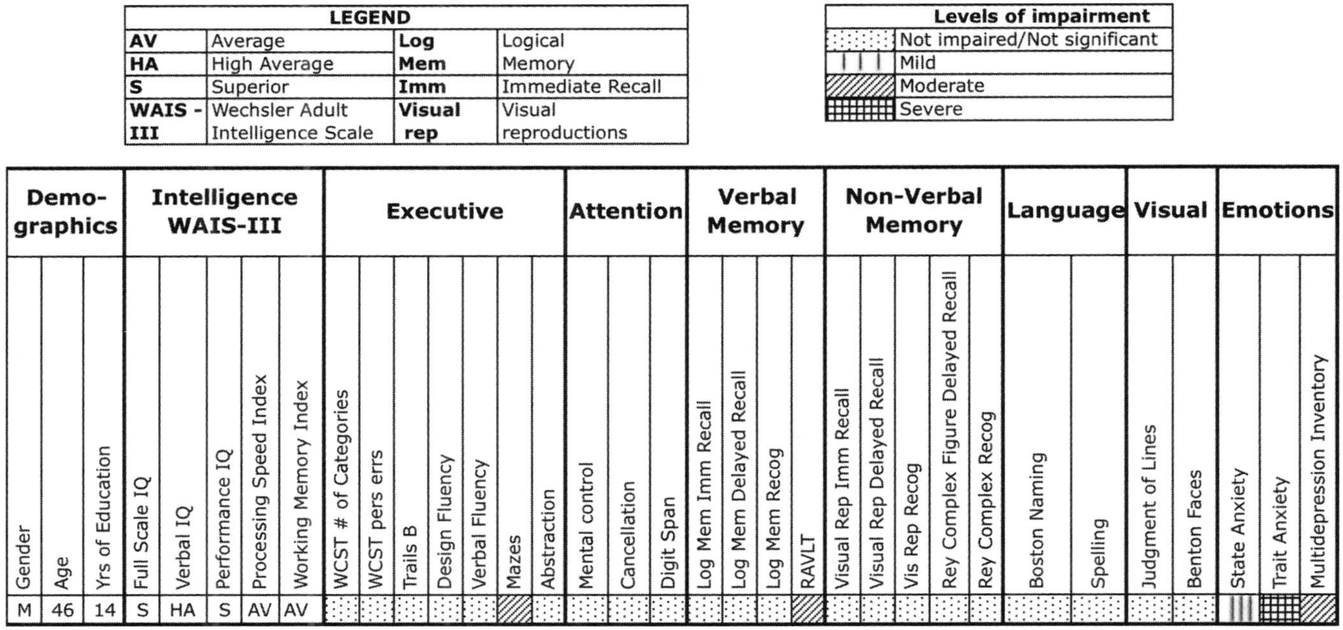
LEGEND
AV Average
HA High Average
S Superior
WAIS - III Wechsler Adult Intelligence Scale
Log Mem Logical Memory
Imm Immediate Recall
Visual rep Visual reproductions
Levels of impairment
Not impaired/Not significant
Mild
Moderate
Severe
Demo-graphics
Intelligence WAIS-III
Executive
Attention
Verbal Memory
Non-Verbal Memory
Language
Visual
Emotions
Gender
Age
Yrs of Education
Full Scale IQ
Verbal IQ
Performance IQ
Processing Speed Index
Working Memory Index
WCST # of Categories
WCST pers errs
Trails B
Design Fluency
Verbal Fluency
Mazes
Abstraction
Mental control
Cancellation
Digit Span
Log Mem Imm Recall
Log Mem Delayed Recall
Log Mem Recog
RAVLT
Visual Rep Imm Recall
Visual Rep Delayed Recall
Vis Rep Recog
Rey Complex Figure Delayed Recall
Rey Complex Recog
Boston Naming
Spelling
Judgment of Lines
Benton Faces
State Anxiety
Trait Anxiety
Multidepression Inventory
M
46
14
S
HA
S
AV
AV

FIGURE 7–3. Data from a neuropsychological test battery for a 46-year-old male who presented 3 years previously with cogniform disorder.

On the Personality Assessment Inventory (PAI), a more comprehensive and detailed measure of psychopathology and personality, he demonstrated a degree of defensiveness about his shortcomings. He exaggerated some of his problems, but this exaggeration was combined with positive impression management in an attempt to portray himself in a more favorable light. This tendency to exaggerate was interpreted as either a cry for help or an extremely negative evaluation of his life. The PAI also identified frequent physical complaints, suicidal thoughts, a pattern of short-lived relationships, a preoccupation with being abandoned or rejected, social isolation, maladaptive behavioral patterns aimed at controlling anxiety, a negative self-concept, and harsh self-criticism. He had a tendency to dwell on past failures and lost opportunities.

The computer-generated PAI diagnostic considerations were as follows:

Axis I: major depressive episode, somatization, dysthymic disorder
Axis I rule out: bipolar II disorder
Axis II: deferred, rule out borderline personality disorder. Based on his presentation, narcissism was considered to be present as well.

During the feedback session, he took out his notebook and said that he wanted to know the numerical value of his IQ because he was certain that Mensa would want to know. He thought his score had dropped, and he seemed discouraged by the information when given. His wife, who was present for the feedback session, wanted a copy of the neuropsychological report for her relatives and planned to place it on the wall of the house. Time was spent on educating the couple about how cognitive abilities can be affected by mood, stressors, and interpersonal dynamics.

Discussion

This patient presented with persistent cognitive difficulties 15 months after a motor vehicle accident. These difficulties were a major source of distress and focus of concern and contributed to his inability to work. They were occurring in the setting of moderate levels of depression and a previous history of a depressive illness. His neuropsychological profile was well preserved, with overall intellectual functioning in the superior range (93rd percentile). Executive capacities and attention were unimpaired. Working memory and processing speed were relatively weak given his overall superior intellectual ability, but his performance on these measures did not convey significant impairment. Although his symptoms had occurred as a consequence of a motor vehicle accident, external incentives such as compensation seeking were not confounds because all litigation linked to his accident had been settled. The magnitude of his symptoms, the level of distress related to them, and his compromised functioning were also not accountable on the basis of a closed head injury, which at worst was minor. Moreover, findings from neurodiagnostic investigations were negative. His symptoms were seemingly progressive, which is inconsistent with a traumatic brain injury 15 months previously in the absence of an identifiable intracranial progressive complication such as hydrocephalus. The differential diagnosis thus lies between the cognitive impairment associated with depression (*depressive pseudodementia*) and the recently described *cogniform disorder*.

The cognitive impairment associated with depression includes difficulties with attention, processing speed, memory, and aspects of executive functioning (Gotlib and Joormann 2010; McClintock et al. 2010). These capacities were intact in this patient. His processing speed was relatively weak but still average and thus unlikely to account for the magnitude of his cognitive complaints.

Cogniform disorder is a described syndrome for those individuals who report excessive cognitive complaints and/or obtain low scores on objective cognitive testing not accounted for by medical, psychiatric, or developmental conditions. There is evidence for noncredible cognitive performance as demonstrated by an implausible symptom report, including delayed onset of symptoms or worsening of symptoms over time in the context of a discrete injury; or inconsistencies between test scores and activities of daily living or observed behavior, inconsistencies in test scores across sequential evaluations, or inconsistencies in symptoms over time. Individuals with cogniform disorder present and behave as if sick; that is, they report cognitive failure that causes subjective distress and disrupts function, consistently feeling and behaving as if compromised by an involuntary disturbed state of their brain function affecting the domain of cognitive ability (Delis and Wetter 2007). This case best fits the diagnosis of cogniform disorder, with contributions from his depression and his personality in which he highly valued his cognitive abilities.

Cogniform disorder and cogniform condition are new subtypes of somatoform disorder in which psychological mechanisms are responsible for symptoms of cognitive failure (Delis and Wetter 2007). Similar to classical motor-sensory conversion symptoms, cogniform disorder is rightfully considered a nonconscious, conversion reaction defined as a somatic presentation that involves any aspect of the CNS over which voluntary control is exercised (Hurwitz 2003). Like psychogenic motor-sensory deficits and all other conversion reactions, cogniform disturbances are identified when the cognitive deficits are not accountable for on the basis of the known damage patterns of brain failure from intrinsic structural injury (e.g., stroke), general medical conditions (e.g., uremia), or primary functional psychiatric disorders (e.g., schizophrenia).

Cogniform disorder or condition is a much-needed diagnostic category for patients with otherwise unexplained cognitive symptoms and complaints and, importantly, is socially neutral without the accusatory implications of conscious faking and interpersonal manipulation as in malingering or factitious disorders. As pointed out by others (Binder 2007; Boone 2007; Larrabee 2007), there is a need for refinements to the Delis and Wetter (2007) descriptions, with stricter defining neuropsychological criteria.

Cogniform disorder is amenable to treatment by psychotherapy. Pharmacotherapy is combined with psychotherapy when moderate-to-severe anxiety and depression are identified as being responsible for somatization and the cogniform presentation.

A neuropsychological evaluation can be therapeutic as well as diagnostic. During testing, patients may be surprised by their good performance. Feedback sessions following an assessment can be vital in allowing patients to gain insight into the relationship between their psychological status and cognitive symptoms as well as the severity of their depression and anxiety.

Key Clinical Points

- A cogniform disorder is an important diagnostic consideration when a patient's primary complaints focus on cognitive changes or decline, especially when associated with a history of or there is evidence for chronic depression and anxiety. A neuropsychological assessment can contribute to diagnostic clarification between cogniform disorder and other causes of cognitive failure.

- The clinician should not overlook the possibility of a cogniform disorder because of a known organic brain injury. Cogniform disorder can be the primary presentation of known organic conditions such as traumatic brain injury.

- Retained leisure time activities, hobbies, and work capacity are useful indicators of intact cognitive ability and can be important clues to a mismatch between reported cognitive failure and preserved functioning.

- In the setting of a cogniform disorder, a comprehensive interview should include a review of financial and psychosocial stressors and concerns about previous diagnostic formulations. Patients may have been advised that psychological factors are causing or contributing to their symptoms but may not be able to recognize or accept a psychiatric diagnosis.

Further Readings

Heilbronner R, Sweet J, Morgan J, et al: American Academy of Clinical Neuro-psychology Consensus Conference statement on the neuropsychological assessment of effort, response bias, and malingering. Clin Neuropsychol 23:1093–1129, 2009

Lamberty GJ: Understanding Somatization in the Practice of Clinical Neuropsychology. New York, Oxford University Press, 2008

Sachdev P, Smith JS, Angus-Lepan H, et al: Pseudodementia twelve years on. J Neurol Neurosurg Psychiatry 53:254–259, 1990

References

Binder LM: Comment on cogniform disorder and cogniform condition: proposed diagnoses for excessive cognitive symptoms. Arch Clin Neuropsychol 22:681–682, 2007

Boone KB: Commentary on "Cogniform disorder and cogniform condition: proposed diagnoses for excessive cognitive symptoms" by Dean C. Delis and Spencer R. Wetter. Arch Clin Neuropsychol 22:675–679, 2007

Delis DC, Wetter SR: Cogniform disorder and cogniform condition: proposed diagnoses for excessive cognitive symptoms. Arch Clin Neuropsychol 22:589–604, 2007

Gotlib IH, Joormann J: Cognition and depression: current status and future directions. Annu Rev Clin Psychol 6:285–312, 2010

Hurwitz T: Somatization and conversion disorder. Can J Psychiatry 49:172–178, 2003

Larrabee GJ: Commentary on Delis and Wetter, "Cogniform disorder and cogniform condition: proposed diagnoses for excessive cognitive symptoms." Arch Clin Neuropsychol 22:683–687, 2007

McClintock S, Husain M, Greer T, et al: Association between depression severity and neurocognitive function in major depressive disorder: a review and synthesis. Neuropsychology 24:9–34, 2010

ALTERATIONS IN CONSCIOUSNESS

Alterations in Consciousness

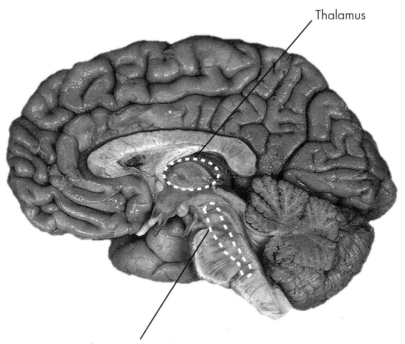

Thalamus

Reticular Activating System

Introduction

Depending on severity and underlying etiology, failing consciousness has a variety of presentations—from stupor to delirium to distractibility. Patients may report difficulties with concentration, multitasking, and tolerating environments with an overabundance of sensory stimuli. They experience variable degrees of cognitive-intellectual failure and perceptual disturbances. They may be confused or unresponsive to the point of stupor and coma. The underlying neuroanatomy is complex and includes the ascending reticular activating system and thalamus (responsible for alertness) and the prefrontal cortex and posterior parietal cortex with a nondominant specialization (responsible for psychomotor focusing). Many neurotransmitters are involved, but acetylcholine in particular has been implicated.

Hashimoto's Encephalopathy

Trevor A. Hurwitz, M.B.Ch.B., M.R.C.P. (U.K.), F.R.C.P.C.

A 31-year-old right-handed woman had a 4-month history of intermittent neurological symptoms. These symptoms had started with transient numbness and tingling in one leg lasting for a few hours. Thereafter she experienced intermittent location-changing numbness that included the side of her face, her fingers, and her arms. She had intermittent double vision, which led her to misjudge distances when reaching for objects and bump into walls when walking. She experienced episodic unsteadiness.

On the day of presentation she awoke feeling fatigued. Later when driving, she experienced a visual hallucination, lasting for seconds, of a man holding a coffee cup and standing in the road in front of her oncoming car. This hallucination recurred three times. There were no associated visual disturbances such as blurred vision and no associated headache.

Her functional inquiry was unremarkable other than a deliberate 50-pound weight loss over the preceding several months.

Previous medical history was significant for a mitral valve prolapse diagnosed at age 8 years and prompting a 1-week hospitalization. At age

10 years she was diagnosed with hypothyroidism. A diagnosis of Hashimoto's thyroiditis was made at age 15–16 years. Two years prior to presentation, she was diagnosed with a chronic fatigue syndrome.

She had a strong family history of autoimmune disease. Her mother had insulin-dependent diabetes mellitus and either rheumatoid arthritis or systemic lupus erythematosus. An uncle had juvenile diabetes mellitus. There was no family history of psychiatric illness.

She had no prior psychiatric history other than a single psychiatric assessment 4 months prior to her presentation. This was done at the behest of her insurer, who wanted to ensure that her chronic fatigue problem was not due to a masked depression.

She was living with a common-law husband. She had no children. She had a college diploma in culinary arts but had worked in sales before going on long-term disability in the preceding 2½ years because of chronic fatigue. She smoked half a pack of cigarettes a day but did not use alcohol or drugs. She was allergic to sulfa drugs. Her only medication was thyroxine 125 mcg/day.

On physical examination she was alert with normal speech and language. Her vital signs were stable, other than a sinus tachycardia of 100 beats/minute, and the results of her general examination were normal. Her thyroid was not enlarged. She scored 26/30 on the Montreal Cognitive Assessment, having lost 2 points on serial 7s, 1 point on the Alternating Trail Making, and 1 point for failing to provide the exact date. The results of her neurological examination were normal other than minimal heel-to-shin dysmetria and minimal gait ataxia. The admitting diagnosis was a mild encephalopathy.

Laboratory test results, including a complete blood count, electrolytes, random blood sugar, and renal and liver chemistries, were all normal. Normal results were also found for anticardiolipin antibody immunoglobulins IgG and IgM, c-ANCA, C3 and C4, anti-double-stranded DNA antibodies, C-reactive protein, thyroid-stimulating hormone, adrenocorticotropic hormone, and morning cortisol. Antinuclear antibody was weakly positive, with a titer of 1:80. Erythrocyte sedimentation rate was normal at 9. Anti–thyroid peroxidase antibodies (anti-TPO) were markedly elevated at 3,546 U/mL (normal range 1–60 U/mL). Cerebrospinal fluid (CSF) analysis showed normal sugar and protein values; there was one white cell and no red cells. Oligoclonal banding was negative. Urinalysis showed pus in the urine, but the culture was negative.

Computed tomography (CT) and magnetic resonance imaging (MRI) of the brain and a single-photon emission computed tomography (SPECT) scan all had normal findings. Findings from nerve and muscle electrodiagnostic studies were also normal. She had two electroencephalograms

(EEGs), both of which had normal findings with no evidence of slowing or focal epileptiform activity.

The patient was given a diagnosis of Hashimoto's encephalopathy and was treated with intravenous (IV) methylprednisolone 1 g/day for 3 days followed by oral prednisone 60 mg/day. Her other medications were levothyroxine 150 mcg/day, alendronate 70 mg/week, calcium carbonate 1,500 mg/day, vitamin D 3,000 IU/day, clonazepam 1 mg tid, and quetiapine XR 50 mg at night. Clonazepam was added for anxiety, and quetiapine was added to help suppress her perceptual symptoms.

She had a positive response to steroids. Most of her symptoms improved by the time of discharge. The discharge treatment strategy was to continue to suppress antibody production through immunomodulatory agents but with a planned gradual taper of her prednisone.

However, 6 weeks after discharge she experienced an exacerbation of symptoms, which included depersonalization, irritability, and personality change. This relapse in symptoms occurred despite a documented fall in her anti-TPO titer to 2,204 U/mL. She received another single pulse of methylprednisolone 1 g followed by an increase in her oral prednisone dosage to 50 mg/day. At the time of her relapse, the dosage had been reduced to 30 mg/day. Following a rheumatological consultation and as a steroid-sparing strategy, she was started on azathioprine. This allowed her prednisone to be once again tapered, at a rate of 2.5 mg/week. The dosage of azathioprine had to be reduced from 150 mg/day to 100 mg/day because of nausea and dizziness and elevated transaminases.

Her presentation now centered on complex perceptual and cognitive-intellectual symptoms followed by affective symptoms. She had a variety of visual distortions. These distortions included seeing a black dot move across her visual field, silhouette transfers in which the outline of a perception moved to a different location in extrapersonal space, and color transfers in which a color in her visual field moved to another object, as well as seeing heatlike waves in front of her. All such experiences lasted for a few seconds and maximally 10–15 seconds. At all times, she maintained insight that such experiences were the product of her mind and understood that they were likely due to Hashimoto's encephalopathy. Cognitive-intellectual symptoms included word-finding difficulties with cognitive derailment, patchy recent verbal and nonverbal memory, impaired calculation, impaired skill memory, impaired problem solving, and impaired stimulus barrier with an inability to tolerate environments with an overabundance of sensory stimulation.

Over the next 6 months, mood symptoms became increasingly dominant and were associated with severe fatigue. Formal neuropsychological assessment done at this time demonstrated difficulties with divided attention, nonverbal intellectual ability, and nonverbal memory associated with severe depression and anxiety. Her subjective complaints about cognitive-intellectual compromise were significantly worse than her objective performance on testing and likely reflected a negative distortion of self-appraisal caused by her fatigue and emotional distress and especially depression.

Her escalating depression was associated with irritability and a fear of loss of psychobehavioral control. She had a single episode of catatonia. Her eyes began to blink and then locked onto a spot in space, followed by total motor inhibition in which she felt that she could not move. She began to slump and drool out of the side of the mouth. She was found in this frozen state by her husband. The catatonic episode resolved over a period of 30 minutes.

Her depression continued to intensify. She started to have suicidal ideation, starting with passive ideation in which she felt that she would not mind if she were not alive. This was followed by self-injurious behaviors in which she made multiple cuts to her thighs. She had no prior history of self-injury. Her self-injurious behavior and worsened depression precipitated an admission to the neuropsychiatry inpatient unit.

Immunosuppression had lowered her anti-TPO titers from a high of 3,546 to the still substantially elevated level of 2,172 U/mL (Figure 8–1), yet her symptoms had worsened by virtue of the added burden of moderate-to-severe affective symptoms. The goal of immunosuppression is to suppress the production of autoantibodies, targeting known and unknown central nervous system (CNS) antigens. These autoantibodies are presumed to be responsible for an immune-mediated inflammatory cascade producing organic damage via either vasculitis or encephalitis. The risks and side effects of immunosuppressants are justifiable if the goal is to arrest and reverse demonstrable and progressive inflammatory brain damage, but extensive and repeated neurodiagnostic investigations had definitively and repeatedly excluded any such pathology in this case. None of her investigations had demonstrated any structural or inflammatory changes in her brain. Clinically, there was also no evidence of focal neurological deficits, seizures, or progressive decline in cognitive-intellectual functioning. Her fluctuating perceptual and cognitive-intellectual symptoms and now dominant affective symptoms were more indicative of a disturbance of brain function rather than structure and highly reminiscent of a typical functional psychiatric illness. Autoantibodies, rather than initiating a destructive inflammatory cascade, may cause an antineurotransmitter/synaptic encephalopathy by compromising neurocellular functioning via interference with normal neural signaling (Moscato et al. 2010). Standard psychoactive medications thus become treatment options by virtue of their actions that either augment or inhibit intercellular communication.

Her treatment strategy was thus altered to emphasize the energetic use of standard psychoactive medications rather than immunosuppression. A complex and prolonged treatment regimen was begun on an inpatient basis and continued on an outpatient basis; this regimen utilized the full spectrum of the psychiatric pharmacological armamentarium. She was maintained on azathioprine and low-dose prednisone, to which was added citalopram, combined first with desipramine and then with atomoxetine and dextroamphetamine. Quetiapine was continued to suppress her perceptual symptoms but also for its benefit on mood. Her symptoms began to stabilize over the ensuing months but have never gone into remission, notwithstanding an ongoing decline in her anti-TPO titers (Figure 8–1).

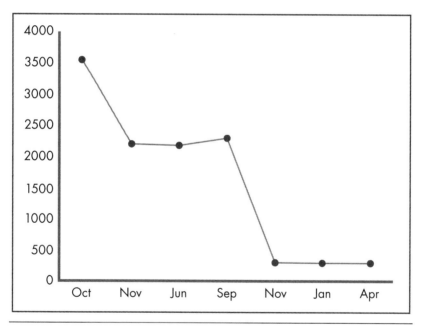

FIGURE 8–1. Anti–thyroid peroxidase antibodies titer (U/mL).

Discussion

Hashimoto's encephalopathy forms part of the spectrum of autoimmune encephalopathies that may be broadly divided into paraneoplastic and nonparaneoplastic forms (Caselli et al. 2010). Hashimoto's encephalopathy is a nonparaneoplastic autoimmune encephalopathy occurring in the setting of thyroid antibodies with or without thyroid hormone fluctuations; it is also known as steroid-responsive encephalopathy associated with autoimmune thyroiditis (SREAT) or nonvasculitic autoimmune inflammatory meningoencephalitis (NAIM) (Schiess and Pardo 2008).

Clinical manifestations of Hashimoto's encephalopathy are highly variable. The onset may be acute or insidious. In the acute form (type I), the presentation is stroke-like with focal neurological deficits, alterations in consciousness, and partial or generalized seizures. In the insidious form (type II), mental status changes predominate and include psychosis and progressive cognitive-intellectual failure that may end in coma; type II is associated with seizures, tremor, myoclonus, and ataxia (Kothbauer-Margreiter et al. 1996).

The average age at onset is 44 years, with a female predominance. Patients are usually euthyroid or hypothyroid and have underlying Hashimoto's thyroiditis. Hashimoto's thyroiditis is an autoimmune disorder in which antithyroid antibodies attack the thyroid gland, usually leading to hypothyroidism. The antibody most commonly associated with Hashimoto's encephalopathy is anti-TPO, previously known as antimicrosomal antibody. Thyroid peroxidase is the main antigen within the thyroid microsome. Importantly, there is no correlation between illness severity and anti-TPO titers (Kothbauer-Margreiter et al. 1996). Other antibodies that are elevated in Hashimoto's encephalopathy include antithyroglobulin antibodies directed against thyroglobulin and anti–alpha-enolase antibodies, which may be directed against the alpha-enolase expressed in vascular endothelium (Schiess and Pardo 2008).

Cerebrospinal fluid (CSF) analysis usually demonstrates an elevated protein level without pleocytosis. Oligoclonal bands are occasionally present (indicating IgG synthesis within the CNS), but the IgG index is usually normal. There are no characteristic neuroimaging findings. The MRI scan is usually normal but may show changes that mimic an ischemic stroke, multiple tumors or granulomas, or a degenerative process. White matter changes, if present, are diffuse, with multiple abnormal confluent areas of varying sizes and shapes located in the periventricular and deep hemispheric subcortical regions but possibly also extending into the cortical gray matter. Brain SPECT may demonstrate focal areas of hypoperfusion. The frontal lobes may be selectively prone to display SPECT perfusion abnormalities. Frontal hypoperfusion has been demonstrated in patients with Hashimoto's thyroiditis who were euthyroid and neurologically and psychiatrically asymptomatic. Electroencephalographic findings consist mainly of diffuse slow-wave abnormalities that reflect the degree of severity of the underlying encephalopathy.

The target neuronal epitope of the autoantibodies remains uncertain. Moreover, the pathogenetic mechanism may not be due to the antithyroid antibodies themselves but to co-occurring antineuronal antibodies such as

N-methyl-D-aspartate receptor (NMDAR) antibodies or antibodies directed against voltage-gated potassium channels (Tüzün et al. 2011).

The underlying pathology also remains uncertain because pathological studies are limited. Case studies have shown an inflammatory vasculitis, an inflammatory encephalitis, demyelination, or no pathology. Pathological cases showing vasculitis are typically associated with MRI changes. Such findings lend confirmatory support to the division of Hashimoto's encephalitis into two types. Type I presents with stroke-like episodes and is presumed to be due to an autoimmune vasculitis. The EEG shows diffuse slowing but may also reveal focal abnormalities and epileptic discharges. Cerebrospinal fluid findings are abnormal in most cases, but nonspecific. The MRI scan may show multifocal hyperintense signals in the white matter. Type II is a noninflammatory, diffuse, progressive encephalopathy. The EEG shows diffuse slowing, rarely associated with epileptic discharges. The MRI or CT scan usually shows normal findings. Type II is presumed to be due to antineuronal autoantibodies directed against antigens that are shared by thyroid and brain.

Insights into how antineuronal antibodies may cause symptoms in the absence of inflammation can be drawn from emerging data about anti–neurotransmitter receptor autoimmune encephalopathies such as anti-NMDAR encephalitis (Moscato et al. 2010). In classical paraneoplastic autoimmune encephalitis, the target antigens are intracellular and symptoms arise from neuronal death mediated by cytotoxic T cells. By contrast, in anti–neurotransmitter receptor autoimmune encephalopathies, symptoms arise from antibodies that bind to autoantigens that are on the cell or synaptic surface. Here several mechanisms may account for symptom production. These mechanisms include agonizing or antagonizing the receptor or causing receptor cross-linking and internalization with subsequent receptor degradation. Autoantibodies may also stimulate complement-mediated neuronal damage. The end result of all such actions is diminished receptor function and a failure of synaptic function and trafficking (Hughes et al. 2010).

The clinical presentation of Hashimoto's encephalopathy overlaps with many other neurological conditions, including CNS infections such as herpes simplex encephalitis, stroke, demyelinating disease, and other autoimmune diseases. These conditions need to be excluded by appropriate investigations.

Treatment of Hashimoto's encephalopathy consists of levothyroxine to ensure an euthyroid state, anticonvulsants in the event of seizures, and immunomodulatory agents. At diagnosis, all patients should be given a trial of corticosteroids, which typically consists of IV methylprednisolone (1 g/day) for 3–7 days, often followed by oral prednisone 60 mg/day, with a slow taper over months.

Response to corticosteroids does not always occur. In the absence of a corticosteroid response or if symptoms resurface after an initial response, other immunomodulatory treatments are added; these treatments include IV immunoglobulin (IVIG), plasma exchange, the hydroxychloroquine sulfate preparation Plaquenil, azathioprine, methotrexate, cyclophosphamide, and mycophenolate mofetil (Marshall and Doyle 2006).

The treatment of patients such as the patient in this case remains a challenge and without literature guidance. These patients present with a diffuse encephalopathy with mostly mental status changes but excluding any alteration in level of consciousness (a variant of Hashimoto's encephalopathy type II). Their symptoms are an admixture of affective disturbances, psychosis, and fluctuating but stable perceptual and cognitive-intellectual difficulties. It is of critical importance that such patients show no clinical or laboratory markers of CNS inflammatory activity or progressive organic structural damage, as reflected in stable neurological functioning and measured neuropsychological capacities and in repeatedly normal CSF analyses, EEGs, and MRI scans. Such patients are assumed to have a version of anti–neurotransmitter receptor encephalopathy with disrupted synaptic trafficking. This assumption is the rationale for using the same treatments indicated in functional psychiatric illnesses to ultimately augment or block synaptic neurotransmission—antidepressants for depression, mood stabilizers for affective and especially manic-type states, anxiolytics for anxiety, antipsychotics for psychosis, and CNS stimulants for impaired attention (which often underlies the cognitive-intellectual and perceptual disturbances found in these patients).

Key Clinical Points

- Autoimmune encephalopathies should be considered in all patients with complex neuropsychiatric presentations.
- Autoimmune screens should include measurement of anti–thyroid peroxidase titers.
- Anti-TPO titers do not correlate with symptom severity.
- All patients who are considered to have Hashimoto's encephalopathy should receive an initial course of high-dose corticosteroids.
- Not all patients with Hashimoto's encephalopathy will respond to corticosteroids, and some will need augmentation with other immunomodulatory agents.
- Patients with Hashimoto's encephalopathy type II may benefit from standard psychiatric therapies with a goal of enhancing or blocking synaptic neurotransmission.

Further Readings

Ferracci F, Carnevale A: The neurological disorder associated with thyroid auto-immunity. J Neurol 253:975–984, 2006

Mahad DJ, Staugaitis S, Ruggieri P, et al: Steroid-responsive encephalopathy associated with autoimmune thyroiditis and primary CNS demyelination. J Neurol Sci 228:3–5, 2005

References

Caselli RJ, Drazkowski JF, Wingerchuk DM: Autoimmune encephalopathy. Mayo Clin Proc 85:878–880, 2010

Hughes EG, Peng X, Gleichman AJ, et al: Cellular and synaptic mechanisms of anti–NMDA receptor encephalitis. J Neurosci 30:5866–5875, 2010

Kothbauer-Margreiter I, Sturzenegger M, Komor J, et al: Encephalopathy associated with Hashimoto thyroiditis: diagnosis and treatment. J Neurol 243:585–593, 1996

Marshall GA, Doyle JJ: Long-term treatment of Hashimoto's encephalopathy. J Neuropsychiatry Clin Neurosci 18:14–20, 2006

Moscato EH, Jain A, Peng X, et al: Mechanisms underlying autoimmune synaptic encephalitis leading to disorders of memory, behavior and cognition: insights from molecular, cellular and synaptic studies. Eur J Neurosci 32:298–309, 2010

Schiess N, Pardo CA: Hashimoto's encephalopathy. Ann N Y Acad Sci 1142:254–265, 2008

Tüzün E, Erdag E, Durmus H, et al: Autoantibodies to neuronal surface antigens in thyroid antibody–positive and –negative limbic encephalitis. Neurol India 59:47–50, 2011

Dissociative Disorders

Joseph Tham, M.D., F.R.C.P.C.

A married, female, 42-year-old right-handed occupational therapist of Asian descent was found unresponsive on the lawn of a public park one August afternoon. The event was unwitnessed. By the time the ambulance arrived, her Glasgow Coma Scale score had recovered to 14 and vital signs were found to be normal, with a blood sugar level of 5. She was brought to the emergency room, where she appeared embarrassed by the whole situation, with no memory of any unusual symptoms prior to "blanking out." The last things she remembered were jogging in the park and waking up surprised that she was being attended to by the ambulance crew.

While in the emergency room, the neurological consultant queried about the possibility of a seizure. The patient was referred for an EEG, which showed normal findings with no epileptiform activity. The rest of her medical screen, including a complete blood count and differential, electrolytes, liver and renal function tests, and electrocardiography, had normal results. Urine screen for illicit substances and intoxicants was negative. An MRI brain scan showed normal findings. She was discharged home with her husband, with the plan to follow up in 3 months with the neurologist.

Two months after this initial event, she was brought back to the emergency room. According to her husband, when he awoke at approximately 1:00 A.M., she was no longer in bed. He noticed that her jacket was still hanging in the closet and her outdoor shoes were still at home, but he could not locate her in the house. Alarmed, he contacted the police department and started driving around the neighborhood to locate her. Eventually he found her sitting on a park bench down the street from where they lived (a different park from the initial event), in her bare feet and wearing only her pajamas. She appeared cold and was shivering, and she did not seem to recognize him. She remained quiet with her eyes closed for the next 10 minutes until the ambulance arrived. She was brought to the local emergency room, where she avoided eye contact and refused to speak to staff. She became agitated and aggressive when prevented from leaving the hospital. Medications, including lorazepam 2 mg with haloperidol 1 mg, were given intramuscularly to help her settle. Blood work was unremarkable, with normoglycemia, normal blood counts, and stable electrolytes.

Having slept through the night medicated, she appeared calm and alert the next morning, claiming no memory of the night before. She requested to be discharged from the hospital as soon as possible. A repeat EEG showed normal findings. An outpatient neurology appointment was arranged, and she was advised to take some time off work (she normally remained quite busy with occupational therapy clients).

About 3 weeks later, shortly after an argument with her daughter, she left the house unannounced. As in previous events, her husband found her sitting on a bench in another local park. She refused to speak to him. She was brought to the emergency room, and once again the medical workup did not demonstrate any evidence of organic pathology. She was referred to the psychiatry department to help with treatment of these episodes of unexplained behaviors. When told that she was to be transferred to the care of psychiatry, she became agitated, demanding discharge. Because of remaining questions around an underlying neurological diagnosis, she was transferred to the acute neuropsychiatry ward.

Initial assessment on admission revealed a physically healthy female appearing her stated age. She was generally compliant with the admission process and had no difficulty providing the admission history. The findings of her physical examination were completely normal. Cognitive-intellectual screen with the Mini-Mental State Examination yielded a score of 30/30. She had no difficulty with other cognitive-intellectual tasks such as digit span (7 forward and 5 backward), reproducing a clock-face diagram, remembering 5 words after 5 minutes of distraction, and providing over 1 minute 15 words beginning with the letter *f.*

The differential diagnosis of her recurrent transient amnestic episodes included possible neurological diagnoses (seizure disorder, transient global amnesia, and a rare form of amnesia with migraine) and a psychogenic disorder, given the repeatedly normal findings of medical investigations.

For safety, the hospital seizure protocol was initiated (oxygen available in her room, side rails available for her bed, no tub baths). She was checked every 30 minutes. She was seen daily by the neuropsychiatry team, one member of which became the primary interviewer/therapist with the goal of developing a strong rapport with her while in the hospital, given the likelihood of the need for regular outpatient follow-up.

No unusual amnestic episodes were observed while she was in the hospital, but in the first 72 hours it became clear that she avoided talking about emotional topics. For example, she refused to comment on the "fight" that she had had with her daughter just prior to the most recent episode of confusion and wandering. She would explain that she was "fine now" and "I'm all right; if I just focus on learning my piano, my memory will get better." She requested that her husband bring her electric keyboard to the hospital so that she could practice her fingering. She also began rereading some old books that she had brought with her, feeling this would also prevent memory lapses. She appeared consistently alexithymic—demonstrating an apparent inability to express herself in emotional ways. She would talk about feeling "upset" rather than about what appeared to be sadness or disappointment as expressed in her body language and facial expression. She admitted to a deteriorating relationship with her husband. However, she described her attitude toward him as "unhappy" even though she seemed visibly angry when talking about his busy work schedule and how she felt when he would often dismiss her.

Over the next 2 weeks, the primary psychiatrist spent hours exploring her life story. The focus was on the index event when she was first found in the park. This location seemed significant given that subsequent events seemed to lead her back to local public parks. In one of the meetings, she acknowledged a fear of going to sleep when the topic of dreams came up. During this hour-long session, she started to reveal details of recurrent nightmares of being harmed in her sleep. She spoke of dreams of physical and sexual abuse. It was in the course of this session that, for the first time, she openly became tearful and used words like *sad, angry,* and *scared.*

Daily meetings from that point on focused on her emotions and allowing her to talk about memories from the past and any recent concerns. Slowly, memories emerged and a narrative could be constructed. On the day when she first lost awareness, she was jogging in the park along a wooded path when she was confronted by a male figure. As she approached, he shockingly exposed himself to her, making lewd sexual gestures. She denied that he had made any attempt at physical contact, and she had run away as fast as she could. She lost awareness shortly after reaching an open field in that park.

Subsequent meetings with the psychiatrist provided further details about her past history. She admitted to numerous episodes of inappropriate touching while growing up in Asia, perpetrated by her elder brother. These events always happened at night and went on sporadically when she was between the ages of 10 and 16 years. She learned to "block out" these events and did not tell anyone for fear of bringing shame to the family. Once, at the age of 14, she found the courage to bring up a complaint against the brother but minimized this to her mother by stating that he was "just" going into her room at night. She did not receive any support from her mother. She never brought up the issue again. By the age of 18, she felt "rescued" by her future husband, escaping the home through marriage.

During the last week before discharge, she wondered why she was "targeted by men" and was able to see the encounter with the exhibitionist as a trigger for emotions that she thought had long been forgotten.

Apart from the psychological work above, she was treated with lorazepam 0.5–1 mg sl prn, as her anxiety level was increased, especially after difficult sessions recounting her memories. An empirical trial of sertraline 150 mg/day was started for an emergent sad mood. Olanzapine 5–10 mg hs was added for a few days after she began experiencing short-lived vague whispers, reminiscent of her brother's voice at night while she was trying to sleep. These events occurred, especially after talking about memories of her brother entering her room, and represented either auditory illusions (possibly a misinterpretation of the voices of people talking on the ward) or hallucinations. The olanzapine was successful in terminating those perceptual experiences.

In total, she spent approximately 6 weeks on the neuropsychiatry unit. She was discharged much improved and, although still emotional about experiences in the past, was able to speak openly to her primary psychiatrist without strong avoidance of emotionally laden topics. She denied thoughts of self-harm or homicidal ideation. She was discharged on sertraline 150 mg qhs but discontinued this after 2 weeks with complaints of headaches. She was also given olanzapine 5 mg hs and lorazepam 0.5 mg sl prn, which she continued to use intermittently.

She was referred to an outpatient psychotherapist to continue work around past sexual abuse. The therapist involved her husband at her request to help him understand her past experiences and improve their communication.

Three years have passed since her admission. She has continued to see her therapist regularly and has continued psychiatric follow-up (about every 3 months) with the neuropsychiatry program. She has been successful in returning to work as an occupational therapist. Other than one episode of threatened self-harm after a verbal altercation at home, she has been stable with no further episodes of amnesia or wandering from home.

Discussion

Among the conditions that can mimic neuropsychiatric disorders including unresponsive states is the group of "dissociative disorders." These conditions are believed to be associated with severe psychological disturbance causing significant instability in mental functions, leading to behavioral, cognitive, and emotional distress. In 1889 Pierre Janet described the psychological formulation around dissociation, or *désagrégations psychologiques*. Although the scope of this concept has evolved over the years, the underlying phenomenology is often described as a "vertical split" (Kohut 1971) in consciousness between concurrent centers of awareness—each with altered memory access, knowledge of the world, and sense of self. This vertical split is in contrast to the "horizontal split" of repression, where emotions and memories are "pushed down" into the subconscious. Work using factor analysis of dissociation has suggested a phenomenological triad of components: absorption-imaginative involvement (markedly narrowing or expanding attention, at times blurring the boundary between self and the world), amnesia, and depersonalization-derealization (Ross et al. 1991).

Although long described in the literature, dissociative disorders became part of the DSM diagnostic system with DSM-III (American Psychiatric Association 1980). Severe cases of dissociative disorder (especially dissociative identity disorder [DID]) were considered rare; there were only 8 cases of multiple personality disorder (the former name for dissociative identity disorder) or DID reported in the literature from 1945 to 1969 and 36 reported in the literature between 1970 and 1979 (Greaves 1980). However, through the 1980s–1990s, the literature suggested an "epidemic" of DID cases not only in number but also in severity (e.g., escalating number of alter egos). This reported increase in number and severity of cases has resulted in controversy and skepticism about dissociative disorders, raising questions around diagnostic validity especially for DID. Over the years extensive research has been conducted on use of the Structured Clinical Interview for DSM-IV Dissociative Disorders (Steinberg 1994) as a diagnostic tool to capture features of dissociation.

Diagnostically, this patient's episodes would be classified as fugue states. A *psychogenic fugue* is defined as a dissociative condition characterized by wandering for hours or, in more severe situations, unplanned traveling lasting days. During the dissociative episode, patients demonstrate loss of identity (as in this case) or in severe cases even assume an alternate identity. Upon resolution of the dissociative state, patients appear to have complete retrograde amnesia of the episode with no anterograde amnesia. Fugue states are believed to be rare, with only case reports in the literature (MacDonald and MacDonald 2009).

The neurobiology of dissociative states remains poorly understood. Studies exploring the core feature of dissociative amnesia have reported neuroimaging findings suggestive of changes in frontal-subcortical activity (Hennig-Fast et al. 2008).

As suggested in this case, psychological dysfunction secondary to pathological stress has historically been seen as a major contributor to the development of dissociation. Models such as the "trauma-memory argument" (Kihlstrom 1995) suggest that dissociation is the result of the deployment of powerful psychological defenses to block awareness of the trauma, resulting in features such as psychogenic amnesia and diminished accessibility to autobiographical memory. The effect of trauma has played such a significant role that some authors have considered the possibility of dissociative disorder being a severe form of posttraumatic stress disorder (PTSD). However, this remains controversial because trauma history has been absent in some cases (Dalla Barba et al. 1997).

Similarly, treatment of dissociative disorders remains uncertain. Specifically in regard to this case, there is at present no systematic outcome study of dissociative amnesia or dissociative fugue. It is believed that most patients spontaneously recover from prolonged fugue or amnestic states, and retrieval cues may hasten the process. Studies in patients with DID have generally focused on a psychodynamic framework for understanding the disorder and have incorporated elements of psychoeducation, cognitive-behavioral therapy, and clinical hypnosis in therapy. In the case presented, it was felt that developing a consistent therapeutic relationship early was essential in undertaking treatment. The therapist in the course of the treatment was able to explore issues with the patient around her past sexual abuse during the inpatient stay, which gave her a safe environment to "recover" memories that had not been shared for decades and offered her the freedom to disclose and work through recent emotional events (i.e., exposure to the exhibitionist). Understandably, retrieval of these memories resulted in emotional distress, hence the empirical use of medications such as antidepressants, benzodiazepines, and low-dose antipsychotics for the respective emergent psychopathology. Unfortunately, the literature is remarkably silent on pharmacological treatment of dissociative disorders other than in the context of comorbid treatment for conditions like PTSD with refractory depression (Kaplan and Klinetob 2000).

Key Clinical Points

- Although relatively rare, dissociative disorders should be considered in the differential diagnosis of conditions presenting with acute onset of altered awareness after ruling out organic conditions.
- The etiology, epidemiology, and neurobiology of dissociative disorders remain poorly understood.
- The diagnosis of dissociative disorders can be extremely difficult, and controversies persist around the diagnostic validity of these disorders.
- The treatment of dissociative disorders as currently understood continues to be based primarily on a psychodynamic framework. Because there is a strong psychological component to these disorders, clinicians should consider comorbidities, including Axis II conditions.
- The role of pharmacological therapy for dissociative disorders is poorly characterized and remains uncertain.

Further Readings

Dell PF, O'Neil JA: Dissociation and the Dissociative Disorders: DSM-V and Beyond. New York, Routledge, 2009

Michelson LK, Ray WJ (eds): Handbook of Dissociation: Theoretical, Empirical, and Clinical Perspectives. New York, Plenum, 1996

Vermetten E, Dorahy M, Spiegel D (eds): Traumatic Dissociation: Neurobiology and Treatment. Washington, DC, American Psychiatric Publishing, 2007

References

American Psychiatric Association: Diagnostic and Statistical Manual of Mental Disorders, 3rd Edition. Washington, DC, American Psychiatric Association, 1980

Dalla Barba G, Mantovan MC, Ferruzza E, et al: Remembering and knowing the past: a case study of isolated retrograde amnesia. Cortex 33:143–154, 1997

Greaves GB, Multiple personality: 165 years after Mary Reynolds. J Nerv Ment Dis 168:577–596, 1980

Hennig-Fast K, Meister F, Frodl T, et al: A case of persistent retrograde amnesia following a dissociative fugue: neuropsychological and neurofunctional underpinnings of loss of autobiographical memory and self-awareness. Neuropsychologia 46:2993–3005, 2008

Kaplan MJ, Klinetob NA: Childhood emotional trauma and chronic posttraumatic stress disorder in adult outpatients with treatment-resistant depression. J Nerv Ment Dis 188:596–601, 2000

Kihlstrom JF: The trauma-memory argument. Conscious Cogn 4:63–67, 1995

Kohut H: The Analysis of the Self. New York, International Universities Press, 1971

MacDonald K, MacDonald T: Peas, please: a case report and neuroscientific review of dissociative amnesia and fugue. J Trauma Dissociation 10:420–435, 2009

Ross CA, Joshi S, Currie R: Dissociative experiences in the general population: a factor analysis. Hosp Community Psychiatry 42:297–301, 1991

Steinberg M: Interviewer's Guide to the Structured Clinical Interview for DSM-IV Dissociative Disorders (SCID-D). Washington, DC, American Psychiatric Press, 1994

Anti–NMDA Receptor Encephalitis

Warren T. Lee, M.D., Ph.D.

Trevor A. Hurwitz, M.B.Ch.B., M.R.C.P. (U.K.), F.R.C.P.C.

A 16-year-old right-handed girl was brought to a family physician because of fever, giddiness, and anxiety that had started 2 weeks prior. The fever had since abated. She was given hydroxyzine 25 mg bid for symptomatic relief. However, her symptoms worsened and in the following week her parents found her increasingly restless, pacing up and down in their home and talking to herself. Her high school teacher called her parents after noticing similar behaviors at school and advised her parents to take her to the hospital.

Prior to this episode, she was an above-average student, quiet but studious. She was active in sports and well liked by her teachers and friends. Up until the onset of this illness, there were no medical problems. Neither were there any past psychiatric or substance abuse problems. Alarmed at her increasingly inexplicable behaviors, the parents brought her to the psychiatric hospital emergency room. During the hospitalization in a child and adolescent unit, she was noted to be very anxious and restless, and she screamed out for no apparent reason. There was loss of eye contact and little spontaneous speech. Given her mental state, it was impossible to assess her orientation and cognitive-intellectual functioning.

Since admission to the hospital she had been afebrile and her vital signs had been stable. A MRI scan of the brain and routine blood investigations, including a toxicology screen done upon admission, were all unremarkable. The diagnostic impression at that time was possible first-episode psychosis. She was treated with lorazepam 1 mg bid and risperidone 1 mg bid. She was noted to be slightly stiff and so risperidone was switched to olanzapine 5 mg hs, but there was no perceptible improvement. Instead she became more quiet and withdrawn and refused to talk or to eat. On day 5 of the admission she had a witnessed generalized tonic-clonic seizure, and she was emergently transferred to the neurology service of a general hospital.

In the neurology ward, she was started on IV sodium valproate. However, she continued to have a series of seizures. The EEG showed left temporal focus spreading into the left hemisphere (Figure 8–2). She was transferred to the neurological intensive care unit and was intubated prophylactically and also given intravenous levetiracetam and midazolam. There were no more overt seizures. Another MRI scan showed only a small focus of T2/FLAIR (fluid-attenuated inversion recovery) hyperintensity in the subcortical white matter. A complete blood count showed mildly elevated leukocytes. Lumbar puncture revealed clear, colorless CSF with 0 red blood cells and 5 nucleated cells/mm^3 with 83% lymphocytes and 8% monocytes. The CSF glucose level was 62 mg/dL, and the protein level was mildly elevated at 47 mg/dL (normal level ≤45 mg/dL). Subsequent CSF studies were essentially unchanged.

The results of renal, hepatic, thyroid, and autoimmune panels were normal, as were erythrocyte sedimentation rate and C-reactive protein level. Other laboratory investigations initiated after admission into the neurology service included CSF and blood serology and Gram stain and cultures testing for *Cryptococcus*, varicella, *Toxoplasma*, cytomegalovirus, herpes simplex, Japanese encephalitis, measles, mumps, syphilis, Epstein-Barr virus, enterovirus, HIV, Lyme disease, West Nile virus, and acid-fast bacillus. In addition to the usual paraneoplastic screen, antibodies to *N*-methyl-D-aspartate receptors (NMDAR) in blood and CSF and antibodies to voltage-gated potassium channels and P/Q- and N-type calcium channels were ordered.

While these laboratory investigation results were pending, and because of the possibility of a CNS infection, she was started empirically on intravenous acyclovir and ceftriaxone.

Clinically she exhibited a frightening and baffling series of fluctuating neuropsychiatric symptoms, including confusion, restlessness, irritability,

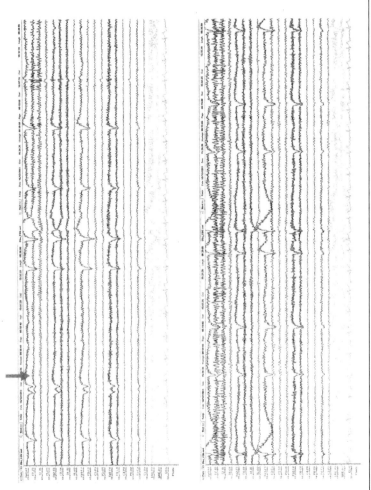

FIGURE 8–2.   Electroencephalogram from a 16-year-old girl showing left temporal focus spreading into the left hemisphere.

rigidity, and dystonic posturing. She appeared at times to be responding to internal stimuli and at other times to be engaging in purposeless repetitive activity. A series of medications were tried, including benzodiazepines, typical and atypical antipsychotics, and antiepileptic medications, but there was minimal improvement. Electroconvulsive therapy (ECT) was considered a possibility.

The results of all investigations were negative except for the NMDAR antibody tests, which yielded positive antibodies to the NR1/NR2 subunits of the NMDAR. She was then started on IVIG 0.4 g/kg/day and methylprednisolone 1 g/day for a week.

An extensive search for tumors was also undertaken. Ultrasound of the pelvis and CT of the pelvis revealed a 6 cm×5.5 cm×4 cm dermoid cyst (teratoma) in the right ovary and another 4 cm×5 cm×3.4 cm cyst in the left ovary. Because she was a minor and in any case was unable to give informed consent, consent for surgical removal was given by her parents. She underwent bilateral ovarian cystectomy. Histopathological findings confirmed the benign nature of the cysts.

Postoperatively she slowly improved, becoming less confused, and her orientation to person, place, and date returned over a protracted course. Prior to surgery her Montreal Cognitive Assessment score was 12/30 during a lucid period; 6 weeks postcystectomy her score improved to 24/30. During the recovery phase, she was started on speech therapy, occupational therapy, physical therapy, and cognitive therapy with a psychologist.

She was discharged after a total of 4 months of hospitalization, and she made a slow and gradual recovery. Seven months after first presentation she was able to return to school, but she was given a reduced workload and special assistance. She had no recollection of the episode surrounding her hospitalization and early recovery. Her grateful parents reported that she was about 80% of her premorbid self, and they were hopeful for further improvement.

Discussion

Autoimmune limbic encephalitis refers to a spectrum of neuropsychiatric disorders that predominantly affect the medial temporal lobes (hippocampus, amygdala) and the orbitofrontal and frontobasal regions of the brain. These disorders are typically described as paraneoplastic and nonparaneoplastic, but this distinction is becoming less tenable as progress is made in the identification of comorbid neoplasia. Autoimmune limbic encephalitis is now better understood, and some researchers have classified it into two broad categories by their pathogenetic mechanisms (Tüzün and Dalmau 2007):

1. *With antibodies directed against intracellular antigens.* The more common ones are anti-Hu (associated with small cell lung carcinoma), anti-Ma (associated with testicular germ cell tumors), anti-CV2/CRMP5 (associated with thymoma and small cell lung carcinoma), and antiamphiphysin (associated with breast carcinoma). These are the conventionally described paraneoplastic encephalitides.

2. *With antibodies directed against cell membrane antigens.* These include anti-NMDAR antibodies and antibodies to voltage-gated potassium channels, AMPA receptors, and gamma-aminobutyric acid (GABA) type B receptors. Other antigens are expected to be elucidated in the future (Vincent et al. 2011). In this second group, the association with tumors is less clear except for anti-NMDAR encephalitis, which is associated with ovarian teratomas in about 60% of the cases (Dalmau et al. 2008). However, given the significant number of cases where no tumor has ever been found, some researchers feel that these conditions would be better described as neuroautoimmune disorders, whereby autoantibodies that cross-react with synaptic proteins are formed in response to a number of possible stimuli (including tumors and infection). The prodromal infection may act as the antigenic trigger in what is described as infection-induced molecular mimicry (Peery et al. 2012).

Anti–NMDAR encephalitis associated with ovarian teratomas was first reported in 2005 (Vitaliani et al. 2005), and the term was coined by those authors (Dalmau et al. 2007). NMDARs are ligand-gated cation channels that are involved in synaptic transmission and plasticity. They are made up of two subunits, NR1 and NR2. Subsequent studies identified specific autoantibodies directed against the NR1 subunit of the NMDAR as the pathogenic cause. Additional work has demonstrated that these autoantibodies cause a decrease in the number of NMDARs in target cells by inducing cross-linking and internalization of the receptors by autophagy (Hughes et al. 2010).

In a seminal paper, Dalmau and his coworkers (2008) reported a case series of 100 patients, mean age 23 years, with confirmed anti-NMDAR encephalitis; 91 were women. All patients presented with psychiatric symptoms or memory problems. Of the 100 patients, 76 had seizures; 88 had unresponsive states; 69 had autonomic instability; 66 had hypoventilation; and 58 had identified tumors, of which ovarian teratomas were the most common. Three-quarters of the patients recovered completely or had mild deficits, whereas one-quarter had severe deficits or died.

Anti-NMDAR encephalitis typically occurs in sequential phases (Peery et al. 2012): prodromal phase, psychotic and/or seizure phase, unresponsive phase, and hyperkinetic phase. The first phase is often a flulike illness with fever, malaise, headache, and fatigue. This is followed by the phase of florid psychiatric symptoms with a wide range of fluctuating psychiatric manifestations, including anxiety, apathy, mood dysregulation, confusion, agitation, phobic preoccupations, paranoid delusions, hallucinations, sleep dysregulation, obsessive-compulsive behaviors, and disinhibition. In this phase, patients often present to psychiatrists or at psychiatric emergency rooms. They may also have seizures, most commonly generalized tonic-clonic; the onset of seizures then brings them to immediate neurological attention and identifies the illness as organic. In the unresponsive phase, those who are not already admitted into hospitals may present with akinetic or catatonic symptoms. The hyperkinetic phase is characterized by autonomic instability, hypertension, hypoventilation, dyskinesias, and stereotypies. Here clinicians are at risk of erroneously attributing the dyskinesias to antipsychotic medications that may have been given for behavioral management. Although this sequence is typical, a wide range of presentations have been reported.

Anti-NMDAR encephalitis can be challenging to diagnose, especially in the earlier phases, and a broad differential diagnosis has to be considered. In the early phase, patients may be diagnosed with acute drug intoxication or first-episode psychosis (as was done for this patient). In the later phases, and concomitantly with antipsychotic treatment, patients may develop rigidity, autonomic instability, and an increase in muscle enzymes, raising the possibility of a neuroleptic malignant syndrome (NMS). Viral encephalitis is an early presumptive diagnosis given the mental status change and CSF abnormality; hence patients are started, with good reason, on antiviral and antibacterial agents. MRI findings are normal in 50% of patients, and for the other 50% T2/FLAIR signal hyperintensity might be seen in the hippocampi or in the cerebral or cerebellar cortices (Figure 8–3). Follow-up MRI scans are usually unchanged (Dalmau et al. 2008, 2011). Electroencephalograms usually show abnormal findings, exhibiting nonspecific, slow, continuous activity interspersed with seizure patterns. Cerebrospinal fluid findings include moderate lymphocytic pleocytosis, normal or mildly raised protein concentration, and, in 60% of patients, CSF-specific oligoclonal bands (Dalmau et al. 2011). Another barrier to accurate and speedy diagnosis is the limited availability of sensitive and specific laboratory tests for these autoantibodies. Outcomes can be improved by early diagnosis via indirect immunofluorescence or cell-based assays (Peery et al. 2012).

Once the diagnosis is made, the current treatment protocols involve immunotherapy: IVIG, high-dose IV corticosteroids, plasma exchange, rituximab, azathioprine, and cyclophosphamide are employed sequentially or in combination. A whole-body search for tumors should take place simultaneously, and the tumor should be resected if one is found.

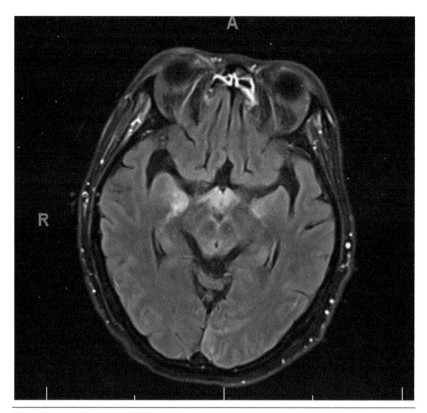

FIGURE 8–3. Axial FLAIR (fluid-attenuated inversion recovery) magnetic resonance image from another patient with anti–NMDA receptor encephalitis showing increased signal in the medial temporal lobes, right much worse than left, for illustration.

Chemotherapy for identified tumors may also be indicated. Meanwhile, anticonvulsants for seizures and antipsychotics (low-dose atypical antipsychotics) for psychotic symptoms or delirium may be used. Patients are usually monitored and treated in an intensive care setting for autonomic instability, hypoventilation, and recurrent seizures.

The recovery process is slow, taking place over several months or longer, and may be incomplete. Episodes of acute illness may recur, especially if no tumor is found. In fact, if no tumor is found despite an assiduous effort, repeat screening for tumors is recommended at regular intervals. Tumors are not commonly found in male patients reported thus far. A majority of all patients will have some persistent cognitive-intellectual impairment, especially with respect to memory and executive function (Finke et al. 2012). Those who receive early immunotherapy or have early tumor resection fare better. A characteristic feature of patients who recover is a persistent amnesia of the entire acute illness episode. This finding would be compatible with a theorized disruption of the mechanisms of synaptic plasticity underlying learning and memory, in which NMDARs play a pivotal role, and the preferential involvement of the hippocampus in the immune-mediated encephalitis (Dalmau et al. 2008).

Anti-NMDAR encephalitis is only one of the disorders of the CNS associated with autoantibodies. The diagnosis can now be made with confidence, and treatment is available. In a recent prospective study of patients with encephalitis in the United Kingdom, 4% of patients with encephalitis were found to have had anti-NMDAR encephalitis (Granerod et al. 2010). This and related disorders may account for a sizable percentage of encephalitides that would otherwise have been classified as of unknown etiology. There are other antigens and antibodies yet to be identified or characterized, and this is an exciting area for future research.

Key Clinical Points

- Anti–NMDA receptor encephalitis is a recently characterized disorder that typically presents with a wide range of florid psychiatric symptoms and memory problems.

- Abrupt changes in behavior, altered levels of consciousness, cognitive-intellectual or memory problems, autonomic dysfunction, dyskinesias or dystonias, and seizures should raise the index of suspicion.

- Definitive diagnosis is made by the presence of anti-NMDAR (NR1) antibodies in blood or cerebrospinal fluid.

- An assiduous search for tumors is necessary. Ovarian teratomas are the most commonly associated tumor. In some cases a tumor cannot be found because it is too small or may have been destroyed by the immune process. However, ongoing tumor surveillance is recommended.

- Early treatment with immunotherapy—typically, IVIG, high-dose IV corticosteroids, and plasma exchange—and tumor resection and chemotherapy improves outcome.

Further Readings

Dalmau J, Lancaster E, Martinez-Hernandez E, et al: Clinical experience and laboratory investigations in patients with anti-NMDAR encephalitis. Lancet Neurol 10:63–74, 2011

Vincent A, Bien CG, Irani SR, et al: Autoantibodies associated with diseases of the CNS: new developments and future challenges. Lancet Neurol 10:759–772, 2011

References

Dalmau J, Tüzün E, Wu HY, et al: Paraneoplastic anti–N-methyl-D-aspartate receptor encephalitis associated with ovarian teratoma. Ann Neurol 61:25–36, 2007

Dalmau J, Gleichman AJ, Hughes EG, et al: Anti-NMDA-receptor encephalitis: case series and analysis of the effects of antibodies. Lancet Neurol 7:1091–1098, 2008

Dalmau J, Lancaster E, Martinez-Hernandez E, et al: Clinical experience and laboratory investigations in patients with anti-NMDAR encephalitis. Lancet Neurol 10:63–74, 2011

Finke C, Kopp UA, Prüss H, et al: Cognitive deficits following anti-NMDA receptor encephalitis. J Neurol Neurosurg Psychiatry 83:195–198, 2012

Granerod J, Ambrose HE, Davies NW, et al: Causes of encephalitis and differences in their clinical presentations in England: a multicentre, population-based prospective study. Lancet Infect Dis 10:835–844, 2010

Hughes EG, Peng X, Gleichman AJ, et al: Cellular and synaptic mechanisms of anti–NMDA receptor encephalitis. J Neurosci 30:5866–5875, 2010

Peery HE, Day GS, Dunn S, et al: Anti–NMDA receptor encephalitis: the disorder, the diagnosis and the immunobiology. Autoimmun Rev 11:863–872, 2012

Tüzün E, Dalmau J: Limbic encephalitis and variants: classification, diagnosis and treatment. Neurologist 13:261–271, 2007

Vincent A, Bien CG, Irani SR, et al: Autoantibodies associated with diseases of the CNS: new developments and future challenges. Lancet Neurol 10:759–772, 2011

Vitaliani R, Mason W, Ances B, et al: Paraneoplastic encephalitis, psychiatric symptoms, and hypoventilation in ovarian teratoma. Ann Neurol 58:594–604, 2005

Neuroleptic Malignant Syndrome

Catherine Chiles, M.D., D.F.A.P.A., F.A.P.M.

A 45-year-old white man, a nursing home resident with a 20-year history of paranoid schizophrenia, was admitted to the medical service of the hospital because he was increasingly belligerent toward the nursing home staff and was refusing food and fluids, which resulted in his losing weight (15 pounds) and becoming dehydrated. He had lived at the nursing home for the last 3 years, had a conservator of person and finance appointed due to mental disability, and had not held employment for over 5 years; he was formerly employed as a maintenance worker. His psychiatric treatment was managed by the facility's consulting psychiatrist, and outpatient medications included divalproex sodium 1,500 mg po qhs, quetiapine 300 mg po bid, and a multivitamin tablet daily. He had a history of multiple long-term hospitalizations, several due to prior episodes of psychogenic polydipsia, but no known suicide attempts. Substance use was confined to alcohol abuse during his early 20s. His past medical history was notable for eosinophilia, which was recently attributed to the divalproex sodium, and hypertension. Baseline functioning at the facility included disorganized behavior, long-term management issues related to food and medication refusals, and limited interactions with other residents and staff.

Following 3 days of rehydration, he was transferred to the hospital's inpatient psychiatric unit, where he was notably delusional about food intake, stating that he "no longer needed to eat." He isolated himself from others and required special nursing care. Vital signs were stable, with borderline low blood pressure (101/70 mm Hg) relative to his baseline. Valproate level on admission was 73 mcg/mL (50–100), and thyroid-stimulating hormone was 0.85 mcIU/mL (0.35–5.5). Results of the complete blood count were in the normal range except for persistent eosinophilia at 24% (0–7), and chemistries were negative. Body mass index was 27.

Therapeutic adjustments in the psychiatric medications targeted the psychosis (quetiapine titrated to 300 mg po qam and 500 mg po qhs) and the eosinophilia (divalproex sodium decreased to 750 mg qhs), but with little improvement in either. With the onset of worsening agitation, the outpatient divalproex sodium dose was resumed. After a few days of behavioral interventions and efforts by nutritionists, he was noted to be increasingly in a state of inanition (exhaustion due to lack of food or fluid intake). Inquiries by care providers about his eating prompted his immediate social withdrawal and refusal to speak. Episodes of posturing were noted at times. On day 5 of the psychiatric admission, he became febrile to 103°F, with a low glucose level (55 mg/dL) and low blood pressure (95/60), and required emergent transfer back to the medical service.

On the medical service, treatment was coordinated with consent of the conservator. He emergently received parenteral hydration and medical examination. A panel of tests was performed, including further assessment of thyroid and adrenal functions and a search for infection (including HIV, syphilis, and Lyme disease). The findings of computed tomography (CT) head imaging were negative. An additional search for underlying medical conditions revealed a left lower lobe infiltrate on chest X ray that correlated with rales on physical examination of the chest. Laboratory investigations revealed leukocytosis at 15.2 K/mm^3 (4.5–11) in the presence of a continued fever of 102.5°F. He was presumed to have a hospital-acquired pneumonia, and broad-spectrum antibiotics were instituted; however, the fever did not fully resolve.

A psychiatry consultation was obtained the day after the transfer to assist the medical service with psychotropic medication management. In the setting of high fever, dehydration, inanition, and long-term antipsychotic use with recent increases in dosages, concern was raised about a possible neuroleptic malignant syndrome. Although the neurological examination did not show severe muscle rigidity, the prior episode of posturing was considered significant. Serum creatine kinase (CK) level was obtained for the first time since admission and found to be elevated at 2,053 U/L (30–200). Cessation of the antipsychotic (quetiapine) now became a priority because of the combination of fever, abnormal movements, leukocytosis, and the recent change in antipsychotic dosing. No myoglobinuria was detected, but the patient received additional hydration to protect his kidneys from rhabdomyolysis. An electrocardiogram recorded a prolonged QTc interval of 550 milliseconds, which provided further impetus for discontinuation of the antipsychotic. Serial CK tests were instituted twice daily, and the levels trended upward, with a peak of approximately 10,000 U/L after 2 days, and thereafter drifted down over several more days after quetiapine treatment was halted. In retrospect, the onset of NMS could be linked temporally to the escalation of quetiapine dose during the hospitalization.

Interim pharmacological management included the use of a benzodiazepine (lorazepam), in standing doses and as needed for agitation, in combination with standing doses of divalproex sodium. These agents did not adequately address the worsening psychosis that compelled the patient to refuse food and fluid except for very sporadic tastes of ice cream and sips of water. The medical team consulted the gastroenterology service for an assessment of possible dysphagia or other gastrointestinal conditions as a cause of inanition, as well as assessment of the need for feeding tube placement. The latter was deferred since a malignancy evaluation was in progress. The endocrinology service was also consulted about possible adrenal insufficiency to account for his decreased oral intake, hypotension, hypoglycemia, and eosinophilia. Respective diagnostic evaluations by both services were limited, but neither found evidence of malignancy or endocrine disturbance.

The negative medical test results pointed to the underlying primary psychosis as the cause of his inanition. With continued weight loss and glucose dysregulation and without the option of antipsychotic treatment, the problem became urgent. Reintroducing an antipsychotic agent was not considered a safe or timely option because of the likelihood of exacerbating the NMS and QT interval prolongation. Strategies to manage the patient's behavior with benzodiazepines and divalproex sodium had proved ineffective in treating the now life-threatening psychosis. In the opinion of the psychiatry consultant, no less-intrusive treatment than ECT was available for inanition due to psychosis. The local probate court granted permission to conduct involuntary ECT, and the treatments began within 8 days following the transfer to the medical service.

In preparation for conducting ECT on a thrice-weekly basis, divalproex sodium was lowered to 750 mg nightly and was held the night before ECT to allow the induction of seizure activity. During the first five treatments with ECT, the patient continued to voice no need for food, and made statements such as "I only need fresh air" and "You will not need food in the future." However, nursing and nutrition notes documented a mild improvement in intake, with occasional consumption of breakfast or a snack. After the sixth treatment with ECT, he returned from the recovery room and abruptly stated, "I want food!" Thereafter he resumed a regular intake of meals and was medically stabilized. Concern for hypoadrenalism remained, and follow-up tests for occult malignancy were also pursued. The pneumonia began to resolve, and antibiotics were discontinued after a full course.

After 25 days on the medical service, he was accepted for transfer back to the inpatient psychiatry unit to continue ECT and for more intensive treatment of the underlying schizophrenia. During an additional 2 weeks in this unit, he completed two more sessions of ECT, making a total of eight treatments. He had begun eating regularly and eventually regained most of his lost weight. The QTc normalized at 450 milliseconds, and risperidone was added to the outpatient regimen of divalproex sodium as a long-term strategy for management of the residual psychotic symptoms. There was no evidence of an NMS relapse. He returned to the nursing home where he resided, and his care was continued by the outpatient psychiatrist. Divalproex sodium was tapered off at the nursing home with resolution of the eosinophilia.

Discussion

The constellation of symptoms that constitute NMS is largely derived from clinical settings. The syndrome is studied primarily by case reports because it is rare (1–2 cases/10,000 patients [0.01%–0.02%] treated with antipsychotics) and therefore difficult to study prospectively. The incidence of NMS has declined due to increased awareness and earlier intervention, but it remains a lethal condition with a mortality risk of approximately 10% (Strawn et al. 2007).

NMS occurs in the context of recent treatment with an antipsychotic agent (Strawn et al. 2007). Cardinal features include fever and severe muscle rigidity, with a range of other physical findings, derangements in autonomic system regulation, and supportive laboratory abnormalities. Mental status changes and rigidity often precede the hyperthermia and autonomic dysfunction that is seen in NMS (Velamoor et al. 1994). From a neurological standpoint, the presentation of NMS may be difficult to distinguish from otherwise benign extrapyramidal side effects of antipsychotics and from other general medical and substance-induced conditions (Strawn et al. 2007).

Populations at risk for NMS include patients with schizophrenia, bipolar disorder, and delirium, with those in the last category at highest risk due to antipsychotic exposure to both high doses and parenteral administration. Additional risk factors are male sex, dehydration, agitation, and a prior episode of NMS. The highest-potency neuroleptics (e.g., haloperidol and fluphenazine) are implicated most frequently, and depot preparations of these medications necessitate a longer period of recovery than oral medications (Seitz and Gill 2009; Strawn et al. 2007). In this case, the patient had been prescribed oral antipsychotics on a long-term basis for schizophrenia, in a supervised setting in which medications were reliably administered.

Laboratory investigations are critical in resolving the broader differential diagnosis, often by the process of exclusion because there is no diagnostic test specific for NMS. Several findings are, however, strongly associated with NMS. Rhabdomyolysis elevates serum CK and aldolase levels. Creatine kinase level is often very high and is the most commonly used marker to track muscle injury. Lactate dehydrogenase and transaminase elevations can also occur. Leukocytosis is often present, widening the differential diagnosis to include infective causes such as viral encephalitis. Results of laboratory tests of CSF are generally normal (Strawn et al. 2007).

Hyperthermia in NMS, with an average temperature of 39.5°C (103.1°F), approaches the temperatures that pose dangerous physiological consequences for neuronal cells, most sensitively the proteins in mitochondrial and plasma membranes that become vulnerable to irreversible changes at temperatures around and above 40°C (104°F) (Gillman 2010). Other conditions that may present with hyperthermia are heatstroke (symptoms include flaccid muscles, dry skin, and a history of heat exposure); malignant hyperthermia (develops intraoperatively in patients with a genetic predisposition); and serotonin syndrome (agitated delirium with myoclonus, seen with exposure to serotonergic agents such as selective serotonergic reuptake inhibitors, tricyclic antidepressants, and monoamine oxidase inhibitors) (Strawn et al. 2007).

Treatment of NMS is based on the theory that NMS represents an acute dopamine deficiency state from central dopaminergic system blockade by antipsychotic agents. Discontinuation of the antipsychotic or other dopaminergic agent that is putatively causing NMS is the first step. Admission to intensive care is often needed for parenteral hydration and supportive care to regulate temperature, manage autonomic derangements, and protect the kidneys from the toxic effects of myoglobinuria. The dopamine agonist bromocriptine and the muscle relaxants dantrolene and benzodiazepines may be helpful, although evidence for their efficacy or even safety in NMS is limited. Electroconvulsive therapy has been used in severe cases of NMS that are refractory to these initial measures (Seitz and Gill 2009; Strawn et al. 2007). Concurrent medical conditions such as pneumonia need to be treated, with the recognition that leukocytosis and fever could also be due to NMS.

After NMS has resolved, antipsychotics may be needed to treat persistent symptoms of the underlying conditions, such as schizophrenia, mood disorders, and delirium due to other conditions. The generally accepted practice is to allow a 2-week interval before restarting an antipsychotic. Atypical antipsychotic agents may have some advantages over typical agents, and the second antipsychotic medication should be different from the antipsychotic implicated in the initial NMS episode (Seitz and Gill 2009; Strawn et al. 2007). Continued vigilance for NMS in a patient who has recovered from NMS in the past is prudent, because the risk of recurrence is higher.

In this patient, elevated CK serum levels were the first evidence that his altered mental status could be attributed to NMS. The CK levels demonstrated a classic crescendo pattern before resolving, well after the antipsychotic was discontinued. He had several medical comorbidities, including pneumonia and inanition, collectively making the cardinal symptoms of NMS harder to detect. Cessation of the antipsychotic and hydration settled the physical manifestations of NMS. Bromocriptine was not deemed safe, for fear of exacerbating the underlying psychosis, and muscle relaxants were not given because muscle rigidity was not prominent, nor was there evidence of renal compromise from myoglobinuria. Involuntary treatment with ECT was used because it was the least harmful intervention for inanition from psychosis as well as safe for persistent NMS.

Key Clinical Points

- Neuroleptic malignant syndrome is rare (0.01%–0.02% of antipsychotic-treated patients) and lethal (10% mortality). NMS generally includes altered mental status and rigidity that may clinically precede hyperthermia and autonomic dysregulation.
- There are no biomarkers or specific laboratory tests for NMS. Extreme elevations in creatine kinase may occur from rhabdomyolysis, which, via myoglobin release, can cause acute kidney injury. Elevated white blood cell count is common.
- The differential diagnosis of NMS is extensive and includes extrapyramidal symptoms, heatstroke, malignant hyperthermia, serotonin syndrome, and general medical conditions (e.g., viral encephalitis).
- Treatment includes cessation of antipsychotics, supportive therapy in an intensive care setting for hydration and autonomic stabilization, ad hoc use of muscle relaxants (e.g., dantrolene), dopamine agonist strategies (e.g., bromocriptine), and ECT in severe cases.
- After a minimum 2-week interval off the initial agent and resolution of NMS, an alternative antipsychotic agent can be started cautiously, if clinically warranted.

Further Readings

Strawn JR, Keck PE, Caroff SN: Neuroleptic malignant syndrome. Am J Psychiatry 164:870–876, 2007

Velamoor VR, Norman RM, Caroff SN, et al: Progression of symptoms in neuroleptic malignant syndrome. J Nerv Ment Dis 182:163–173, 1994

References

Gillman PK: Neuroleptic malignant syndrome: mechanisms, interactions, and causality. Mov Disord 25:1780–1790, 2010

Seitz DP, Gill SS: Neuroleptic malignant syndrome complicating antipsychotic treatment of delirium or agitation in medical and surgical patients: case reports and a review of the literature. Psychosomatics 50:8–15, 2009

Strawn JR, Keck PE, Caroff SN: Neuroleptic malignant syndrome. Am J Psychiatry 164:870–876, 2007

Velamoor VR, Norman RM, Caroff SN, et al: Progression of symptoms in neuroleptic malignant syndrome. J Nerv Ment Dis 182:163–173, 1994

Neuropsychiatric Systemic Lupus Erythematosus

Warren T. Lee, M.D., Ph.D.

A 25-year-old right-handed, single woman who worked as a waitress was diagnosed with systemic lupus erythematosus (SLE) 4 years prior to admission to the hospital. She had been coping fairly well with her illness, continuing with her job and adhering to her treatment, which was limited to low-dose prednisone. For about 4 days prior to admission, her mother and sister had found her confused, emotionally labile, and having poor sleep.

The attending rheumatologist called for an urgent neuropsychiatric consult. There was no preceding history of illness or substance use, nor did she have prior psychiatric problems. The team agreed that she should be treated presumptively for delirium. An extensive workup for precipitating medical causes, especially infection and vasculitis, was done. Her physical examination and blood and CSF cultures all had negative findings. Her autoimmune markers were positive for antinuclear and anti-double-stranded DNA (dsDNA) antibodies. Other blood, urine, and CSF laboratory investigations revealed no significant abnormalities other than mild anemia. Chest X ray and MRI scans of the brain showed normal findings. There was no radiological evidence of cerebral vasculitis. An electroencephalogram showed nonspecific diffuse slowing but no epileptiform activity.

On examination, she was found lying on the bed in hospital clothing, awake but inattentive—she could focus only very briefly before drifting away. She was restless and agitated and was unable to engage in a conversation. A detailed cognitive-intellectual examination could not be performed because of her inattention and disorientation. Her affect was labile and at times inappropriate. At other times, she would stare blankly for long stretches of time. Moreover, she demonstrated textbook echolalia, repeating the final few words spoken to her, and had occasional stereotypies, such as rocking her head as she lay in bed. The diagnostic impression at this juncture was delirium and catatonia.

The rheumatologists increased the oral prednisone to 10 mg qd, and she was started on lorazepam as the primary treatment of catatonia, but she did not respond to the latter medication at dosages up to 10 mg/day. Subsequently haloperidol was added since her clinical picture was also consistent with delirium. But then she became stiffer and was still confused and agitated, so the haloperidol was switched to quetiapine and ratcheted up to 600 mg/day (in divided doses). There was no discernible improvement except for some sedation. On day 11 of hospitalization she was started on IV pulse methylprednisolone, and on day 20 she was started on IV pulse cyclophosphamide.

Despite high doses of potent immunosuppressant and psychotropic medications, her symptoms remained refractory. Other neuropsychiatrists were consulted, and an extensive literature search on treatment options was conducted. Her mother and sister were consulted about the possible use of ECT, and after a few lengthy discussions her mother gave consent as the substitute decision maker. On day 31 of hospitalization she was started empirically on an ECT regimen. In total, she received six ECT treatments over a 2-week period; ECT was administered utilizing a bilateral electrode placement.

There was marked clinical response to ECT. At the end of the course of treatment, she was calmer and was oriented to person and place. She denied mood or psychotic symptoms, and was able to engage in simple conversations. She was finally able to tolerate neuropsychological testing, although it was administered with some difficulty and taking into account the confounding effects of her recent course of ECT. She showed significant impairments in fluid reasoning ability, visuospatial and visuoconstruction skills, speed of information processing, language, and memory. Her performance was significantly affected by her impaired attention, and thus interpretation of the results was cautiously made. There was guarded optimism that these deficits would ameliorate with time. On day 49, she finally went home. Her family commented that she was around 70% of her usual self. Her discharge medications were prednisone 2 mg qd, quetiapine 100 mg qam and 200 mg qhs, and diazepam 10 mg qhs.

After discharge from the hospital, she was followed up as an outpatient by the neuropsychiatry and rheumatology services. At the first outpatient visit, she was visibly brighter and more animated, but then it became quite obvious that she was too animated. She fidgeted constantly and talked incessantly, with most of what she said being irrelevant to the conversation. More disturbingly, she would move her face inappropriately close to the clinician and, when told not to do so, would apologize and back off. However, within a minute or so she would move her face within inches again, as if she was testing her limits. Although she denied feeling sad or happy, her affect was labile and she would fluctuate between tears and laughter. Her mother reported that she appeared never to tire and slept only a few hours a night. In view of these prominent manic symptoms, quetiapine was increased to 100 mg qam and 400 mg qhs. The possible diagnoses of "frontal lobe disinhibition syndrome" and "manic symptoms" were added to the chart. Another MRI scan was ordered and again yielded normal findings, including the gradient echo sequence, which is sensitive to the microhemorrhages that may occur in vasculitis. Close consultation with rheumatologists led to the reinstitution of high-dose prednisolone and commencement of azathioprine, all the while mindful that these medications could affect her mood further.

Over the course of a few months, she seemed to improve. Her hyperactivity and prolixity were somewhat muted, and she no longer invaded others' interpersonal space. Her sleep improved, and she began to help out a lot more in the home. However, she was still largely housebound and remained dependent on her mother and sister for instrumental activities of daily living. She could not manage her finances, and she needed the help of her family for shopping, transport, food preparation, and taking medications. She appeared sedated in the daytime, and her quetiapine dose was reduced to 200 mg qhs at the family's request.

She was seen every 6–8 weeks, accompanied by her mother and sister. She was largely adherent to appointments but in a couple of instances simply refused to come in.

Six months after discharge, on a subsequent follow-up visit, she was very quiet and appeared withdrawn. Her affect was constricted and stable. In addition to depressed mood, negative symptoms of psychosis and frontal lobe apathy were considered in the differential diagnosis. She denied having any hallucinations or delusions and did not appear to be responding to internal stimuli. When probed, she acknowledged feeling down. Her sister was concerned because she had mentioned that her life did not seem worth living. However, she did not verbalize or acknowledge any suicidal thoughts or plans. For the first time she appeared to have some insight into her predicament. In view of her previous manic symptoms, antidepressants were withheld. She continued in this state for two subsequent visits. Then escitalopram 10 mg qd was added, with a reduction of quetiapine to 100 mg qhs. She also attended weekly supportive psychotherapy sessions with a psychologist, and she was seen by an occupational therapist for vocational rehabilitation.

Over the course of the following year, her mental status remained largely unchanged. She was, for the most part, euthymic but her thinking remained concrete and vacuous. Her neuropsychological testing 1½ years after the initial presentation was slightly, but not significantly, improved. Although she had become more active in her vocational rehabilitation, she was still unable to find even sheltered employment.

Discussion

Neuropsychiatric systemic lupus erythematosus (NPSLE) is a quintessential neuropsychiatric disorder. It encompasses neurological syndromes of the central, peripheral, and autonomic nervous systems and a variety of psychiatric syndromes. These manifestations can be the initial symptoms of the disease before the patient is diagnosed as having SLE.

The American College of Rheumatology (ACR) nomenclature for NPSLE provides case definitions for 19 neuropsychiatric syndromes ("The American College of Rheumatology" 1999). Manifestations of these syndromes include acute confusional state, cognitive dysfunction, and anxiety, mood, and psychotic symptoms. One of the diagnostic steps is to exclude a primary psychiatric disorder. The estimated cumulative incidences of NPSLE syndromes in white populations are as follows: cognitive dysfunction, 10%–20%; severe cognitive dysfunction, 3%–5%; mood disorders, 10%–20%; anxiety disorders, 4%–8%; acute confusional state, 3%–4.5%; and psychosis, 2.5%–3.5% (Bertsias and Boumpas 2010). The wide range of neuropsychiatric manifestations, necessitating 19 case definitions, reflects the multiplicity of the underlying pathophysiological mechanisms.

Three mechanisms have been proposed to account for NPSLE (Hanly and Harrison 2005):

1. Autoantibodies, including antineuronal, anti–ribosomal P, and antiphospholipid antibodies; antiphospholipid autoantibodies can increase the likelihood of thrombosis in cerebral blood vessels but may also directly bind to neurons and cause neuronal injury
2. Vascular abnormalities, including vasculitis and noninflammatory vasculopathy
3. Inflammatory mediators, such as interleukins, interferons, and tumor necrosis factor

Although not on the ACR list, catatonia in SLE has been well reported in the literature and includes symptoms of catalepsy, stupor, excessive motor activity, negativism, mutism, posturing, stereotypies, mannerisms, and echophenomena (echolalia and/or echopraxia). Use of ECT for catatonia in NPSLE is not well established. In literature searches, there have only been two previous reports of its use (Ditmore et al. 1992; Fricchione et al. 1990). In both cases, the first course of ECT was associated with some improvement, but the results were not sustained.

Mood symptoms are found in 10%–20% of SLE patients and can represent a psychological reaction to the severe illness and/or overt damage to the brain parenchyma. These cannot be easily teased apart, and a combination of the two is likely. Cognitive dysfunction is prevalent in SLE, with a wide range of estimates that reflects the diversity of definitions of cognitive-intellectual dysfunction, SLE disease characteristics, demographics, and neuropsychological tests employed. Ainiala et al. (2001) found that as many as 81% of SLE patients had some cognitive-intellectual dysfunction.

Standard laboratory testing includes antinuclear antibody, anti–extractable nuclear antigen (anti-ENA), anti-dsDNA and antihistone antibodies, and C3 and C4. The anti-dsDNA test is highly specific for SLE and tends to reflect disease activity. However, there are no well-established markers to monitor pathological activity in the CNS or NPSLE per se. Experimental approaches to monitor NPSLE include anti-NMDAR antibodies in the CSF (Arinuma et al. 2008) and CSF interleukin-6 (Hirohata and Miyamoto 1990). Another putative marker is anti–ribosomal P protein antibodies (Toubi and Shoenfeld 2007).

Brain MRI is commonly ordered for NPSLE patients and may reveal small focal lesions concentrated in the periventricular and subcortical white matter (Karassa et al. 2000) or the presence of microhemorrhages in the event of an inflammatory vasculitis. This patient had severe NPSLE with delirium, catatonia, mania, and depression, and treatment approaches employed a wide variety of psychotropics and ECT. Resolution of catatonic symptoms came only when the patient was treated with ECT combined with cyclophosphamide. From these observations, it can be postulated that in treating catatonic NPSLE, there is a need to suppress the underlying autoimmune process and also to normalize the neurochemical dysfunction in concert. Moreover, the patient's initial delirium persisted despite intense immunosuppression. In retrospect and based on her subsequent mania, her initial delirium may have been a manic delirium with catatonia either caused directly by an immune mechanism from her SLE or caused by a comorbid primary bipolar disorder. Her abnormal electroencephalographic results point to NPSLE and not bipolar disorder. The EEG showed diffuse slowing that was consistent with an organic encephalopathy, which is not seen in bipolar manic delirium with catatonia (Hurwitz 2011).

After the delirium and catatonia abated, this patient exhibited the whole range of psychiatric symptoms over the course of 2 years, including manic, depressive, and perhaps apathetic symptoms and persistent cognitive dysfunction. This again raises the question of etiology and one that is not easily answered—is it NPSLE following an undulating course or an independent psychiatric disorder?

The rheumatologists had assiduously followed this patient throughout the course of her fluctuating illness with a standard series of blood markers to measure SLE activity together with MRI scans. The results of these tests did not change significantly with the changes in her mental status. Hence she had to be treated empirically with powerful immunosuppressants. She had a history of mild joint pain and malar rash, but there was no clinical or biochemical evidence of cardiopulmonary or renal involvement. Her successive scans were negative despite florid and severe persistent symptomatology; this remains a puzzle but could be accounted for on the basis of an independent bipolar disorder (Rovaris et al. 2000). Alternatively, one could postulate a non-inflammatory encephalopathy mediated by SLE-generated autoantibodies that interact with neuronal epitopes causing synaptic or cellular dysfunction but not cellular death (another variation of anti-neurotransmitter autoimmune encephalopathy).

Such patients are complex, and their care is managed in conjunction with a rheumatologist. For emergent neuropsychiatric symptoms, immunosuppression is the primary intervention where there is evidence of inflammatory activity in the CNS as reflected in abnormalities on MRI and EEGs and in CSF changes. The psychiatrist's role is to provide symptomatic management of emergent psychopathology if this fails to settle with immunosuppression. In the absence of overt CNS inflammation, the psychiatrist is the primary intervener, using standard therapies that target anxiety, depression, mania, and psychosis while not knowing with any degree of certainty whether the psychopathology is part of NPSLE or an independent but comorbid primary psychiatric disorder.

Key Clinical Points

- Neuropsychiatric involvement in systemic lupus erythematosus is common, and psychiatric symptoms can manifest across a wide spectrum in the same patient. These symptoms include cognitive dysfunction, delirium, depression, mania, psychosis, and, rarely, catatonia during SLE flares.
- Cognitive dysfunction is the most commonly reported central nervous system symptom and may persist when SLE is quiescent.
- There are presently no established biomarkers to track CNS disease activity in neuropsychiatric NPSLE; hence clinical assessment is still the current standard.
- Aggressive treatment of underlying SLE is likely to prevent or reduce permanent damage of the CNS and should be instituted early.
- Treatment of psychiatric manifestations of NPSLE should address specific symptoms and include psychotropic medications, psychotherapy, and electroconvulsive therapy if appropriate.

Further Readings

Bertsias GK, Boumpas DT: Pathogenesis, diagnosis and management of neuropsychiatric SLE manifestations. Nat Rev Rheumatol 6:358–367, 2010

Hanly JG, Harrison MJ: Management of neuropsychiatric lupus. Best Pract Res Clin Rheumatol 19:799–821, 2005

References

Ainiala H, Hietaharju A, Loukkola J, et al: Validity of the new American College of Rheumatology criteria for neuropsychiatric lupus syndromes: a population-based evaluation. Arthritis Rheum 45:419–423, 2001

The American College of Rheumatology nomenclature and case definitions for neuropsychiatric lupus syndromes. Arthritis Rheum 42(4):599–608, 1999

Arinuma Y, Yanagida T, Hirohata S: Association of cerebrospinal fluid anti–NR2 glutamate receptor autoantibodies with diffuse neuropsychiatric systemic lupus erythematosus. Arthritis Rheum 58:1130–1135, 2008

Bertsias GK, Boumpas DT: Pathogenesis, diagnosis and management of neuropsychiatric SLE manifestations. Nat Rev Rheumatol 6:358–367, 2010

Ditmore BG, Malek-Ahmadi P, Mills DM, et al: Manic psychosis and catatonia stemming from systemic lupus erythematosus: response to ECT. Convuls Ther 8:33–37, 1992

Fricchione GL, Kaufman LD, Gruber BL, et al: Electroconvulsive therapy and cyclophosphamide in combination for severe neuropsychiatric lupus with catatonia. Am J Med 88:442–443, 1990

Hanly JG, Harrison MJ: Management of neuropsychiatric lupus. Best Pract Res Clin Rheumatol 19:799–821, 2005

Hirohata S, Miyamoto T: Elevated levels of interleukin-6 in cerebrospinal fluid from patients with systemic lupus erythematosus and central nervous system involvement. Arthritis Rheum 33:644–649, 1990

Hurwitz TA: Psychogenic unresponsiveness. Neurol Clin 29:995–1006, 2011

Karassa F, Ioannidis JP, Boki K, et al: Predictors of clinical outcome and radiologic progression in patients with neuropsychiatric manifestations of systemic lupus erythematosus. Am J Med 109:628–634, 2000

Rovaris M, Inglese M, Viti B, et al: The contribution of fast-FLAIR MRI for lesion detection in the brain of patients with systemic autoimmune diseases. J Neurol 247:29–33, 2000

Toubi E, Shoenfeld Y: Clinical and biological aspects of anti-P-ribosomal protein autoantibodies. Autoimmun Rev 6:119–125, 2007

MEMORY FAILURE

Memory Failure

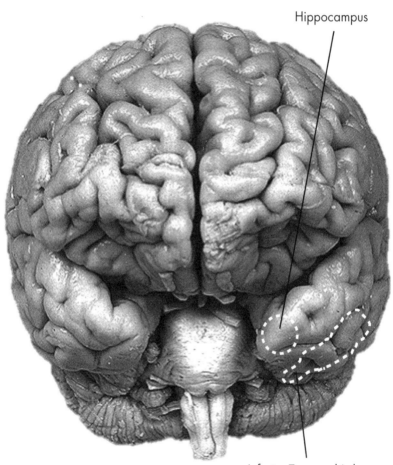

Hippocampus

Inferior Temporal Lobe

Introduction

In some patients, the predominant or only complaint is memory failure, but the impact may be devastating. Memory is not a unitary concept, and the classification of memory disorders has grown increasingly complex. At its simplest level, memory can still be divided into recent (episodic) and remote (semantic) memory. The neuroanatomy has become clearer and focuses on the temporal lobe—the hippocampus and Papez circuit for episodic memory and inferior lateral temporal lobes for semantic memory. The most important neurotransmitters are the excitatory amino acids, especially glutamate and the N-methyl-D-aspartate receptor, which play a critical role in learning via long-term potentiation.

Amnesia Associated With Epilepsy

Aaron Mackie, M.D., F.R.C.P.C.

A 34-year-old man was referred for assessment of a problem with his memory. He lived with his wife and two children and was employed as a business analyst for a financial firm. His wife also worked in the business world, and the two had initially met during their M.B.A. program.

Until 1 year previously, he had had no medical problems. He then developed new nocturnal seizures, which were first noted by his wife. They tended to occur about once a week, within 15 minutes of falling asleep, and were characterized by his suddenly sitting up in bed, eyes open, with unresponsive staring. He would occasionally rock backward and forward with side-to-side head movements or fidgeting, but he had no other automatic behaviors. A typical event lasted 30–60 seconds; he would then return to sleep and would have complete amnesia for the episode. There was no history of focal tonic or clonic activity or secondary generalization.

There were also at least three episodes that occurred at work, in which he stared blankly for approximately 1 minute, with amnesia for the details of the conversation happening at the time. These daytime events were much less frequent, occurring only once every 3 months.

On further questioning, he recalled that over the preceding few months he had experienced more frequent episodes of déjà vu, depersonalization, and derealization; these occurred a few times per week.

A referral was made to a neurologist, and a subsequent electroencephalogram (EEG) demonstrated intermittent left anterior temporal and occasional left frontal sharp and spike discharges. Two magnetic resonance imaging (MRI) brain scans with coronal temporal slices showed normal findings. Screening blood work had normal results and did not demonstrate any underlying medical condition associated with seizures. He was treated with levetiracetam, and his episodes ceased.

He had no history of trauma, infection, or autoimmune or inflammatory processes. He did not drink alcohol, and he denied the use of recreational drugs. He had no history of seizures as a child and no family history of epilepsy.

He provided a history of a normal pregnancy and delivery, with normal milestones. He was a gifted student in school, graduating at the top of his class through high school and university. He went on to complete an M.B.A. degree and finished at the top of his class in this program.

A few months following the successful treatment with levetiracetam, he and his family went on a trip to Hawaii to attend a large family reunion. They spent about 1 week in Hawaii before returning home. Approximately 1 week later, while sitting at the breakfast table, he blurted out, "I thought we were supposed to go to Hawaii last week!" Perplexed, his wife responded, "We did go, remember? We were there with your entire family?" It quickly became apparent that he had no recollection of the trip to Hawaii. His wife gathered photos from the trip, and on reviewing them he could not recall any of the events captured in photos. At work that week, he found that he had no memory of any of the projects that he had been working on, and he reviewed a number of documents that he himself had created and notes he had written, without any recollection of having written them.

Distressed by this, he returned to his neurologist, who arranged for him to be admitted to a video-electroencephalographic monitoring unit. The EEG showed frequent low-amplitude spikes and sharp waves, seen maximally over the left midtemporal region; they were more pronounced in drowsiness and sleep but were also present in the awake state. Occasional similar discharges were seen in the right midtemporal hemisphere most prominently over T4.

During the video-electroencephalographic monitoring, he experienced a number of his typical auras, consisting of depersonalization, derealization, and déjà vu. These were correlated with a buildup of anterior temporal rhythmic activity, characterized by sharply contoured theta and delta waves lasting between 10 and 60 seconds. Most originated in the left anterior temporal region, and then frequently spread to high-amplitude right anterior temporal rhythmic activity. Four nocturnal seizures were captured on an EEG (Figure 9–1). Buildup of sharply contoured theta activity was seen in the left anterior and midtemporal region, frequently spreading to the contralateral anterior temporal regions. Two daytime seizures were characterized by loud sighs followed by activity arrest and side-to-side head movements, as well as hand fidgeting and some leg movements, with confusion. The EEG again demonstrated buildup of rhythmic, sharply contoured alpha and theta activity in the left anterior temporal region.

A further medical workup was undertaken. A computed tomography (CT) scan of the abdomen and pelvis showed two hypodense lesions in the liver, too small to characterize but thought to be cystic. The right kidney had a 7-mm lesion in the upper pole, again thought to be cystic. A right hydrocele with a scrotal pearl was identified. No lymphadenopathy was identified, and the results of subsequent paraneoplastic antibody testing were negative. A CT scan of the chest had normal findings, and the results of blood investigations showed normal. Anti–thyroid peroxidase antibody was elevated at 537 IU/mL but returned to normal during repeat testing a few months later. Cerebrospinal fluid studies had normal results, with no oligoclonal banding, negative VDRL (Venereal Disease Research Laboratory), negative cryptococcal antigen, and negative Lyme studies.

He was continued on levetiracetam, and carbamazepine was added; this combination resulted in a significant decrease in the apparent seizure activity, as evidenced by a lack of auras and nocturnal seizures. Blood investigation confirmed a therapeutic carbamazepine level, but unfortunately his memory did not improve.

Neuropsychological testing was performed twice, before and after the addition of carbamazepine. The testing demonstrated isolated autobiographical memory impairment, with otherwise high-average to superior range of intellectual functioning on testing.

He scored 11 out of a possible 63 (not depressed) on the Beck Depression Inventory scale. Clinical screening for depressive symptoms was negative. He described his mood as "worried," particularly with respect to his current impairment and the implications for the future. He denied that his worries were excessive. The results of screening for other symptoms of anxiety, including those consistent with obsessive-compulsive disorder, phobias, and panic disorder, were negative. Likewise, the results of screening for psychotic symptoms were negative. He reported that he was no longer experiencing any symptoms of depersonalization, derealization, or déjà vu.

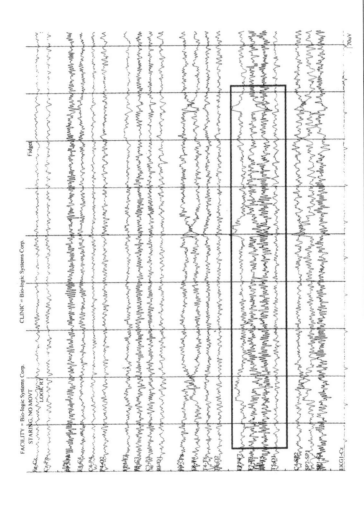

FIGURE 9–1.   Electroencephalographic recording of temporal lobe seizure in a patient with transient epileptic amnesia. Outlined area shows polyspike activity in the left temporal lobe associated with a brief episode of unresponsive staring.

He denied any personality changes. However, he noted that he had become more self-conscious when speaking with people, often prefacing his statements with "Have I already asked you this?" There was no evidence of change in religious interests, increased emotionality or viscosity, altered sexual interest, or hypergraphia.

He described the personal experience of his memory problems as being "like a picture that is fading." As an example, he reported that now he could not conjure up a mental image of what his office looked like, and he was unsure of the name of the building, even though he had worked in this building for over a decade. He thought that there were perhaps two towers, but he did not know which tower his office was in or which floor it was on; he had a feeling that it was "higher up."

He began to keep a notebook with him at all times, maintaining a commentary of the events of each day. His functioning at work suffered as a result of his memory impairment, as well as the time required to maintain his notes. Ultimately, he found it necessary to go on indefinite medical leave.

Following the consultation, further investigations were arranged, many of them a repeat of the initial investigations. Additional investigations included single-photon emission computed tomography scan, an ambulatory EEG, thyroid ultrasound, and repeat MRI brain scan. There were no abnormalities found on any of these investigations, and specifically the ambulatory EEG did not demonstrate any ongoing seizure activity. In spite of apparently good seizure control, he continued to experience a slow degradation of any new memories, which faded over a span of about a week; this degradation of new memories continues today.

Discussion

The association between amnesia and temporal lobe epilepsy (TLE) has been recognized for over a century, and in certain cases, amnesia has been the only manifestation of a temporal lobe seizure seen. The concept of transient epileptic amnesia (TEA) was first described in 1888 by neurologist John Hughlings-Jackson, who reported a case of a colleague physician, "Dr. Z" (Hughlings-Jackson 1888). Dr. Z had a history of seizures, at the time termed "the dreamy state," which he was able to describe in his own words:

> I was attending a young patient whom his mother had brought me with some history of lung symptoms. I wished to examine the chest, and asked him to undress on a couch. I thought he looked ill, but have no recollec-

tion of any intention to recommend him to take to his bed at once, or of any diagnosis. Whilst he was undressing I felt the onset of a petit mal. I remember taking out my stethoscope and turning away a little to avoid conversation. The next thing I recollect is that I was sitting at a writing-table in the same room, speaking to another person, and as my consciousness became more complete, recollected my patient, but saw he was not in the room. I was interested to ascertain what had happened, and had an opportunity an hour later of seeing him in bed, with the note of a diagnosis I had made of "pneumonia of the left base."

In 1894, following Dr. Z's death from an overdose of chloral hydrate, his brain biopsy showed a "small patch of softening in the left uncinate gyrus" (Taylor 1958).

The term *transient epileptic amnesia* is used to describe a subtype of TLE whose principal manifestation of seizures is recurrent episodes of isolated memory loss. Whether amnesia associated with TLE is an ictal or a postictal phenomenon remains a matter of controversy. Many authors have provided specific case reports suggestive of both phenomena.

In one case during video-EEG monitoring, a brief episode of bilateral mesial temporal epileptiform activity occurred at the exact time the patient was speaking on the telephone. The patient was not aware that she was experiencing a seizure at the time it happened, but following the telephone conversation she had no recollection of having made the phone call (Palmini et al. 1992). In another case, a unilateral hippocampal seizure was shown to disrupt recall of a previously learned word list (Bridgman et al. 1989).

Furthermore, researchers have demonstrated that brief bilateral stimulation of mesial temporal structures either during acquisition of memories or at the time of retrieval can cause amnesia as an isolated symptom (Halgren et al. 1985).

There are additional case descriptions in the literature that suggest the persistence of amnesia even in the absence of ongoing epileptiform activity, somewhat analogous to a Todd's paralysis (Morrell 1980).

One of the challenges in assessing memory in epilepsy is that performance on neuropsychological tests may not necessarily correlate with the subjective report of memory dysfunction. Additionally, patients with TEA may complain of persistent memory difficulties (Butler and Zeman 2011). As described in the case above, they often describe a rapid decay of newly acquired memories over a period of days to weeks, in addition to the loss of specific memories of personal events like weddings or holidays that have occurred in the remote past. Some studies have even demonstrated patients as manifesting memory impairment for events that occurred decades prior to the onset of their seizures (Butler and Zeman 2011).

Standard neuropsychological testing tends to test for decay of information over minutes to hours, and thus frequently fails to show any deficit. However, some studies that have examined memory over extended intervals have demonstrated a phenomenon of accelerated long-term forgetting (ALF) over a period of weeks (Butler and Zeman 2011).

Patients with TEA can have subtle atrophy of the medial temporal lobes on studies using voxel-based morphometry, which tends to correlate with performance on standard tests of anterograde memory. However, the degree of atrophy in the medial temporal lobes fails to correlate with deficits in autobiographical memory or measures of ALF (Butler and Zeman 2011). This atrophy tends to be subtle; one study quantified a loss of about 8% of total hippocampal volume, with atrophy predominantly isolated to the body of the hippocampus (Butler and Zeman 2011). Older studies have found volume changes predominantly localized to the hippocampal head. Overall, there is poor correlation between the severity of amnesia and the degree of atrophy.

The pathophysiology of ALF remains uncertain. Some have proposed that ALF is a direct result of damage to the mesial temporal lobes. To date, studies have not been able to correlate mesial temporal lobe damage with ALF, or with any other neuroanatomical structure, and the case for mesial temporal damage being responsible for ALF remains unproven.

Others have proposed that there may be intermittent dysfunction of neurons in the mesial temporal lobes, producing subclinical epileptic activity specifically during the sleep-wake transitions, disrupting the consolidation of memories (Stickgold 2005). Still others have hypothesized that the memory impairments are a direct effect of antiseizure medications; however, this is generally less accepted, because better seizure control tends to correlate with improvement in memory dysfunction.

Because of a paucity of data, we do not have a clear understanding of autobiographical memory loss. The generally accepted theory of remote memory formation is that memories eventually become independent of the hippocampus. Therefore, pathology of the mesial temporal structures should have no effect on autobiographical memories. The multiple trace theory of remote memory alternatively proposes that recall of episodic memories continues to rely on the hippocampus while such memories retain their vividness and detail. Over time, memories lose detail and become more semantic and, only then, hippocampus independent (Moscovitch et al. 2006). Accordingly, impairment in autobiographical memory has been shown to correlate with mesial temporal lobe volumes in both TLE and Alzheimer's dementia.

In this patient's case, adequate seizure control did reduce the number of distinct seizure episodes associated with amnesia for the events at the time of the seizure. However, he continued to suffer from a rapid decay of newly acquired memories, as well as a loss of certain autobiographical events from the remote past.

Key Clinical Points

- Temporal lobe epilepsy may present as transient epileptic amnesia, a manifestation of seizures characterized exclusively by recurrent episodes of isolated memory loss.
- Patients with transient epileptic amnesia often describe a rapid decay of newly acquired memories over days to weeks, and they may lose memories of personal events from the remote past, possibly even from a period of time prior to the onset of the seizures.
- Adequate treatment of seizures will reduce or eliminate recurrent episodes of isolated memory loss.
- Adequate treatment of seizures will often have no effect on the decay of new information or loss of remote memories.
- There is currently poor correlation between findings from clinical neuroimaging techniques and memory impairment, both autobiographical memory deficits and accelerated long-term forgetting.

Further Readings

Butler CR, Graham KS, Hodges JR, et al: The syndrome of transient epileptic amnesia. Ann Neurol 61:587–598, 2007

Butler CR, Bhaduri A, Acosta-Cabronero J, et al: Transient epileptic amnesia: regional brain atrophy and its relationship to memory deficits. Brain 132:357–368, 2009

References

Bridgman PA, Malamut BL, Sperling MR: Memory during subclinical hippocampal seizures. Neurology 39:853–856, 1989

Butler C, Zeman A: Transient epileptic amnesia. Adv Clin Neurosci Rehabil 11:10–12, 2011

Halgren E, Wilson CL, Stapleton JM: Human medial temporal lobe stimulation disrupts both formation and retrieval of human memories. Brain Cogn 4:287–295, 1985

Hughlings-Jackson J: On a particular variety of epilepsy ("intellectual aura"), one case with symptoms of organic brain disease. Brain 11:179–207, 1888

Morrell F: Memory loss as a Todd's paralysis (abstract). Epilepsia 21:185, 1980

Moscovitch M, Nadel L, Winocur G, et al: The cognitive neuroscience of remote episodic, semantic and spatial memory. Curr Opin Neurobiol 16:179–190, 2006

Palmini AL, Gloor P, Jones-Gotman M: Pure amnestic seizures in temporal lobe epilepsy. Brain 115:749–769, 1992

Stickgold R: Sleep-dependent memory consolidation. Nature 437:1272–1278, 2005

Taylor J (ed): The Selected Writings of John Hughlings Jackson. New York, Basic Books, 1958

Memory Loss Associated With Herpes Simplex Encephalitis

William J. Panenka, M.Sc., M.D., F.R.C.P.C.
Trevor A. Hurwitz, M.B.Ch.B., M.R.C.P. (U.K.), F.R.C.P.C.

In 1982 a 23-year-old white male developed a flu-like illness, accompanied by vomiting, headache, disorientation, and insomnia. His past medical history was unremarkable aside from a past right knee surgery. He was married but without children. He had a master's degree and was employed in the Canadian federal government, in the Ministry of Labor. He was admitted to the hospital, and a lumbar puncture revealed herpes simplex antibodies in cerebrospinal fluid, along with lymphocytosis. He was diagnosed with herpes simplex virus (HSV) encephalitis. He was treated with cytosine arabinoside, since acyclovir was not yet available. He stabilized medically and his delirium cleared.

As the fluctuations in consciousness settled, profound memory problems became apparent. His short-term memory of life events was most affected. He could not recount any recent events, and despite having been in the hospital for months, he was convinced that he had only been there for a few days. He could not recall any word from a list of three words after an interval of 2 minutes. Long-term memory was less affected. He correctly gave his own birth date but could not remember his wife's birthday. His memory of American presidents was limited to John F. Kennedy and of Canadian prime ministers to Pierre Trudeau. He confabulated extensively, making up names of political figures and describing his caregivers as coworkers. Attention and working memory were relatively unaffected. Digit span was 6 forward and 4 backward. He was unable to remember the location of the bathroom or the way back to his room. He could do calculations with ease, and abstraction as judged by similarities was intact.

Funduscopy and cranial nerve examination were unremarkable. Frontal release signs were present, with snout, suck, and mild grasp reflexes bilaterally. Graphesthesia, double simultaneous extinction, and two-point discrimination were normal. Deep tendon reflexes were 2+ and symmetrical. Tone, power, sensation, and coordination were all normal.

A CT head scan done in the hospital a few weeks after admission showed normal findings. Repeat CT 4 months later showed enlargement of lateral and third ventricles with bilateral extensive temporal lobe encephalomalacia. The first MRI scan of his brain in 2002 showed dramatic cystic encephalomalacia involving the anterior two-thirds of the right temporal lobe and approximately one-half of the anterior left temporal lobe (Figure 9–2). The tissue destruction also extended into the cingulate gyri and orbitofrontal cortices bilaterally.

After 3 months in the hospital he was placed in a transitional care facility, but after 9 months of attempted semi-independence it became clear that he required permanent custodial care in a locked mental health facility. Ten years later he was successfully placed into a residential long-term-care facility, his safety assured with the help of a locating bracelet and a modified elevator. He has been living in this facility ever since.

Over the past three decades, there has been some mild improvement in his memory. He is now able to recognize his treating neuropsychiatrist on most occasions. He has learned new rules to the card game Solitaire, one of his favorite pastimes. He still believes he lives in the mental health facility where he was initially hospitalized some 30 years ago. He can identify pictures of his wife and old friends. His attention is mostly intact, with a digit span of 7 forward and 4 backward. Recent verbal and non-verbal memory remain impaired. Recall is 0/3 words after distraction, occasionally improving to 1/3 with forced choice. Memory for shapes is also 0/3, improving to 1/3 with forced choice. He can name common objects but cannot name or describe the function of modern devices such as computers, CDs, or cellphones. Some behavioral interventions have been moderately successful. A sign placed where he will see it as he enters his bathroom reads "Brush your teeth"; this has led to an improvement in his dental hygiene. He chooses his own clothes and dresses himself. However, he is unable to remember what he wore the previous day, resulting in minor hygiene issues. He cannot, when asked, place himself into yesterday by providing details of what he did or the circumstances in which he found himself. Similarly he cannot, when asked, imagine a tomorrow by providing any immediate or long-term plans or desires. He has neither

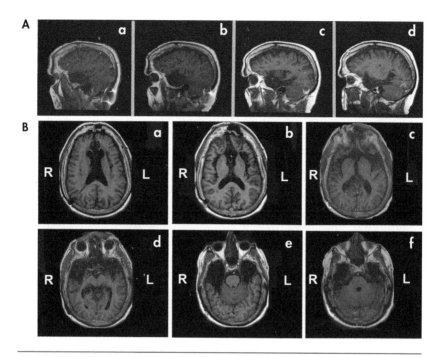

FIGURE 9–2. Sagittal (A) and axial (B) T1 inversion recovery magnetic resonance imaging sequences demonstrating extensive cystic encephalomalacia involving the anterior two-thirds of the right temporal lobe and approximately one-half of the anterior left temporal lobe.

recent memories nor future hopes; he exists entirely in the present. He is not angry, anxious, or sad; rather, he is perpetually content in the now.

Pharmacological interventions for his memory problems included a trial of anticholinesterase inhibitors, but these demonstrated no benefit.

The results of his comprehensive neuropsychological test battery are shown in Figure 9–3. He has severe impairment in verbal and nonverbal memory and significant executive function difficulty, with relative preservation of other cognitive-intellectual capacities. Other neuropsychological testing (not shown) indicates that he has greater problems with memory encoding than with retrieval.

Discussion

HSV is the most frequent causative agent among infectious encephalitides, with an incidence rate of 1–3 cases/million per year (Steiner 2011). Serologically, HSV-1 is the culprit in over 90% of HSV encephalitis cases,

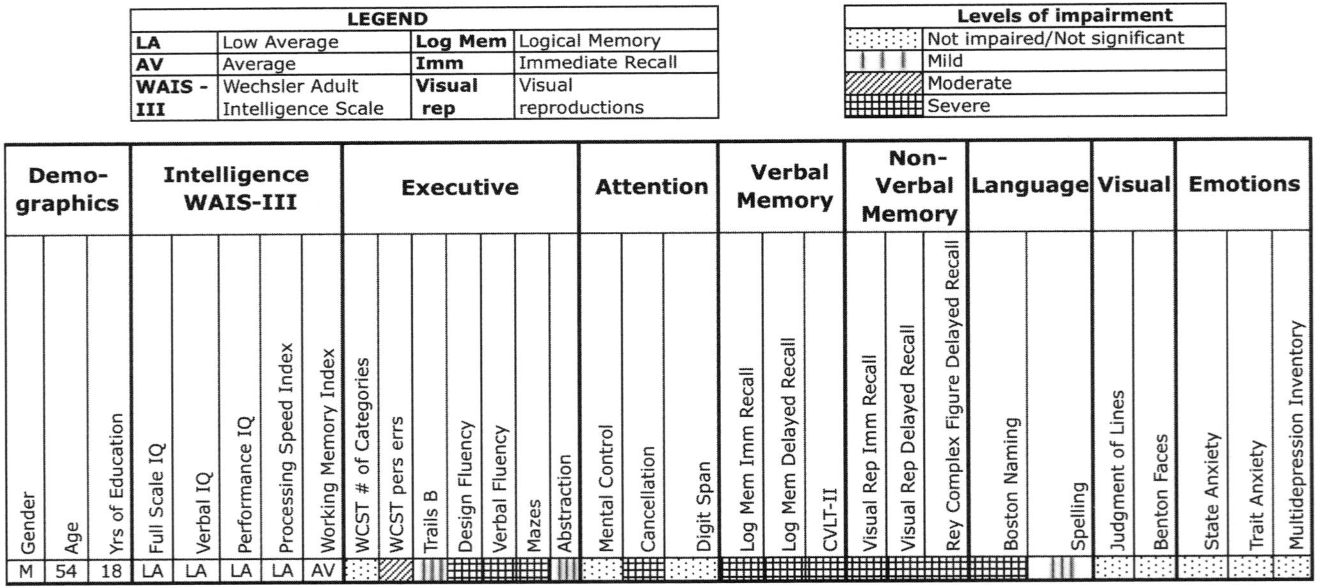

FIGURE 9–3. Data from a neuropsychological test battery from a 54-year-old male with bitemporal injury from herpes simplex encephalitis showing severe impairment in verbal and nonverbal memory with patchy severe executive function difficulty in the context of relatively spared overall IQ.

with the exception being neonatal HSV, which is predominantly HSV-2 (Steiner 2011). As seen in this case, the herpes virus has a proclivity for the frontal and temporal lobes, usually bilaterally. The reason for this localization is unknown, although proximal spread from the trigeminal ganglion along the trigeminal nerve and possible entry of the virus through the olfactory epithelia are presumed factors.

HSV encephalitis is a neuropsychiatric emergency. Fever and headache are the most common presenting features, followed by confusion, behavioral change, seizures, and other symptoms of gray matter dysfunction. The lack of fever should trigger a reevaluation of the differential diagnosis, except in the case of immunocompromised individuals (Steiner 2011). When HSV encephalitis is suspected, antiviral treatment with intravenous acyclovir 10 mg/kg tid should be instituted immediately (Baringer 2008), and a lumbar puncture for HSV by polymerase chain reaction should be pursued. Without treatment, the mortality from HSV encephalitis approaches 70%; with early use of acyclovir, this figure is reduced to approximately 10%, although over 50% still suffer severe neurological impairment (Steiner 2011). As with this case, memory, especially anterograde memory, is one of the cognitive-intellectual domains most affected. The focus of the remainder of this chapter is thus concentrated on our understanding of memory systems.

Memory is a complex process that cannot be reduced to a single neuroanatomical or genetic locus. The study of memory is challenging. Through the first half of the twentieth century, very little was understood. An epiphanic moment came after the unfortunate and unexpected loss of memory suffered by patient Henry Gustav Molaison (originally known as H.M. in the literature) after bilateral medial temporal lobe (including bilateral hippocampi) resection for intractable epilepsy (Scoville and Milner 1957). This case and other contemporary seminal work have led to the wider adoption of a previously described neuroanatomical model of memory—the Papez circuit (Papez 1937/1995). This early neuroanatomical paradigm, and later refinements, highlighted the central importance of the temporal lobe, and especially the hippocampus, in memory systems.

Memory is now understood to be a nonunitary complex process that is subdivided into different capacities. The terminology and a basic framework of memory systems that has clinical utility and is simple to remember are summarized in Table 9–1 (Budson and Price 2007).

In this schema, memory is divided into *explicit* (conscious) and *implicit* (unconscious) components. Memory can also be divided into two large categories based on whether it can or cannot be verbalized. Declarative memory can be spoken, whereas nondeclarative memory cannot.

TABLE 9–1. Terminology and constructs of a basic framework of memory systems that have clinical utility: a modified excerpt

Memory system	Examples	Duration of memory	Main neuroanatomical structures
Episodic memory (fixed to time and place)	Remembering a conversation you had yesterday or 5 minutes ago, remembering the events of last New Year's Eve, remembering your children being born	Minutes to years (generally more recent than semantic memories)	Medial temporal lobes, Papez circuit, prefrontal cortex, parietal lobe
Semantic memory (acontextual, your general fund of knowledge)	Knowing which states make up a given country, knowing former heads of state, knowing your date of birth	Minutes to years (generally more remote than episodic memories)	Inferior lateral temporal lobes
Procedural memory (skill memory)	Knowing how to play an instrument, ride a bike, throw a ball, dress yourself, or open a door	Minutes to years	Basal ganglia, cerebellum, supplementary motor area
Working memory (attention plus processing)	Reciting the alphabet backward, rotating a mental image in your mind	Seconds to minutes; information consciously held (very recent)	Phonological: prefrontal cortex, Broca's area, Wernicke's area Spatial: prefrontal cortex, visual association areas

Source. Adapted from Budson AE, Price BH: "Memory Dysfunction in Neurological Practice." *Practical Neurology* 7:42–47, 2007. Used with permission.

These rather unwieldy distinctions have theoretical and research value, but for simplicity we take the approach found in much of the literature, which considers explicit memory synonymous with declarative, and implicit memory as synonymous with nondeclarative.

Explicit memory is then further divided into episodic, semantic, and working memory. Implicit memory is also known as procedural memory. However, it should be noted that there are other types of implicit memory, such as priming, classical conditioning, and emotional conditioning.

Procedural memory is skill memory. It can be conceptualized as the mind's ability to learn a sequence or task, usually motoric in nature. With repeated practice one learns to drive a car, throw a football, ride a bike, or operate a television remote without conscious participation; the underlying neuromuscular programming completes the task. Not surprisingly, the anatomical structures that subserve this memory system are also integral to modifying motor activity—namely, the cerebellum, the basal ganglia, and the supplementary motor cortex (Budson and Price 2005). Conditions that affect procedural memory include Parkinson's disease, Huntington's disease, progressive supranuclear palsy, forms of frontotemporal dementia, degenerative diseases, insults to the cerebellum, and brain trauma (Budson and Price 2005).

Working memory is the most transient of the memory systems and likely the most neuroanatomically widespread. The terms *short-term memory* and *working memory* are used interchangeably in much of the older literature, but more recently the term *working memory* has evolved to mean a composite of the attentional matrix (consciously holding the information in mind) and memory manipulation (performing some form of mental operation on the consciously held information; this is the "working" part)—in short, attention plus processing. Since conscious effort is needed to keep and manipulate the thought, this type of memory system falls into the declarative/explicit category. Working memory is diffusely located cortically and subcortically, in a modality-specific pattern. Memory for a verbal list, for example, will involve different structures than remembering a map or other visuospatial information. One neuroanatomical commonality, however, is the dorsolateral prefrontal cortex. A multitude of imaging and lesion studies reproducibly demonstrate its involvement in all forms of general working memory.

Episodic memories are recallable experiences that are fixed to a specific time and place. Episodic memory is the memory we have of the *episodes* that we've been through and the temporal order in which they occurred. Remembering conversations you just had, what you did on your last holiday, your wedding night, and your children being born are examples of episodic memories. Episodic memory is centered in the hippocampus,

with significant contributions from other medial temporal lobe structures, the Papez circuit, the prefrontal area, and the parietal lobes (Wagner et al. 2005).

Autonoetic consciousness is intimately tied to episodic memory and is
critical in determining selfhood. Autonoetic consciousness is a concept
that was originally advanced by Endel Tulving; it denotes the uniquely human capacity to place ourselves in time, self-reflect using past memories,
imagine ourselves in the future, and thus influence our behavior (Tulving
1985). Failure of autonoetic consciousness erases not only past recollec-
tions but also the ability to place oneself in an imagined future. When this
ability is lost, hopes and ambitions cease to have meaning.

Neuroanatomically, the hippocampus and the parietal lobes are critical
for autonoetic consciousness (Lou et al. 2004; Wagner et al. 2005). A recent elegant study of patients experiencing transient global amnesia demonstrated that impaired episodic memory and autonoetic consciousness
localized specifically to area CA1 of the hippocampus (Bartsch et al. 2011).

Source memory is the recollection of the context around a specific
memory, and it is unique to the episodic memory system. An example of
source memory is remembering what you had for dinner (the memory
event) and remembering the surroundings that night (the memory source).
The frontal lobes are integral to source memory (Budson 2009; Johnson
et al. 1997). Frontal lesions result in memories that lack context; the
memories become difficult to link with other memories, or to an internal
time sequence. It is thought that confabulation, which is a prominent feature of frontal lobe damage, is an unconscious compensatory attempt to
create context around these decontextualized memories.

When a memory can no longer be clearly recollected, but still main-
tains an element of *familiarity*, then it shifts from the episodic to the *semantic* memory system. *Semantic memory* broadly describes the process
of remembering and using decontextualized facts (Saumier and Chertkow 2002). More simply, it denotes our reservoir of knowledge of the
world. Unlike episodic memory, semantic memory has no associated self
or source, meaning that we remember the fact or figure, but we do not
associate it with any specific time period or episode in our life. Examples
include knowing which countries make up North America, the date of
your birth, remembering how to count to 10, or the alphabet. The inferior-
lateral temporal lobes are the main storage sites for the semantic memory
system (Budson and Price 2005). Disorders that can specifically affect the
semantic system include the semantic variant of frontotemporal dementia, corticobasal degeneration, and ischemic or space-occupying lesions in
the inferior-lateral temporal lobes. In later stages of diseases such as Alzheimer's dementia or dementia with Lewy bodies, as the pathology pro-

gressively spreads from the medial to lateral aspects of the temporal lobes, the semantic memory deficit correspondingly worsens.

Remembering the unique roles of the various anatomical structures involved in memory is clinically useful. This is especially true of the division between the frontal and temporal lobes, because they are readily distinguishable on mental status examination and accurate localization can significantly inform diagnosis and management.

In medial temporal lobe disorders, the impairment is mainly one of encoding. Memories cannot be transferred from the attentional matrix into the neural substrate. This patient is a typical case: his ability to recite digits forward and backward is normal, but any appreciable delay or distraction erases the memory.

The frontal lobes, in contrast, are mainly involved in accessing stored memories. With damage to this area, encoding of new memories does occur but there is a marked deficit in the ability to retrieve the information. In addition, as mentioned earlier, frontal lobe damage leads to ineffective source memory, resulting in a fragmented and poorly contextualized recollection.

This patient had very limited benefit from cuing. Cuing is a simple bedside strategy to help localize the memory defect. With medial temporal lobe injury, the memory is not encoded, so cuing the memory with memory aids or clues has no effect. In contrast, frontal memories are simply "misplaced" and difficult to access, and therefore cues that aid in recall are very effective.

In this case, the encephalitis spared his cerebellum, basal ganglia, and supplementary motor cortex. Thus, his procedural memory was seemingly unaffected within the context of his highly custodial environment. He was still able to dress and groom himself and use a toothbrush and bathing facilities. He had severe, bilateral involvement of his medial temporal lobes, which resulted in maximal impact on his episodic memory system. He also had a superimposed semantic memory deficit, attributable to either the damage to his inferior-lateral temporal lobes or the long-term effect of persistent profound episodic memory failure, preventing the transfer into and hence the formation of updated semantic memory. His decline in executive functioning is due to the extension of encephalomalacia into the frontal lobes, with some contribution from the massive bilateral temporal lobe destruction. His tendency to confabulate is likely a problem with source memory, stemming also from his frontal injury. Albeit severely compromised, this patient continues to be able to learn new information, as evidenced by his playing of Solitaire and now being able to name his treating neuropsychiatrist. How this is possible is open to debate, but it highlights caveats about the reductionist approach to memory. Memory systems are much more interconnected than this approach would suggest, and other nonclassical memory structures can make compensatory contributions.

Key Clinical Points

- Severe cases of herpes encephalitis can result in extensive damage to medial temporal lobe and frontal lobe structures.
- Memory can be divided into explicit (further subdivided into episodic, semantic, and working) and implicit (procedural) memory systems.
- The hippocampus and medial temporal lobe are most critical to the episodic memory system.
- The inferior-lateral temporal lobes are involved with the semantic memory system.
- The basal ganglia, cerebellum, and supplementary motor cortex subserve the procedural memory system.

Further Readings

Blumenfeld H: Limbic system: homeostasis, olfaction, memory, and emotion, in Neuroanatomy Through Clinical Cases, 2nd Edition. Edited by Blumenfeld H. Sunderland, MA, Sinauer Associates, 2010, pp 819–879

Kandel ER, Kupfermann I, Iverson S: Learning and memory, in Principles of Neural Science, 4th Edition. Edited by Kandel ER, Schwartz JH, Jessell TM. New York, McGraw-Hill, 2000, pp 1227–1247

Shohamy D, Foerde K: The role of the basal ganglia in learning and memory: insight from Parkinson's disease. Neurobiol Learn Mem 96:624–636, 2011

References

Baringer JR: Herpes simplex infections of the nervous system. Neurol Clin 26:657–674, 2008

Bartsch T, Döhring J, Rohr A, et al: CA1 neurons in the human hippocampus are critical for autobiographical memory, mental time travel, and autonoetic consciousness. Proc Natl Acad Sci U S A 108:17562–17567, 2011

Budson AE: Understanding memory dysfunction. Neurologist 15:71–79, 2009

Budson AE, Price BH: Memory dysfunction. N Engl J Med 352:692–699, 2005

Budson AE, Price BH: Memory dysfunction in neurological practice. Pract Neurol 7:42–47, 2007

Johnson MK, Kounios J, Nolde SF: Electrophysiological brain activity and memory source monitoring. Neuroreport 8:1317–1320, 1997

Lou HC, Luber B, Crupain M, et al: Parietal cortex and representation of the mental self. Proc Natl Acad Sci U S A 101:6827–6832, 2004

Papez J: A proposed mechanism of emotion (1937). J Neuropsychiatry Clin Neurosci 7:103–112, 1995

Saumier D, Chertkow H: Semantic memory. Curr Neurol Neurosci Rep 2:516–522, 2002

Scoville WB, Milner B: Loss of recent memory after bilateral hippocampal lesions. J Neurol Neurosurg Psychiatry 20:11–21, 1957

Steiner I: Herpes simplex virus encephalitis: new infection or reactivation? Curr Opin Neurol 24:268–274, 2011

Tulving E: Memory and consciousness. Can Psychol 26:1–12, 1985

Wagner AD, Shannon BJ, Kahn I, et al: Parietal lobe contributions to episodic memory retrieval. Trends Cogn Sci 9:445–453, 2005

INTELLECTUAL FAILURE

Intellectual Failure

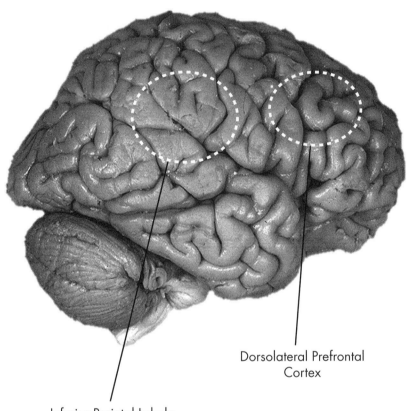

Inferior Parietal Lobule

Dorsolateral Prefrontal
Cortex

INTRODUCTION

Patients may experience a breakdown of their fundamental computational capacities, in addition to memory problems. This loss of ability may be confined to one domain, such as executive functioning. In the postconcussive syndrome, the difficulties involve multiple computational domains but are relatively mild. A dementia syndrome becomes manifest when the deficits are acquired, widespread, and severe. If the deficits are present since birth, the diagnosis of intellectual disability is made. The neuroanatomy includes the dorsolateral prefrontal cortex (executive ability), the nondominant inferior parietal lobule (visuospatial ability) and the dominant inferior parietal lobule (calculation ability), the anterior and inferior temporal lobes (semantic memory), and the mesial temporal structures (episodic memory). Multiple neurotransmitter systems are involved.

Frontotemporal Dementia

Joseph Tham, M.D., F.R.C.P.C.

A 53-year-old right-handed widow who lived alone was referred by her family physician for assessment of "depression" and with more recent concerns about her cognitive-intellectual functioning. She attended the initial neuropsychiatric assessment with her son.

Approximately 1 year prior to assessment, the owner of the restaurant where she had worked as a cook died from metastatic cancer. She grieved the sudden loss of her employer and close friend and appeared depressed. She had early-morning awakenings and admitted to concentration difficulties. She was anhedonic, and she did not seem to be vigilant with her appearance or the upkeep of her home, which contrasted with her previous immaculate standards of cleanliness. She was also failing to deposit her rental checks on a regular schedule. For the past 7 years she had rented the basement of her home to a young couple, who noticed that she was no longer managing her garden and yard work as she had before. In the 6 months prior to her assessment, her son and daughter were having to come by her home on a weekly basis to help with some of the household chores, such as stocking the refrigerator with food after they noticed that the refrigerator was almost empty on several of their visits. Their mother did not seem to be aware of the problems with personal and household management and did not show any concern when informed.

According to the family, she had no past psychiatric history of depression and was overall in good health. There was no history of alcohol or substance use. Both her children were born by cesarean section, but there were no other surgeries. There was no history of head injury, seizures, central nervous system infections, or strokes. The family history was significant for both her parents dying from stroke but when well into their 80s. There was no family history of psychiatric disorders or degenerative neurological conditions.

During the initial assessment she appeared calm and in no distress, and she was unconcerned about the issues raised by her family. She admitted that she was "not happy" but denied any major challenges in life despite what appeared to be a clear functional deterioration according to the collateral sources. She answered questions in brief sentences but often could not elaborate, suggesting some degree of poverty of thought content. Her thought form was goal oriented. She described her mood as "normal," but the range of affect in the office seemed diminished, almost flat. She denied feeling anxious, and there was no evidence of perceptual disturbances like auditory or visual hallucinations. There were no delusional beliefs noted.

A Mini-Mental State Examination (MMSE) conducted on the initial visit yielded a score of 27/30. She scored 2/3 on the three-word delayed recall. She was disoriented to the date and day of the week. There was no evidence of apraxia, aphasia, or agnosia.

General physical examination was unremarkable. She was a mildly disheveled woman appearing her stated age, with no evidence of respiratory, cardiovascular, or abdominal abnormalities. Neurological exam showed normal cranial nerve functioning, full motor strength, normal sensation, and normal deep tendon reflexes.

Baseline blood work was done for electrolytes, complete blood count (CBC) and differential, thyroid screen, liver and renal functions, fasting glucose, and serum cholesterol level. An electrocardiogram was done. The results all came back negative.

The initial diagnosis was that she was depressed, with possible cognitive-intellectual symptoms secondary to her mood disorder ("pseudo-dementia") leading to poor motivation and concentration. The antidepressant sertraline was prescribed, starting at 50 mg hs and increased to 100 mg hs over 1 month.

At 3-month follow-up, she was seen at the clinic to assess the antidepressant medication trial. The family advised that she was not compliant with the sertraline and indicated ongoing concerns about her cognitive-intellectual abilities and behavior. For example, on a few occasions when they went into her home, she was playing music by the Backstreet Boys and 'N Sync—these were popular "boy bands" of the time that were generally aimed at a much younger demographic. Furthermore, the family had heard from the tenants downstairs that on a number of occasions this music was playing loudly at 3 A.M. At this follow-up appointment, she was unable to explain these behaviors but cheerfully stated, "I love the Backstreet Boys." She could not explain when she became interested in this music, but clearly her family felt that her recent appreciation of this genre of music was unusual. Her mental state did not suggest a manic episode in that there was no psychomotor acceleration, her speech was of normal rate, and sleep disturbance was not an identified concern. Her family continued to do her grocery shopping, and her son helped with maintaining the garden.

Computed tomography (CT) of the head was requested because of the atypical features in her presentation. The CT scan demonstrated significant frontotemporal atrophy, enlarged sylvian fissures, and disproportionately enlarged anterior horns of the lateral ventricles (Figure 10–1). Vitamin B_{12} level was normal, and syphilis serology (VDRL [Venereal Disease Research Laboratory]) was negative.

Given the clinical features and CT scan findings, the most likely diagnosis was a frontotemporal dementia (FTD). She was referred to the local dementia clinic for further assessment and treatment. Over the next 12 months, arrangements were made for a private caregiver and eventually she was admitted to a nursing facility. A number of medications were tried. Selective serotonin reuptake inhibitors (SSRIs) (first sertraline and then citalopram) seemed to improve her mood. Low-dose antipsychotics (first quetiapine and then olanzapine) helped to calm her when she became more irritable and agitated, including when she exhibited "catastrophic reactions"—explosive frustration upon realizing that she could not perform many basic activities of daily living. The cholinesterase inhibitor medications donepezil and then galantamine were added, but any improvement was either minimal or short-lived.

Two years after the initial assessment, her MMSE score had dropped to 18/30. Her memory was now obviously worse and verbal production had dropped off significantly, with severe word-finding difficulties. She would often resort to pointing at objects, saying "that one" to identify items. Questions were answered with brief or overlearned phrases such as "Go away!" or "I'm OK." By this time, she had been admitted to a nursing care facility equipped with a "wander alert" system, which was needed because she was often disoriented and would wander off the ward.

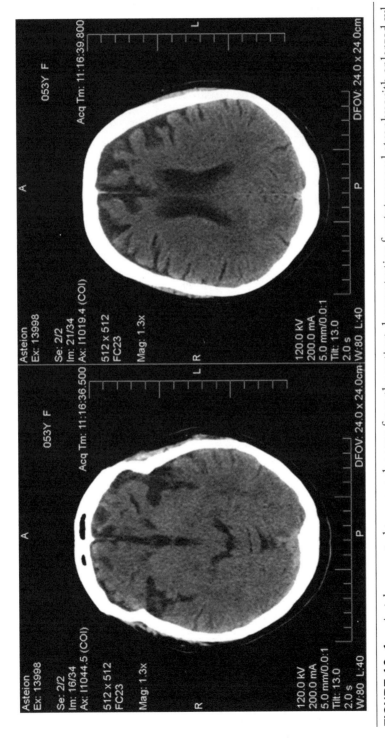

FIGURE 10–1.   Axial computed tomography scan from the patient demonstrating frontotemporal atrophy with enlarged sylvian fissures.

About 5 years after the initial assessment, she developed aspiration pneumonia and died from complications of the infection. At autopsy her brain demonstrated extensive frontal atrophy and numerous Pick bodies, the argyrophilic inclusion bodies characteristic of Pick's disease, which is a common type of FTD.

Discussion

The term *frontotemporal dementia* generally refers to the clinical cognitive-intellectual and behavioral deterioration associated with the pathological changes of *frontotemporal lobar degeneration* (FTLD)—widespread neural network damage affecting frontal and temporal lobar regions (Neary et al. 2005). Postmortem pathology shows extensive volume loss in the frontal and temporal lobes (as was demonstrated by the patient's CT scan). Although at one time FTD was thought to be rare, the prevalence of FTD is about equivalent to that of Alzheimer's disease for those ages 45–64 (Ratnavalli et al. 2002). Histopathology varies but is broadly split between cases with accumulation of tau protein as in Pick's disease (FTLD-tau) and cases with ubiquitin-positive inclusions (FTLD-U). Some cases, however, may lack distinctive pathology (McKhann et al. 2001). Genetic linkages have been demonstrated for chromosomes 3, 9, and 17. More recent studies have identified TAR DNA-binding protein (TDP-43) and fused in sarcoma protein (FUS) as the predominant abnormal intracellular protein aggregates underlying FTLD-U (Mackenzie et al. 2010).

Patients with FTD are also classified based on clinical presentations: behavioral variant FTD (bvFTD), semantic dementia, and progressive nonfluent aphasia. Clinical consensus criteria, known as the Neary criteria, have been developed to identify core and supportive features to use in clinical practice (Neary et al. 1998). Briefly, features of each syndrome are as follows:

1. *Behavioral variant FTD* often starts with impaired motivation and progresses to impulsivity and personality change such as childlike regressive or selfish behaviors, perseveration, repetitive stereotyped behaviors, hyperorality, and unusual punning and humor (*Witzelsucht*). Antisocial-like behaviors such as shoplifting or apparent lack of conscience may occur (pseudopsychopathy). Poor insight at an early stage is common.
2. *Semantic dementia* is a multimodal disorder of meaning in which patients lose the abilities to name and understand words and to recognize the significance of faces, objects, and other sensory stimuli. Although speech remains fluent, patients may demonstrate word-finding diffi-

culties to the point of asking about the names of common objects; sub-
stitution of related words (e.g., "car" when they mean "bus"), known as
semantic paraphasia; verbal comprehension difficulties; loss of facial
recognition (prosopagnosia); and inability to link an object with its
intended function.
3. *Progressive nonfluent aphasia* is characterized by early loss of speech
   fluency and agrammatism. Stuttering and speech hesitancy are obvious features. Phonemic paraphasia, where word sounds become confused (e.g., saying "care" instead of "chair"), can be seen. Combined
   with the loss of ability to construct sentences, this condition leads to
   severely limited language output. Language comprehension will also
   deteriorate in time, but generally later than in semantic dementia.

These presentations overlap in terms of behavioral, cognitive-intellectual, and language deficits, which are determined by the initial localization and subsequent spread of FTD pathology within the frontal and
temporal lobes. The case presented here would be consistent with the
syndrome of bvFTD, given the early presentation of unusual psychiatric
features and late onset of aphasia.

Given the gradually progressive nature of FTLD, onset of symptoms
is slow and insidious. This often leads to a significant delay between presentation and a final neurological diagnosis. Early on in the illness and
especially in cases of bvFTD, the patient presents with features often attributed to psychiatric disorders. For example, anhedonia, apathy, psychomotor slowing, and emotional dysregulation may all suggest an
underlying mood disorder, as they did in this patient's case. Perseverative
behaviors can be misinterpreted as compulsive but are not usually linked
to intrusive thoughts as in obsessive-compulsive disorder. A psychotic
disorder may need to be considered in the differential diagnosis in severe
cases of behavioral and thought disorder (Mendez and Perryman 2002).

Diagnosis requires a thorough history with a focus on family history
and careful review of psychiatric history. In otherwise healthy individuals
with no past psychiatric illness in the family, the onset of mood disorder,
psychosis, and especially personality change in later life (beyond 50 years
old) demands a high index of suspicion around organic etiologies. Physical examination in cases of FTLD may demonstrate frontal release signs
(e.g., palmar, palmomental, and glabellar reflexes). Standard medical investigations, including CBC and differential, electrolyte panel, liver and
renal chemistries, serum vitamin B_{12} level, thyroid-stimulating hormone
(TSH), and infectious disease screen (e.g., for syphilis), would be appropriate to rule out some of the medical causes of cognitive-intellectual
impairment. An electroencephalogram (EEG) and careful medical history

can help rule out delirium. Neuroimaging, including CT and magnetic resonance imaging (MRI) of the brain, may not show much atrophy initially but, in time, will demonstrate progressive frontotemporal volume loss as shown in this case.

The patient's mental state may mimic psychiatric disorders such as depression, mania, or psychosis. Suspicion for an organic condition should be aroused in the presence of unusual features or an atypical combination of symptoms. For example, the patient with FTLD is often remarkably impulsive and disinhibited in a manner that is reminiscent of a bipolar manic state, but without decreased need for sleep, grandiosity, or an increase in goal-directed activities. Unfortunately, commonly used clinical dementia screens such as the MMSE may not pick up the initial subtle cognitive-intellectual changes in the illness compared with cases of Alzheimer's disease, where memory impairment tends to be an early feature. A specialized frontal cognitive battery such as the Frontal Assessment Battery (Slachevsky et al. 2004) or assessment tools like the Frontal Behavioral Inventory (Kertesz et al. 1997) improve detection of frontal clinical features, including disinhibition and executive dysfunction. Ultimately, a formal neuropsychological evaluation could provide the needed sensitivity to detect abnormalities in language and executive function relative to preserved visuospatial and memory abilities.

There is no known cure for FTLD, so the focus is on symptomatic treatment of behavioral symptoms. Nonpharmacological interventions should be attempted first. These interventions usually involve home support to maintain safety and provide assistance in completing activities of daily living. Family and caregiver support are essential to prevent burnout, given the intense emotional strains that are generated by the patient's behavior and failing functionality. Behavioral management strategies may need to be developed as part of the patient care plan, especially around safety and psychobehavioral disinhibition and apathy.

The role of cholinesterase inhibitors and N-methyl-D-aspartate (NMDA) receptor antagonists, commonly used in Alzheimer's disease, remains unclear. As of yet, there are no agents targeting the proteinopathy of FTLD.

Medications for symptomatic treatment of the behavioral dysregulation broadly include antidepressants, mood stabilizers, anxiolytics, and antipsychotic agents (Chow and Mendez 2002). SSRI medications are often used for treatment of depression, perseverative behaviors, and impulsivity. Mood-stabilizing medications such as valproic acid and carbamazepine may help regulate emotional lability. Sedatives, anxiolytics (e.g., benzodiazepines), and antipsychotic medications can decrease the frequency of or help abort severe episodes of aggression. As in other patients with underlying organic conditions, close monitoring is important to rule out significant side effects from these medications, especially delirium.

A large, retrospective, longitudinal study comparing FTLD patients with Alzheimer's disease patients suggested a median survival in FTLD patients of 8.7 years compared with 11.8 years in Alzheimer's disease patients (Roberson et al. 2005).

Key Clinical Points

- Frontotemporal lobar degeneration can be differentiated from other forms of dementia by clinical presentation and neuropathological changes.
- Clinical criteria are helpful in distinguishing between three presentations of FTD: behavioral variant FTD, semantic dementia, and progressive nonfluent aphasia.
- Because of the potential for early presentation of psychiatric and behavioral issues, the diagnosis of frontotemporal lobar degeneration may not be initially obvious.
- At present, only symptomatic treatments are available for FTLD.
- Caregiver burnout can be a major problem and needs to be identified and addressed.

Further Readings

The Association for Frontotemporal Degeneration: Frontotemporal degeneration. Available at: http://www.theaftd.org/frontotemporal-degeneration/ftd-overview. Accessed August 1, 2011.

Hodges JR (ed): Frontotemporal Dementia Syndromes. Cambridge, UK, Cambridge University Press, 2007

Moore DP: Frontotemporal dementia, in Textbook of Clinical Neuropsychiatry, 2nd Edition. Edited by Hodder A. London, Oxford University Press, 2008, pp 341–342

References

Chow TW, Mendez MF: Goals in symptomatic pharmacologic management of frontotemporal lobar degeneration. Am J Alzheimers Dis Other Demen 17:267–272, 2002

Kertesz A, Davidson W, Fox H: Frontal Behavioral Inventory: diagnostic criteria for frontal lobe dementia. Can J Neurol Sci 24:29–36, 1997

Mackenzie I, Rademakers R, Neumann M: TDP-43 and FUS in amyotrophic lateral sclerosis and frontotemporal dementia. Lancet Neurol 9:995–1007, 2010

McKhann GM, Albert MS, Grossman M, et al: Clinical and pathological diagnosis of frontotemporal dementia: report of the Work Group on Frontotemporal Dementia and Pick's Disease. Arch Neurol 58:1803–1809, 2001

Mendez MF, Perryman KM: Neuropsychiatric features of frontotemporal dementia: evaluation of consensus criteria and review. J Neuropsychiatry Clin Neurosci 14:424–429, 2002

Neary D, Snowden JS, Gustafson L, et al: Frontotemporal lobar degeneration: a consensus on clinical diagnostic criteria. Neurology 51:1546–1554, 1998

Neary D, Snowden JS, Mann DMA: Frontotemporal dementia. Lancet Neurol 4:771–779, 2005

Ratnavalli E, Brayne C, Dawson K, et al: The prevalence of frontotemporal dementia. Neurology 58:1615–1621, 2002

Roberson ED, Hesse JH, Rose KD, et al: Frontotemporal dementia progresses to death faster than Alzheimer disease. Neurology 65:719–725, 2005

Slachevsky A, Villalpando JM, Sarazin M, et al: Frontal Assessment Battery and differential diagnosis of frontotemporal dementia and Alzheimer disease. Arch Neurol 61:1104–1107, 2004

Dementia Syndrome of Depression

Robert Stowe, M.D., F.R.C.P.C.

A 71-year-old black male was referred for assessment because of rapidly progressive neurocognitive deterioration, thought possibly to represent Creutzfeldt-Jakob disease (CJD). He had a 9-month history of progressive personality change and deterioration in neurocognitive capacities and functioning. His wife had recently suffered several myocardial infarctions, and he became anxious and ruminative about her health. His memory started to fail, and he became irritable and impulsive. He lost 34 pounds due to anorexia. He became progressively more abulic, ultimately staring vacantly into space, and became incontinent of urine and feces.

Treatment in a community hospital with amitriptyline and an antipsychotic improved apathy and delusions, although he remained incontinent, amnestic, and disoriented. He returned home for several months but became agitated one night, filling anything hollow with water because he was convinced that the house was on fire. At a university psychiatric hospital, there was some improvement on nortriptyline, which was replaced by bupropion because of orthostatic hypotension. He also received perphenazine and benztropine. A pyloric ulcer was treated with ranitidine. Abulia and agitation improved, but confusion persisted. The director of the Alzheimer's Disease Research Center noted myoclonic jerks and suspected CJD. The patient was transferred to a VA neurobehavioral unit for stabilization and placement.

The patient was a Korean War veteran and had experienced frequent nightmares related to posttraumatic stress disorder for years, but there was no past history of depression or psychosis. He had worked in a galvanizing plant for many years, retiring 10 years earlier, but was working as a janitor and custodian when he fell ill. He was stably married for 43 years.

He was treated for syphilis in his 30s, and again several decades later. He took furosemide for mild peripheral edema attributed to chronic venous insufficiency and took stool softeners for constipation. Remote medical history included a perforated peptic ulcer, and a shoulder injury in a motor vehicle accident without head trauma 2 years earlier. There was no substance abuse history. Family history was negative for dementing disorders.

Mental status examination revealed him to be friendly, cooperative, and seemingly attentive, but mostly indifferent. Mood was described as "okay," but affect was constricted, with frequent sighing. Thought processes were impoverished. Delusions and hallucinations were absent. Although effort was good on neurocognitive testing, he appeared indifferent to the results.

Neurocognitive examination demonstrated orientation only to place and person. He repeated 8 digits forward and 5 backward, and he recited months of the year backward correctly. He was vigilant and not impulsive on a go/no-go task. Perseveration was evident in an alternating graphomotor sequence (Figure 10–2) but not in Luria loops. He was extremely slow on a random letter cancellation test, without evidence of hemispatial neglect. Speech was hypophonic, but fluent and grammatical, without paraphasias or word-finding difficulty. Fluency was reduced (seven words beginning with *f* and nine animal names, over 1 minute each). Naming, repetition, comprehension, reading, and writing were normal. Praxis was intact. On clock drawing, number placement was correct, although the hands were not properly drawn, and constructions were impoverished (Figure 10–3). On the Three Words–Three Shapes memory test, copying of internal detail was impaired. He recalled no words, and only the external configuration of one shape incidentally. After one study period, he recalled three words and the external configuration, plus some internal detail, of two shapes. Fifteen minutes later, he recalled no words, while reproduction of the shapes was unchanged. Multiple-choice recognition was two words and three shapes, unchanged after 24 hours. He knew the dates of his wife's myocardial infarctions and his admission date. Interpretation of similarities was very impaired.

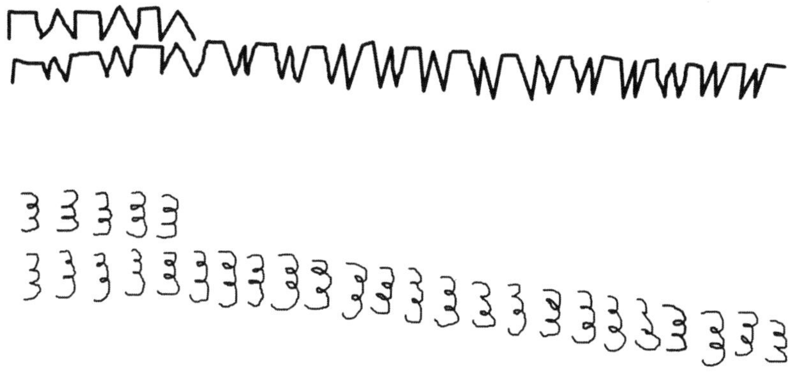

FIGURE 10–2. Reproduction of a graphomotor sequence (top) and Luria loops by a 71-year-old male.

(Top) In an alternating graphomotor sequence task, the patient was asked to "copy and continue this sequence below." Perseverative distortion was evident on this drawing; note the replacement of vertical elements of the square wave component with diagonal edges. (Bottom) In a Luria loops task, he was asked to make "a whole row of these figures with the same number of loops as shown above." He did not add extra loops, which would have been a more extreme example of perseveration.

Neurological examination revealed normal visual acuities and fields, funduscopy, and extraocular movements. Pupils were equal and reactive to light and accommodation. Speech was hoarse and slightly hypophonic. Occasional rapid lapses of extensor muscle tone (suggestive of asterixis); subtle, spontaneous finger/hand myoclonus; and a rapid, fine terminal action tremor were observed. Stimulus-sensitive myoclonus and enhanced auditory startle reflexes were absent. Tone and power were normal. Reflexes were symmetrically brisk (without clonus) except at the ankles, where they were normal. Plantar responses were flexor. There were no release (grasp, snout, suck or glabellar) reflexes. Light touch, vibration, and joint position sense were intact. Gait was mildly bradykinetic with decreased arm swing, mildly decreased stride length, and slight stiffness at the knees.

Blood pressure was 145/85 mm Hg without orthostasis. There were no bruits. Cardiac examination was normal, and lung bases were clear. There was mild pitting edema of both ankles, accompanied by venous stasis changes. Hepatosplenomegaly and abdominal, prostatic, and testicular masses were not detected.

Abnormalities on routine laboratory studies were restricted to slightly low thyroxine (T_4) (4.1; normal range 5–12 mcg/dL) and triiodothyronine by radioimmunoassay (T_3 RIA) (0.7; normal range 0.9–2.2 mcg/L), with a

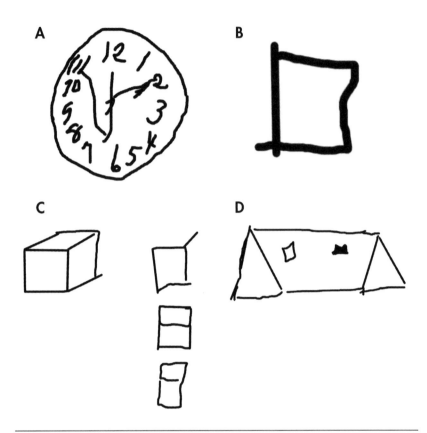

FIGURE 10–3.   Evidence of constructional impairment in the patient's drawings.
(A) He was asked to draw and number a clock face and to set the hands to indicate "10 past 11." (B) He was asked to draw a cube. (C) He was asked to copy the cube drawn on the left by the examiner. (D) He was asked to draw a house, showing two sides and a roof.

normal TSH and a free thyroxine index (FTI) of 5.7. Antithyroid antibodies and antinuclear antibodies were negative. Cerebrospinal fluid (CSF) was acellular with normal glucose and protein, a negative VDRL, and negative cryptococcal antigen. Chest X ray and abdominal CT scan were unremarkable.

Three EEGs were normal. An MRI brain scan showed mildly enlarged ventricles without periventricular edema, and T2 signal hyperintensities typical of mild small vessel ischemic changes. Xenon-133 cerebral blood flow (CBF) showed mild global reduction (5%–10% below normal) without definite focal abnormalities.

Considering his partial improvement on antidepressants, a dementia syndrome of depression was suspected. Benztropine was discontinued and bupropion was increased to 100 mg q8h, with progressive improvement in affective blunting and abulia. The Mattis Dementia Rating Scale score improved from 83/144 to 128/144 (above the cutoff for dementia based on his limited educational background), and repeat neuropsychological testing demonstrated improvement in memory, list learning, and visuointegrative dysfunction. Given these improvements, he was discharged home. His neurocognitive abilities continued to improve, incontinence resolved, and anergia, abulia, and restricted affect remitted. Within 3 months, he had recovered completely and was back at work.

He remained in remission for 5 years but relapsed at age 76, with severe somatic preoccupation following his wife's rehospitalization, and after bupropion was slowly titrated down below 150 mg qd. He developed a morbid fear that she would stop breathing, and he followed her around the house, awakening her at night to ensure that she was still alive. This time, it was harder to reverse his depression. He developed an intermittent resting tremor and an asymptomatic 20 mm Hg drop in orthostatic blood pressure upon reintroduction of perphenazine. A CT scan showed frontal and posterior parietal atrophy, raising the possibility of corticobasal degeneration, although myoclonus was no longer evident, and apraxia, rigidity, and supranuclear ophthalmoplegia had not developed. A specific diagnosis had not been reached by the time he was lost to follow-up.

Discussion

Mild degrees of reversible neurocognitive impairment can be identified on neuropsychological examination in the majority of depressed elderly individuals. Impairment may be largely attributable to psychomotor slowing (Butters et al. 2004). The *dementia syndrome of depression* represents a more severe compromise of neurocognitive function masquerading as a dementing disorder and occurs in a small but clinically important minority of depressed patients. (The term "depressive pseudodementia" is sometimes used to describe this disorder but is ambiguous and misleading, as the term pseudodementia can be used to denote conscious or unconscious elaboration of neurocognitive impairment.) Because depression may presage or accompany mild cognitive impairment (MCI) and early Alzheimer's disease, differentiating between the neurocognitive impairment imparted by depression and a neurodegenerative dementia can be difficult, if not impossible (Potter and Steffens 2007). Indeed, there is considerable evidence that both depression and neurocognitive impairment in many depressed elderly individuals may be mediated by shared risk factors, including ischemic white matter disease, basal ganglia lacunae, and neuronal loss in the hippocampus (Taylor et al. 2006).

Although recent research in the neurobiology of depression has focused on hippocampal atrophy and corticolimbic network changes, the striking reversibility of neurocognitive impairment that can be seen following antidepressant treatment is best explained by dysregulation of bioaminergic systems, predominantly noradrenergic, dopaminergic, and serotonergic—the last via secondary effects of 5-hydroxytryptamine type-2A (5-HT$_{2A}$) receptors on prefrontal dopamine release (Gareri et al. 2002). Via ascending "state-setting" cortical and limbic projections, the brain stem and basal forebrain neurons that synthesize neurotransmitters modulate and "fine-tune" sensory and neurocognitive systems responsible for the speed, planning, execution, and maintenance of movement and speech; and arousal, mood, motivation, and memory retrieval (Mesulam 2000). Disordered interaction and imbalance between these neuromodulatory systems may underlie the neurocognitive and emotional deficits in neuropsychiatric disorders (Briand et al. 2007).

The characteristic presentation of a dementia syndrome of depression typically encompasses the following changes:

1. Psychomotor slowing with increased response latencies; apathy; and decreased generative capacity on tasks such as letter, category, and design fluency. Anomia improving after phonemic or semantic cues may also be seen.
2. Executive dysfunction manifested by deficits in divided/complex attention; divergent thinking/responding; cognitive flexibility; planning; and hygiene and grooming. Disinhibited behaviors and importuning are frequently seen.
3. A frontal-subcortical profile of memory impairment characterized by decreased working memory, a depressed learning curve, and poor uncued retrieval (often accompanied by a negative response bias, in contrast to the confabulation typically seen in Alzheimer's disease and Korsakoff's syndrome). Cued retrieval and/or recognition memory, and autobiographical memory for personally significant recent events, are typically relatively preserved in the dementia syndrome of depression.
4. Visuospatial ability may be impaired secondarily as a consequence of impaired spatial working memory, impaired speed of processing, and executive dysfunction.

The Montreal Cognitive Assessment, the Frontal Assessment Battery, the Modified Mini-Mental State Examination, and the Mattis Dementia

Rating Scale are more sensitive to this profile of impairment than the standard MMSE.

The differential diagnosis includes FTD, extrapyramidal disorders, normal-pressure hydrocephalus, vascular dementia (especially with basal ganglia infarcts), hypothyroidism, and emerging catatonia.

Pointers to a dementia syndrome of depression include a past history of affective disorders; a major prodromal anxiogenic stressor and/or depressive symptoms at onset; a normal EEG (keeping in mind that lithium and atypical neuroleptics can cause background slowing and even sharp waves and spikes in some individuals) (Centorrino et al. 2002); and neuroimaging studies showing only age-related generalized volume loss and/ or minor white matter changes on MRI, which are more common in depressed elderly individuals.

In this patient, the picture at presentation was of fairly rapid neurocognitive deterioration with striking abulia and psychomotor retardation, possible confusional episodes, memory impairment, and executive dysfunction. Given mild ventricular enlargement, decreased stride length, and incontinence, normal-pressure hydrocephalus was an important consideration. However, his gait was not "magnetic," and abulia and gait changes might have been related to treatment with the neuroleptic perphenazine, vascular leukoencephalopathy (given brisk reflexes and MRI findings), and/or cervical spondylotic myelopathy (as the jaw reflex was not enhanced). Although verbal memory was impaired, preservation of recognition memory argued against the accelerated rate of forgetting typical of Alzheimer's disease and paraneoplastic limbic encephalitis. Alzheimer's disease was also felt to be unlikely in the absence of aphasia, apraxia, and agnosia. Parkinsonian features were mild despite perphenazine, and specific features of dementia with Lewy bodies (visual hallucinations, REM [rapid eye movement] sleep behavior disorder, frequent falls) were absent. Normal morning cortisol levels excluded Addison's disease. Absence of supranuclear ophthalmoplegia and specific extrapyramidal findings argued against progressive supranuclear palsy and corticobasal degeneration, and neither MRI nor xenon-133 CBF provided evidence for a frontotemporal degeneration. Cerebrospinal fluid examination excluded neurosyphilis. Low T_4 and T_3 RIA with normal FTI and TSH suggested a "sick euthyroid" profile rather than hypothyroidism.

The presence of asterixis was puzzling, because this is typically associated with toxic-metabolic encephalopathy or anticonvulsant toxicity, but three normal EEGs made metabolic encephalopathy and anticholinergic delirium as well as seizure disorders and Hashimoto's encephalopathy (negative antithyroid antibodies) unlikely. Furthermore, renal and liver function tests, arterial blood gases (to rule out hypercarbia), and ammonia level were normal. Asterixis can be seen with frontal lobe, thalamic, or midbrain pathology, but there were no indications of abnormalities in these regions seen on MRI. Absence of stimulus-sensitive myoclonus and normal EEGs made CJD unlikely (Geschwind et al. 2008). Myoclonus and asterixis ("negative myoclonus") were ultimately attributed to his psychotropic medication regimen (Jiménez-Jiménez et al. 2004), and they resolved after perphenazine was titrated down.

When a dementia syndrome of depression is suspected, even if there is a question of an underlying vascular or neurodegenerative dementia, therapeutic approaches should be exhaustive. Failure to recognize and aggressively treat individuals with a dementia syndrome of depression can lead to the tragedy of unnecessary nursing home placement or death from complications of cachexia and decreased mobility.

Although Class I evidence regarding specific treatments is largely lacking for this syndrome, both theoretical considerations and clinical experience suggest that dual-action antidepressants with low anticholinergic properties, such as venlafaxine, duloxetine, or mirtazapine (when insomnia is severe), often work best, with augmentation from low doses of an atypical antipsychotic in the presence of refractory anxiety, psychotic features, or a prior history suggestive of bipolar II traits. Should SSRIs be preferred because of concerns about the arrhythmogenic potential of serotonin-norepinephrine reuptake inhibitors, sertraline may have an advantage because it is a mild dopamine reuptake inhibitor, whereas citalopram enhances hippocampal acetylcholine release (possibly advantageous if comorbid amnestic MCI is suspected). Electroconvulsive therapy (ECT) is indicated after failed trials of first- and second-line antidepressants and augmentation using atypical antipsychotics (and perhaps lithium), or in the presence of lorazepam-refractory catatonic features. Augmentation with bupropion, stimulants, or dopamine agonists such as pramipexole may be considered when psychomotor slowing persists. Adjunctive cholinesterase inhibitor therapy may be indicated in the setting of comorbid Alzheimer's disease or amnestic MCI, vascular dementia, diffuse Lewy body disease, or Parkinson's disease; when drugs with secondary anticholinergic properties such as tricyclic antidepressants must be used; and when neurocognitive function worsens during ECT, despite improvement in depression. Although the most robust benefit of cholinesterase inhibitors in Alzheimer's disease is improvement in apathy and social engagement, they may be mildly depressogenic in individuals without Alzheimer's disease (Reynolds et al. 2011). Therefore, routine use for neurocognitive enhancement in depressed patients with neurocognitive impairment cannot be recommended.

Key Clinical Points

- Late-life depression can produce a reversible syndrome resembling profound dementia.

- A dementia syndrome of depression typically presents with psychomotor slowing, executive dysfunction, a frontal-subcortical profile of memory impairment, and visuospatial impairment.

- A dementia syndrome of depression can occur in the absence of self-reported sadness and concern over neurocognitive and memory deficits.

- When there is a significant possibility of depression based on the early presentation, atypical features should not prevent aggressive antidepressant treatment.

- Asterixis and myoclonus can be side effects of psychotropic medications.

Further Readings

Marvel CL, Paradiso S: Cognitive and neurological impairment in mood disorders. Psychiatr Clin North Am 27:19–36, 2004

Panza F, Frisardi V, Capurso C, et al: Late-life depression, mild cognitive impairment, and dementia: possible continuum? Am J Geriatr Psychiatry 18:98–116, 2010

References

Butters MA, Whyte EM, Nebes RD, et al: The nature and determinants of neuropsychological functioning in late-life depression. Arch Gen Psychiatry 61:587–595, 2004

Briand LA, Gritton H, Howe WM, et al: Modulators in concert for cognition: modulator interactions in the prefrontal cortex. Prog Neurobiol 83:69–91, 2007

Centorrino F, Price BH, Tuttle M, et al: EEG abnormalities during treatment with typical and atypical antipsychotics. Am J Psychiatry 159:109–115, 2002

Gareri P, De Fazio P, De Sarro G: Neuropharmacology of depression in aging and age-related diseases. Ageing Res Rev 1:113–134, 2002

Geschwind MD, Shu H, Haman A, et al: Rapidly progressive dementia. Ann Neurol 64:97–108, 2008

Jiménez-Jiménez FJ, Puertas I, de Toledo-Heras M: Drug-induced myoclonus: frequency, mechanisms and management. CNS Drugs 18:93–104, 2004

Mesulam M-M: Behavioral neuroanatomy: large-scale networks, association cortex, frontal syndromes, the limbic system, and hemispheric specializations, in Principles of Behavioral and Cognitive Neurology, 2nd Edition. Edited by Mesulam M-M. New York, Oxford University Press, 2000, pp 1–120

Potter GG, Steffens DC: Contribution of depression to cognitive impairment and dementia in older adults. Neurologist 13:105–117, 2007

Reynolds CF 3rd, Butters MA, Lopez O, et al: Maintenance treatment of depression in old age: a randomized, double-blind, placebo-controlled evaluation of the efficacy and safety of donepezil combined with antidepressant pharmacotherapy. Arch Gen Psychiatry 68:51–60, 2011

Taylor WD, Steffens DC, Krishnan KR: Psychiatric disease in the twenty-first century: the case for subcortical ischemic depression. Biol Psychiatry 60:1299–1303, 2006

Psychosis and Cognitive Impairment in an Adolescent[1]

Robert Stowe, M.D., F.R.C.P.C.

A 16-year-old black male was admitted to a child psychiatry unit for evaluation and treatment of psychosis. Over the preceding several months he had experienced paranoid delusions and other ideas of reference, auditory hallucinations of his mother's and sister's voices emanating from the radio, and command hallucinations from the television. He began to sleep erratically and behaved in an increasingly bizarre fashion, isolating himself in his room. He engaged in uncharacteristic compulsive checking and counting behaviors and repeatedly inventoried his possessions and clothing. He made several calls to a "meet a star" call-in line, resulting in phone bills totaling several thousand dollars. One week prior to admission, he became convinced that his mother and sister were "prostituting themselves" and that a peer was planning to cut off one of his fingers.

With the exception of brief exposure to haloperidol in a community hospital prior to transfer, there was no history of exposure to psychotro-

---

[1]This case was previously published as a case report (Campo et al. 1998), and the neuropathological and biochemical findings were included in the series by Natowicz et al. (1995). The author initially evaluated the patient with Dr. Andrea DiMartini, whose consultation report was helpful in the summary of the clinical findings.

pic medications, no history of psychiatric evaluation or treatment, and no evidence of prior mood, anxiety, or conduct difficulties. He also denied alcohol, drug, and inhalant abuse.

Developmental history and milestones were unremarkable. Psycho-educational history suggested average to above-average premorbid intellectual ability. A gradual decline in academic performance and athletic performance began 2–3 years prior to psychiatric presentation. His family expressed concerns about his memory, attention, and motivation. These problems were initially attributed to marital conflict and a tense home environment. Notably, however, over the same period he became increasingly clumsy and uncoordinated.

Pertinent family history included alcohol dependence in his father. A maternal uncle had been hospitalized with "chronic paranoid schizophrenia."

Mental status examination revealed a mostly pleasant and cooperative adolescent with reasonable hygiene and grooming. He attributed his depressed mood to hospitalization. Suicidal ideation was denied. Affect was blunted, but he did laugh and joke spontaneously on occasion. Thought processes were goal directed and not grossly disorganized, but quite concrete. He had mild loosening of associations and some idiosyncratic responses, without ideomotor pressure, tangentiality, or circumstantiality. He appeared somewhat suspicious and guarded at times during the interview. He denied hallucinations and delusions during this interview but had admitted having them to a previous interviewer.

Neurocognitive examination revealed the patient to be alert and oriented to person and location, but 7 days off on the date. His MMSE score was 22/30. Digit spans were 6 forward and 4 backward. He could spell *world* backward but was unable to perform serial 7s or recite months backward, and he took a full minute to recite days of the week backward. Speech was fluent but slightly dysarthric. Repetition was intact but showed perseverative intrusions from a previous task, as he initially attempted to repeat sentences in reverse. He generated 9, 1, and 6 words beginning with the letters *f*, *a*, and *s*, respectively, for each initial letter over 1 minute each and included occasional neologisms. Syntactic comprehension was preserved, but he had difficulty with some "yes/no" questions, likely attributable to loosening of associations. Writing demonstrated poor penmanship, without aphasic dysgraphia. He could not generate a coherent written sentence spontaneously, but he wrote correctly to dictation. On a previous examination, he produced the sentence "My mind has seen the light." Buccofacial, limb, and axial praxis were intact. He drew and numbered a clock correctly on his second attempt. Cube drawing was intact. On the Three Words–Three Shapes memory test, incidental recall was 2 words and 1 shape, with 6/6 stimuli reproduced accurately after one study period.

After 15 minutes of distraction, he recalled 0/3 words and 2/3 shapes, with some confabulation on the remaining items, recognizing 2 words and 3 shapes on multiple choice. He was observed to have difficulty remembering the location of his room on the ward. Impulsive responding was demonstrated on a go/no-go paradigm. Graphomotor sequences were performed without perseveration.

General neurological examination revealed intact visual fields, fundi, pupils, and acuity. There was subtle impairment of downgaze, although vertical and horizontal optokinetic nystagmus was elicited. Cranial nerve examination was otherwise unremarkable except for subtle dysarthria. There was no drift, myoclonus, asterixis, or tremor. Lower-extremity tone was slightly increased. Muscle bulk and power were full throughout. Fine finger dexterity was impaired. Reflexes were brisk, with a few beats of knee and ankle clonus. Plantar responses were flexor. Sensory exam was intact to light touch, pinprick, vibration, and proprioception, and Romberg testing was negative. There was notable difficulty with rapid alternating movements (right>left), and both ataxic and fine terminal action tremors were evident on finger-nose-finger testing. Gait appeared normal except for diminished arm swing. He had mild difficulty with tandem gait and demonstrated bilateral posturing with stressed gait maneuvers.

General physical examination was negative for icterus, thyroid and cardiac abnormalities, and hepatosplenomegaly.

Neuropsychological testing revealed declines over 2 years on the Wechsler Intelligence Scale for Children—Revised in Verbal IQ from 90 to 64, Performance IQ from 70 to 47, and Full Scale IQ from 78 to <45. Naming and basic language functions were preserved, but motor and visuospatial processing skills, memory, conceptual flexibility, and abstract reasoning were significantly impaired.

Initial CT and MRI scans were normal; however, brain single-photon emission computed tomography (SPECT) revealed diffuse bifrontal and posterior parietal hypoactivity. Electroencephalography showed mild slowing and nonspecific posterior abnormalities. Hearing was normal on audiological screening, but brain-stem auditory evoked potentials (BAEPs) were bilaterally delayed. Pattern-shift visual evoked potentials were normal. A sleep study revealed dramatically decreased REM, decreased amplitude in all sleep stages, and very poor sleep continuity for age.

Ophthalmological examination showed no optic atrophy or retinal signs of storage material, and a slit lamp examination for Kayser-Fleischer rings was negative.

Routine hematological and biochemical tests, thyroid functions, B_{12}, folate, lead level, rapid plasma reagin, thyroid-stimulating hormone, erythrocyte sedimentation rate, anti-nuclear antibody, LE cell preparation, ceruloplasmin, urine copper, venous blood gases, serum ammonia, plasma amino and urine organic acid screens, and long-chain fatty acids were unremarkable. Serum total protein was slightly elevated due to a mild increase in globulins, but serum protein electrophoresis, Lyme titers, and HIV screen were normal, as were cerebrospinal fluid tests (cell count and differential, glucose and protein, oligoclonal banding, IgG index, and measles titers to rule out subacute sclerosing panencephalitis). Urinalysis, urine drug screen, and screens for heavy metal toxicity were negative.

Several months prior to hospitalization, he had been evaluated by a pediatric neurologist with particular expertise in metabolic disorders, who ultimately concluded that he most likely suffered from "childhood schizophrenia." However, review of laboratory investigations revealed a number of concerning findings, including occasional vacuolated fibroblasts and rare round, granular bodies enclosed by narrow myelinated membranes, suggestive of axonal spheroids, on electron microscopy of a skin biopsy. There was reduced total leukocyte hexosaminidase activity at 2,281 nmol/mg protein/ hour (normal range 3,013–3,423 nmol/mg protein/ hour), despite normal percentages of hexosaminidases A and B, and reduced sphingomyelinase level at 32 nmol/mg/hour (normal range 56–82 nmol/mg/hour). Assays of other lysosomal enzymes, including alpha-mannosidase, beta-glucosidase, beta-galactosidase, alpha-L-fucosidase, arylsulfatase A, and alpha-neuraminidase, were normal.

The diagnoses entertained at this point included adult-onset Tay-Sachs disease (TSD), possibly due to a deficiency in hexosaminidase activator protein; early Hallervorden-Spatz disease (given axonal spheroids); mucolipidosis II (I-cell disease); and Niemann-Pick type C disease (NPC) based on the axonal spheroids. Further testing ruled out beta-hexosaminidase deficiency. Fibroblast sphingomyelinase activity was reduced at 36 nmol/mg/hour (normal 129±43 nmol/mg/hour). The ability of the patient's skin fibroblasts to esterify exogenous cholesterol was severely reduced (<1% of normal), which is diagnostic of NPC (Natowicz et al. 1995).

Haloperidol 3 mg qd improved paranoia but caused confusion and disorientation, sedation, and bradykinesia. Pimozide was substituted and titrated up to 4 mg bid, with resolution of hallucinations and improvement in sedation and thought disorder. Because of drug-induced parkinsonism, risperidone was substituted for pimozide and benztropine was added. Clonazepam was added at 0.25 mg bid for anxiety. Discontinuation of benztropine was associated with marked gait deterioration. Dysphagia supervened, and progressive ataxia confined him to a wheelchair. A repeat MRI scan showed progression of central and cortical atrophy, and another EEG showed frontally predominant intermittent rhythmic delta activity.

Discussion

The clinical picture at presentation was of a psychotic illness indistinguishable from paranoid schizophrenia on the basis of psychiatric phenomenology. However, neurocognitive deficits, including bradyphrenia (in the absence of drug-induced parkinsonism or catatonic signs), perseveration, paraphasic errors, dyscalculia, and memory impairment (particularly confabulation out of keeping with mild thought disorder), made an uncomplicated primary psychiatric illness such as schizophrenia, a schizoaffective disorder, or psychotic depression unlikely. Abnormalities on SPECT, EEGs, BAEPs, and polysomnography further supported concerns about an organic etiology (Campo et al. 1998).

The differential diagnosis of such a presentation in adolescence (as in adulthood) is extremely broad, encompassing infectious, demyelinating, vascular, toxic-metabolic, endocrine, systemic medical, and congenital/genetic etiologies. Although neurocognitive deterioration may precede the onset of positive psychotic symptoms in adolescent-onset schizophrenia, which often has a poor prognosis, prodromal clumsiness and incoordination are atypical for a primary schizophrenic illness. Neurological abnormalities exceeded "soft neurological signs" described in the early course of schizophrenia (Bachmann et al. 2005) and included mild limitation of downgaze (which, unlike upgaze impairment, could not be attributed to haloperidol); lower-extremity hypertonia and hyperreflexia; and mild appendicular and truncal ataxia, raising the possibility of a multisystem neurodegenerative disorder or lysosomal storage disease. The general neurological findings were not suggestive of the akinetic-rigid (Westphal or juvenile variant) or choreiform (adult-onset) forms of Huntington's disease. There was no history of hallucinogen, cocaine, stimulant, cannabis, or solvent use, and urine toxicological screening was negative. Normal premorbid motor and intellectual development and absence of dysmorphic features argued against a microdeletion of chromosome 22q11.2 (velocardiofacial syndrome).

Although there were no specific pointers to the possibility of an underlying malignancy such as a testicular germ cell tumor, autoimmune-mediated limbic encephalitis—especially anti–NMDA receptor encephalitis and the more recently described anti–AMPA receptor encephalitis—is certainly in the differential diagnosis of this patient's presentation. Today this possibility would warrant consideration of a paraneoplastic antibody panel and appropriate screening procedures to rule out underlying malignancies (Vincent et al. 2011). Specific laboratory testing, including CSF analysis and neuroimaging, ruled out HIV encephalitis and other infectious causes. Serum ammonia, plasma amino acid, and urine organic acid screens helped exclude urea cycle disorders. Absence of abdominal pain, neuropathy, dysautonomia, and proximal motor axonopathy excluded neuropsychiatric porphyria. Absence of cataracts, tendon xanthomas, and characteristic imaging changes ruled out cerebrotendinous xanthomatosis.

The finding of vacuolated fibroblasts on skin biopsy raised suspicion of a lysosomal storage disease. Prominent considerations within this group of disorders of predominantly autosomal recessive inheritance included GM_2 gangliosidosis (hexosaminidase A deficiency), commonly known as Tay-Sachs disease, and NPC. Ashkenazi Jews of Central and Eastern European ancestry are much more likely to develop some of these recessively inherited disorders, especially TSD.

There is an unusually high incidence (up to 50%) of psychosis in both TSD and NPC, and in the largest reported series of NPC cases (Sevin et al. 2007) psychosis was the most frequent presenting feature (in 38% of cases). Neurocognitive deterioration, psychosis, or both can predate neurological signs in NPC by up to 10 years, and, on average, 6–10 years elapse before the correct diagnosis is made (Staretz-Chacham et al. 2010). In TSD, acute psychotic episodes can occur with partial or complete remissions in early disease, with a presentation resembling disorganized schizophrenia in later stages. Less frequently, both NPC and TSD can present with unipolar depressive, schizoaffective, bipolar, or obsessive-compulsive disorder phenomenology (Neudorfer et al. 2005).

Supranuclear gaze palsy (particularly downgaze impairment; upgaze limitation can be seen in drug-induced parkinsonism and hydrocephalus) is a relatively specific pointer to NPC or TSD in a young adult with psychosis, and is thought to reflect involvement of the rostral interstitial nucleus of the medial longitudinal fasciculus. This may be evident first as loss of downward saccades on optokinetic testing. Ataxia, dysarthria, dysphagia, dystonia, pyramidal tract signs, and seizures occur commonly in both NPC and TSD. Cortical atrophy (especially frontal) and cerebellar atrophy are seen in NPC. Severe cerebellar atrophy and prominent ataxia and cerebellar tremor in TSD frequently lead to misdiagnosis of a spinocerebellar degeneration. Additional signs of TSD include lower motor neuron involvement (muscle cramps, weakness and muscle atrophy, and fasciculations), exaggerated tactile startle reflexes, absent triceps and patellar reflexes with crossed adductor responses, and peripheral neuropathy. The diagnosis of TSD is suggested by markedly reduced or absent beta-hexosaminidase A activity (in the face of preserved beta-hexosaminidase B activity) in leukocytes or skin fibroblasts, and it is confirmed by genetic testing (Kaback and Desnick 1999).

Additional pointers to NPC include a history of neonatal cholestatic jaundice; mild splenomegaly (detected on abdominal ultrasound in 45%–92%) (Sevin et al. 2007); and cataplexy. Myoclonic jerks and chorea can also occur. Mild diffuse white matter hyperintensity may also be seen on MRI scans in NPC. As in this case, the diagnosis is frequently challenging; it is usually made by the demonstration of filipin staining and markedly reduced cholesterol esterification capacity in skin fibroblasts. NPC can be confirmed by genetic testing, which is now clinically available in many laboratories worldwide (Patterson 2011).

Recently, building on findings from a transgenic mouse model, liquid chromatographic mass spectroscopy has demonstrated consistent and specific elevation of two oxysterols (cholesterol oxidation products) in plasma from patients with NPC. This method shows promise as a cost-effective screening tool for NPC (Jiang et al. 2011).

The detection of a lysosomal storage disease as the cause of psychosis has important ramifications for prognosis and treatment. Patients with a lysosomal storage disease are more sensitive to extrapyramidal side effects and catatonia with neuroleptic treatment. At the time the patient was evaluated, second-generation antipsychotics were not readily available. Today risperidone or olanzapine, rather than haloperidol, would be tried first. Concern has been raised about the use of neuroleptics, which exacerbate lipid storage in experimental models of NPC and TSD; conversely, valproic acid, a histone deacetylase inhibitor, restores defective cholesterol metabolism and cellular differentiation in a mouse model of NPC (Pipalia et al. 2011). Miglustat, a small iminosugar that reversibly inhibits glucosylceramide synthase and thereby decreases glycosphingolipid synthesis, has been shown to stabilize and sometimes improve neurological deficits in NPC (otherwise a relentlessly progressive and ultimately fatal neurocognitive disorder) in both animal models and recent clinical trials (Wraith et al. 2010).

Key Clinical Points

- While neurocognitive impairment is seen in some patients with schizophrenia, it is usually not prominent early on in the illness, and its presence in early psychosis warrants careful neurocognitive, neurological, and physical examination, and thorough investigation to rule out underlying medical and neurological disorders that can cause both neurocognitive impairment and psychosis.

- Clues to an underlying general medical or neurological condition may include attentional and memory impairment; eye movement abnormalities; unexplained movement disorders and/or marked susceptibility to extrapyramidal side effects of neuroleptics; pyramidal tract, cerebellar, lower motor neuron, and neuropathic findings; ocular abnormalities; and organomegaly and other signs of major organ involvement.
- Impaired vertical eye movements, particularly downgaze, may be a clue to a lysosomal storage disease, particularly adult-onset Niemann-Pick disease type C or Tay-Sachs disease.
- The presence of cerebellar and/or cortical atrophy unexplained by substance abuse may be a pointer to a lysosomal storage disease, although magnetic resonance imaging may be normal early in the course of NPC.
- When unexplained neurocognitive impairment is seen in early psychosis, diagnosis often requires a multidisciplinary approach involving psychiatrists, neurologists, neuropsychologists, laboratory physicians, and medical geneticists/metabolic disease experts.
- While lysosomal storage diseases are rare, the availability of new therapeutic approaches makes early diagnosis important.

Further Readings

Sampson EL, Warren JD, Rossor MN: Young onset dementia. Postgrad Med J 80:125–139, 2004

Sedel F, Baumann N, Turpin JC, et al: Psychiatric manifestations revealing inborn errors of metabolism in adolescents and adults. J Inherit Metab Dis 30:631–641, 2007

Staretz-Chacham O, Choi JH, Wakabayashi K, et al: Psychiatric and behavioral manifestations of lysosomal storage disorders. Am J Med Genet B Neuropsychiatr Genet 153B:1253–1265, 2010

Tang Y, Li H, Liu JP: Niemann-Pick disease type C: from molecule to clinic. Clin Exp Pharmacol Physiol 37:132–140, 2010

References

Bachmann S, Bottmer C, Schroder J: Neurological soft signs in first-episode schizophrenia: a follow-up study. Am J Psychiatry 162:2337–2343, 2005

Campo JV, Stowe R, Slomka G, et al: Psychosis as a presentation of physical disease in adolescence: a case of Niemann-Pick disease, type C. Dev Med Child Neurol 40:126–129, 1998

Jiang X, Sidhu R, Porter FD, et al: A sensitive and specific LC-MS/MS method for rapid diagnosis of Niemann-Pick C1 disease from human plasma. J Lipid Res 52:1435–1445, 2011

Kaback MM, Desnick RJ: Hexosaminidase A deficiency. GeneReviews [serial on-line] March 11, 1999. Available at: http://www.ncbi.nlm.nih.gov/ books/ NBK1218/. Accessed August 10, 2012.

Natowicz MR, Stoler JM, Prence EM, et al: Marked heterogeneity in Niemann-Pick disease, type C: clinical and ultrastructural findings. Clin Pediatr (Phila) 34:190–197, 1995

Neudorfer O, Pastores GM, Zeng BJ, et al: Late-onset Tay-Sachs disease: pheno-typic characterization and genotypic correlations in 21 affected patients. Genet Med 7:119–123, 2005

Patterson M: Niemann-Pick disease type C. GeneReviews [serial online] January 26, 2000. Available at: http://www.ncbi.nlm.nih.gov/books/NBK1296/. Ac-cessed August 10, 2012.

Pipalia NH, Cosner CC, Huang A, et al: Histone deacetylase inhibitor treatment dramatically reduces cholesterol accumulation in Niemann-Pick type C1 mutant human fibroblasts. Proc Natl Acad Sci U S A 108:5620–5625, 2011

Sevin M, Lesca G, Baumann N, et al: The adult form of Niemann-Pick disease type C. Brain 130:120–133, 2007

Staretz-Chacham O, Choi JH, Wakabayashi K, et al: Psychiatric and behavioral manifestations of lysosomal storage disorders. Am J Med Genet B Neuropsy-chiatr Genet 153B:1253–1265, 2010

Vincent A, Bien CG, Irani SR, et al: Autoantibodies associated with diseases of the CNS: new developments and future challenges. Lancet Neurol 10:759–772, 2011

Wraith JE, Vecchio D, Jacklin E, et al: Miglustat in adult and juvenile patients with Niemann-Pick disease type C: long-term data from a clinical trial. Mol Genet Metab 99:351–357, 2010

Cognitive-Intellectual Dysfunction in Multiple Sclerosis

Omar Ghaffar, M.Sc., M.D., F.R.C.P.C.

A 44-year-old right-handed black male was referred to a neuropsychia-try clinic by his family doctor for "anger and difficulty coping." He had been diagnosed with multiple sclerosis (MS) nearly two decades previ-ously. He lived in the suburbs with his wife (who accompanied him to the appointment) and their two teenage children. It had been a decade since he, a machinist by trade, had worked. He was being supported by a government disability pension and by his wife, a registered nurse. Still, he described his MS as "mild," because he could walk without an aid and drive.

His illness began in his late teens as acute episodes of diplopia, vertigo, and paresthesias in the lower extremities. These "attacks" or relapses would occur suddenly, once every year or so. They would typically last a few days before subsiding. In their aftermath, he would experience residual numbness and tingling in his legs for up to 2 days.

His most recent relapse was 4 years ago, the day he was to be best man at his brother-in-law's wedding. On the morning of the occasion, he awoke with vertigo so severe it caused him to vomit and left him almost unable to walk. He and his wife were unable to attend the ceremony. As he described the events of that day, his frustration was palpable. His voice shook, and he gripped his wife's hand tightly. Since missing the wedding, he had stopped attending his annual neurology appointments. He commented that aside from the ever-present numbness and tingling in his legs, he had not had any symptoms since he stopped seeing doctors. He said, "I haven't had an attack for so long that I forget I have MS. I can walk fine. I'm pretty much normal."

But there were problems. He and his son used to enjoy spending Sunday afternoons together, watching sports on television. A much-loved part of the ritual was the banter they would exchange as the action unfolded on screen. In the last few years, according to his wife, he had become an increasingly quiet spectator, immersing himself in the game to the exclusion of all else. When his son made a remark, he would mute the television and ask the boy to repeat himself. In addition to the Sunday trouble, he was having difficulty following conversations. He stopped attending social gatherings unless his wife could be at his side. She reported that his public persona had changed from "life of the party" to "strong, silent type."

Notes were strewn all about the family home—memos he had written to himself in regard to performing routine tasks. Misplacing wallet and keys, losing track of where the car was parked at the mall, and repeating the same stories at the dinner table had all become regular occurrences for him. Sometimes while driving he would forget his destination. Three years ago, there was a minor accident in which he rear-ended another car, ostensibly due to poor visibility. Fortunately, no one was injured.

Although he was generally able to maintain his composure in public, at home he had daily episodes of frustration triggered by forgetting or misplacing something. He ruminated on "mistakes" he had made, often lying in bed for hours before falling asleep. He endorsed other recurring, self-deprecating thoughts—negative cognitions of feeling "useless" and guilt for not financially contributing to his family. He suspected that others doubted his illness and wondered why he did not work. Appetite, weight, and libido were stable. There was daytime fatigue, particularly toward evening, when he reported, "My legs feel tired and my brain feels scrambled," symptoms that were noticeably worse in the summertime. He had difficulty making decisions because "I don't trust myself." However, he denied suicidal ideation and thoughts of self-harm.

The remainder of the psychiatric history was unremarkable. On review of systems, he endorsed that his legs felt "tired" toward the end of the day. He also described a persistent pins-and-needles sensation over both lower extremities that occasionally became anesthetic. There was no bladder, bowel, or sexual dysfunction.

He had one standard drink per month. He did not use tobacco products and had never used recreational drugs. He took no medication and had no drug allergies.

His psychiatric history and medical history were noncontributory. There was no history of head injury, seizure, or toxic occupational exposures.

His sister had lupus and died at the age of 20. There was no additional family neuropsychiatric history, including MS, other autoimmune disorders, or dementia.

He ambulated without aid and did not have any difficulty sitting down or standing up. He was fully cooperative with the assessment, notwithstanding his admission that he would have preferred to avoid the appointment. His affect was marked by worry and frustration. At times, he was reactive to information provided by his wife, arguing about details with her, albeit at a normal volume. His speech was fluent. There were noticeable pauses before he answered questions. Once he began talking, however, he was overinclusive and often had to be gently redirected. He occasionally perseverated on responses to earlier questions. He answered inappropriately at times, seeming to not quite grasp the question; for example, when asked about his current mood, he answered that he was "happy-go-lucky." Thought content was negative for obsessions or delusional material. There was no suicidal ideation. There was no perceptual disturbance. Insight into his difficulties was poor.

His MMSE score was 22/30. He lost 2 points each on orientation, attention, and 5-minute recall. He lost 1 point each on repetition and three-stage command. Clock drawing was normal with respect to contour and number placement; however, "10 after 11" was set at positions 10 and 2, with the hour and minute hands being of the same length. On the Frontal Assessment Battery, he scored 10/18, losing 1 point for similarities, 2 points each for the Luria test and conflicting instructions, and 3 points for go/no-go.

Visual acuity was 20/25 bilaterally. The remainder of the cranial nerve exam was normal. Muscle bulk, tone, and strength were normal. Reflexes were grade 2+ and symmetrical. The left plantar response was extensor. Bilaterally, in the lower extremities, vibration at the medial malleoli was diminished, and joint position sense was impaired at the distal interphalangeal joints. He had difficulty with fine motor dexterity of both hands. There was mild right-leg ataxia. He was unable to manage a tandem gait.

He had cognitive-intellectual dysfunction due to MS. He also had depressive symptoms, which were potentially contributing to his neuropsychological deficits.

Initial psychoeducation was provided to him and his wife regarding cognitive-intellectual dysfunction in MS. Referral to community occupational therapy was made to assess his functioning in the home. Consultation from neuropsychology was requested for detailed testing and recommendations of how he might manage his deficits. He agreed to follow up with his neurologist in the MS clinic. Arrangements were made for contrast-enhanced MRI brain and spine scans to assess disease activity. He and his wife were given the contact information for the local chapter of the MS society.

A trial of an SSRI was initiated for management of his irritability and feelings of frustration. The anticholinergic effects and risk of sexual dysfunction were emphasized to husband and wife so possible side effects would not be mistaken for symptoms of MS.

Local legislation mandated that the Ministry of Transportation of the Province of Ontario be notified of his condition. This legal requirement was discussed at length with him and his wife. The Ministry of Transportation was notified that his safety on the road might be compromised by cognitive-intellectual decline, and a road test was recommended.

At the second visit, he reported that the antidepressant had been well tolerated. Bouts of frustration and ruminative thoughts had significantly diminished. He still had negative thoughts about himself, albeit less frequently. His license was revoked after he failed a road test he had paid to take. Although he described this as a "big blow," he said that failing the road test validated his disability, which actually gave him some comfort. He and his wife had begun attending a monthly support group through the MS society.

He saw his neurologist in follow-up, and the neurologist's report indicated that he had been diagnosed with MS 18 years ago and had had a relapsing-remitting disease course. He had received interferon beta-1a for 2 years. This was replaced with glatiramer acetate, which he discontinued after the first dose due to an injection site reaction. He had declined further disease-modifying treatment. The results of an MRI scan completed since his last appointment at the neuropsychiatry clinic are shown in Figure 10–4. He was now in the secondary-progressive phase of his illness.

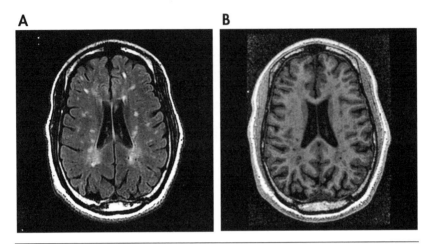

FIGURE 10–4.   Magnetic resonance imaging brain scans of patient with multiple sclerosis.
(A) Fluid-attenuated inversion recovery (FLAIR) image showing periventricular, deep white matter, and juxtacortical white matter hyperintensities. (B) T1 image (unenhanced) showing hypointense lesions.

Detailed neuropsychological testing demonstrated impairment in multiple cognitive-intellectual domains. The neuropsychologist's report commented that on the visual memory task the patient seemed to give up easily, feeling frustrated by difficulties manipulating the pencil. This was not an issue with tests administered orally. Table 10–1 summarizes his cognitive-intellectual performance. At the time of testing, his score on the Beck Depression Inventory—Second Edition was 15, in the "mild" depression range, suggesting that his mood might be exacerbating but not causing his cognitive-intellectual impairment. The neuropsychologist gave detailed feedback to him and his wife, recommending that he use a memory book (and take his time writing in it) to help keep track of things, instead of the haphazard system of notes he had previously used. It was also suggested that he try to give himself more time to process information—for example, by politely asking people speaking to him to slow down. His wife was advised that crucial information might be best conveyed without unnecessary detail. He was also referred to a cognitive support group.

TABLE 10–1. Patient's performance on the Minimal Assessment of Cognitive Function in MS

Cognitive domain	Test	Percentile
Attention and psychomotor speed	PASAT (3-second version)	1
	PASAT (2-second version)	<0.1
	Symbol Digit Modalities Test	<0.1
Learning and memory	CVLT-II total learning	1
	CVLT-II delayed recall	1
	BVMT-R total learning	<0.1
	BVMT-R delayed recall	<0.1
Executive functions	D-KEFS sorting task correct sorts	3
	D-KEFS sorting task description score	3
Visual perception and spatial orientation	Judgment of Line Orientation	10
Verbal fluency	Controlled Oral Word Association Test	32

Note. Percentiles are derived from age-, gender-, and education-corrected z scores (i.e., standardized to the normal population). The five cognitive domains most often affected in multiple sclerosis are represented. BVMT-R=Brief Visuospatial Memory Test—Revised; CVLT-II=California Verbal Learning Test—Second Edition; D-KEFS= Delis-Kaplan Executive Function System; PASAT=Paced Auditory Serial Addition Test.

The occupational therapist recommended a stove alarm, which automatically shuts off the appliance if unattended. Although difficulty with fine motor function of his hands necessitated increased time to dress, he did not regard this as a problem.

Discussion

Cognitive-intellectual deficits affect 40%–60% of MS patients and are closely associated with difficulties in employment, relationships, and activities of daily living (Chiaravalloti and DeLuca 2008). Driving safety may also be compromised (Schultheis et al. 2010). Although the pattern and course of cognitive-intellectual problems vary between individuals, deficits in attention, psychomotor speed, multiple memory systems, and executive function are common (Prakash et al. 2008) and may be present at the earliest stages of the disease. These difficulties are independent of disease course and correlate weakly with physical disability.

In clinical settings, the detection of cognitive-intellectual dysfunction in MS is challenged by the insensitivity of generic screening tools such as the MMSE. The aphasia, agnosia, and apraxia that typify classic "cortical" dementing syndromes are generally absent in MS. The 45-minute Brief Repeatable Battery of Neuropsychological Tests (BRB-N) and 90-minute Minimal Assessment of Cognitive Function in MS (MACFIMS) have good psychometric properties and have been validated in MS populations (Strober et al. 2009). Nonetheless, their routine administration in a busy, general neuropsychiatry clinic without a dedicated psychometrist may be impractical. For small centers with few staff, the Brief International Cognitive Assessment for Multiple Sclerosis (BICAMS) was developed by expert consensus (Langdon et al. 2012). The BICAMS takes only 15 minutes to administer and requires no specialized equipment or expertise in cognitive-intellectual assessment. It consists of the Symbol Digit Modalities Test (SDMT, for attention and information-processing speed), the California Verbal Learning Test—Second Edition (first five recall trials for verbal memory), and the Brief Visuospatial Memory Test—Revised (first three recall trials for visual memory). If only 5 minutes is available for cognitive-intellectual screening of MS patients, the BICAMS committee recommends the SDMT—a sensitive, reliable, easily administered test that correlates with various indices of MRI-elicited brain pathology in MS. Ecological validity of the SDMT is supported by significant associations with current and future employment status (Langdon et al. 2012).

Cognitive-intellectual deficits correlate with various brain imaging metrics in MS (Filippi et al. 2010). Early studies emphasized modest associations with lesion loads. More recently, brain atrophy has emerged as a strong predictor of cognitive-intellectual dysfunction. To what extent these associations can be further refined by measurements of regional volume loss (e.g., cortical atrophy, hippocampal atrophy, thalamic atrophy) is an active area of research. In addition, pathology in normal-appearing brain tissue is now appreciated by diffusion tensor imaging, magnetic resonance spectroscopy, and magnetic transfer imaging. Increased magnetic field strength and double inversion recovery MRI sequences readily reveal cortical lesions, the majority of which had been undetectable with conventional MRI deployed in a clinical setting. Taken together, contemporary neuroimaging techniques offer a plethora of variables, some of which may be associated with cognitive-intellectual dysfunction. A significant challenge to neuropsychiatric inquiry will be to disentangle these highly interrelated magnetic resonance–based measures and identify those of most relevance to behavioral sequelae of the disease.

Evidence-based treatments for cognitive-intellectual dysfunction in MS are lacking. An initial study suggesting a possible role for donepezil was not supported by a subsequent multicenter trial (Krupp et al. 2011). Studies of modafinil and methylphenidate have been small and contradictory, with methodological limitations. Large, multicenter trials of disease-modifying treatment generally do not include neuropsychological function as one of the primary outcome variables. What little data there are tend to favor interferon beta-1a (Patti et al. 2010).

Support for rehabilitative treatment is also sparse. A recent development, however, suggests that cognitive-intellectual reserve (or simply "cognitive reserve"), a theoretical construct defined as the brain's resilience to neuropathological damage (Stern 2009), may protect against cognitive-intellectual compromise. Premorbid intelligence (Sumowski et al. 2010a) and cognitive leisure activities (Sumowski et al. 2010b) are hypothesized to enhance cognitive-intellectual reserve, raising the possibility that engaging in intellectually enriching activities may delay or deter the onset of cognitive-intellectual dysfunction in MS patients. However, it has yet to be demonstrated that an intellectually stimulating lifestyle can protect against neuropsychological dysfunction in MS.

Key Clinical Points

- Neuropsychological deficits affect 40%–60% of multiple sclerosis patients and are closely associated with difficulties in employment, relationships, and activities of daily living.

- Deficits in attention, psychomotor speed, multiple memory systems, and executive function are common and may be present at the earliest disease stages.

- In many patients, cognitive-intellectual deficits do not correlate with indices of physical disability; objective cognitive-intellectual screening is therefore essential.

- The Mini-Mental State Examination is relatively insensitive to cognitive-intellectual deficits in MS. The Symbol Digit Modalities Test is a sensitive and reliable screening test and takes only 5 minutes to administer.

- When screening for cognitive-intellectual dysfunction in MS, it is important to consider depressive symptoms as a possible exacerbating factor that can be treated.

- Evidence-based treatments for cognitive-intellectual dysfunction in MS are lacking, though this is an active area of research. Psychoeducation, identification and treatment of comorbidities (e.g., depression), and development of compensatory strategies ideally involve a comprehensive, multidisciplinary approach.

Further Readings

Benedict RHB, Zivadinov R: Risk factors for and management of cognitive dysfunction in multiple sclerosis. Nat Rev Neurol 7:332–342, 2011

Feinstein A: The Clinical Neuropsychiatry of Multiple Sclerosis, 2nd Edition. Cambridge, UK, Cambridge University Press, 2007, pp 115–213

Langdon DW: Cognition in multiple sclerosis. Curr Opin Neurol 24:244–249, 2011

References

Chiaravalloti ND, DeLuca J: Cognitive impairment in multiple sclerosis. Lancet Neurol 7:1139–1151, 2008

Filippi M, Rocca MA, Benedict RH, et al: The contribution of MRI in assessing cognitive impairment in multiple sclerosis. Neurology 75:2121–2128, 2010

Krupp LB, Christodoulou C, Melville P, et al: Multicenter randomized clinical trial of donepezil for memory impairment in multiple sclerosis. Neurology 76:1500–1507, 2011

Langdon DW, Amato MP, Boringa J, et al: Recommendations for a Brief International Cognitive Assessment for Multiple Sclerosis (BICAMS). Mult Scler 18:891–898, 2012

Patti F, Amato MP, Bastianello S, et al: Effects of immunomodulatory treatment with subcutaneous interferon beta-1a on cognitive decline in mildly disabled patients with relapsing-remitting multiple sclerosis. Mult Scler 16:68–77, 2010

Prakash R, Snook E, Lewis J, et al: Cognitive impairments in relapsing-remitting multiple sclerosis: a meta-analysis. Mult Scler 14:1250–1261, 2008

Schultheis MT, Weisser V, Ang J, et al: Examining the relationship between cognition and driving performance in multiple sclerosis. Arch Phys Med Rehabil 91:465–472, 2010

Stern Y: Cognitive reserve. Neuropsychologia 47:2015–2028, 2009

Strober L, Englert J, Munschauer F, et al: Sensitivity of conventional memory tests in multiple sclerosis: comparing the Rao Brief Repeatable Neuropsychological Battery and the Minimal Assessment of Cognitive Function in MS. Mult Scler 15:1077–1084, 2009

Sumowski JF, Wylie GR, Chiaravalloti N, et al: Intellectual enrichment lessens the effect of brain atrophy on learning and memory in multiple sclerosis. Neurology 74:1942–1945, 2010a

Sumowski JF, Wylie GR, Gonnella A, et al: Premorbid cognitive leisure independently contributes to cognitive reserve in multiple sclerosis. Neurology 75:1428–1431, 2010b

---

Postconcussive Syndrome and Depression After Mild Traumatic Brain Injury

Robert M. Rohrbaugh, M.D.

A 52-year-old married white woman slipped on a wet floor and landed on the back of her head on a concrete floor. Her daughter reported that she was unconscious for about 30 seconds; afterward she was "pretty foggy" but coherent, and had no memory of the event or her activities immediately before and after the event. Characteristically stoic and independent, she refused to go to the hospital: "I'm not even bleeding." She had trouble sleeping that night because of a severe headache.

The next morning, she continued to have a headache and felt dizzy and tired. She was unsure whether she would be able to safely operate the machine that she used in her job and so did not go to work. Over the next few days she continued to have difficulty with balance, slight confusion, and headache. Although her balance slowly improved, she continued to feel unsteady.

Five days after her fall, she went back to work at half-time. Her daughter drove her because she was unsure of her coordination. At work she had to "think extra hard" to remember the sequence of steps that were involved in her job, even though this was routine work for her. By midday her headache had worsened and she felt very tired. The rest of that week was similar and when at home she would rest, instead of cooking and cleaning the house. Because her fatigue continued, she consulted her primary care physician, who diagnosed "symptoms of a concussion" and reassured her that the symptoms were likely to remit. The physician signed a note to her employer suggesting another 2 weeks of working half-time. As another 2 weeks passed, her daughter became resentful that her mother was not contributing to the household chores and that she was obligated to drive her mother to and from work. Her husband began to make comments about "beginning to get lazy in your old age."

She became upset when she was unable to balance the family accounts and so returned to her primary care physician. Because of the cognitive-intellectual symptoms, she was referred to a neurologist. His examination had normal findings, but he did note difficulties with concentration and calculation as measured by serial 7s. The neurologist ordered an EEG and a CT scan, both of which were normal. An MRI brain scan demonstrated "several very small bilateral punctuate regions of hyperintensity in the frontal lobes," thought to be consistent with microhemorrhages. His diagnosis was a "contra-coup frontal lobe syndrome."

She felt increased pressure at work and at home. Her boss frequently reminded her of her lost productivity. Her daughter began openly complaining about the extra work, and her husband commented that she "wasn't keeping herself up." She also lost her libido. She and her husband had not had sexual relations since the time of her accident.

The thought that she might "be this way for the rest of my life" began to preoccupy her. She attempted to work full-time, but both she and her employer found errors in the work she completed in the afternoon, when her fatigue was most prominent. Losing her job was a constant source of worry. Her daughter reported that she was irritable and easily upset. She felt that her daughter was implicitly criticizing her whenever the daughter ran an errand on her behalf, activities that she used to do herself. The mother felt unable to manage her home, which had been a source of great pride for her. These problems made her feel increasingly "stupid," a word her alcoholic father used to berate her when she was growing up. She lay awake at night thinking that what her father had predicted ("you'll never have a happy family or be able to take care of yourself") had come true.

Another 2 months passed. She and her employer decided that she should go on disability. She felt depressed, with daily crying spells, had difficulty sleeping, and had gained weight as a result of, she believed, not being as active as usual. She continued to have problems concentrating, often either skipping or adding ingredients twice when cooking. One day, she reported beginning to hear a scratching sound "like a fingernail on a blackboard" throughout the day and night. No one else heard it. Over the course of a week, the sound became louder and louder. When she talked about it, her family would laugh and call her "crazy." Ten days later, she reported that the house was filled with a swarm of bees that had chewed through a wall.

At this point, she was referred for neuropsychiatric assessment. A screening neuropsychological examination showed mild difficulties with attention and short-term memory. Because many of her symptoms were consistent with depression, and after a screen for medical causes of depression was negative, sertraline 25 mg/day was begun and was increased to 50 mg/day after 2 weeks. She was seen weekly for supportive psychotherapy and medication monitoring. A primary focus was addressing her ruminative cognitive distortions about her life trajectory and helping her to see that in fact, her father's prophecy had not been accurate: she had developed a successful career and had a relatively happy family but unfortunately had sustained a mild traumatic brain injury (MTBI), which was now disrupting her life. Although her husband refused to participate in therapy, she was seen with her daughter on several occasions to discuss their relationship and be provided education that her symptoms, including her hyperacusis, were due to MTBI. She was able to diminish her sensitivity to her daughter's statements about doing errands, and her daughter was able to better understand the etiology of the functional changes that had occurred in her mother.

After 4 weeks of neuropsychiatric treatment, she was referred to a traumatic brain injury (TBI) rehabilitation clinic. After negotiating with her disability insurance company to ensure her benefits would not be affected, she was referred to a state work evaluation program and within 2 months was able to find part-time employment stocking shelves at a drugstore 4 mornings a week. Although she missed her old job, she enjoyed the collegiality of working with others and contributing to her household's income.

Eight weeks after beginning treatment, both she and her daughter reported that she had improved mood, fewer crying episodes, fewer arguments with her daughter, better self-esteem, and mild improvement in sleep. She began wearing earplugs to decrease everyday environmental noise, which she believed contributed to her irritability. She continued to feel fatigued in the afternoons and had difficulty with concentration and poor libido, but she had improvement in the frequency of her headaches. The dosage of sertraline was slowly increased to 150 mg/day, but these symptoms were not reduced. Augmentation strategies for treatment of depression did little to improve her symptoms. The addition of methylphenidate up to 30 mg/day resulted in some initial response but no sustained improvement.

After 3 months of weekly treatment, she began to be seen on a once-per-month basis for medication monitoring, continued supportive psychotherapy, and occasional follow-up sessions with her daughter. One year after the injury, she continued to have mild cognitive-intellectual and depressive symptoms but had improved functioning in her social and new occupational roles. She also had found great solace in an MTBI support group, where she became a mentor to new members.

Discussion

The yearly incidence of TBI in the United States is 180–250 per 100,000 people. Risk factors for sustaining a TBI include age (very young, adolescent, young adult, and old adult), male sex, urban dwelling, and lower socioeconomic class (Williams et al. 2010). Having one TBI is a risk factor for sustaining another head injury. Although fewer than two million unique patients are affected each year, incidence data suggest that TBIs are among the most frequent of neuropsychiatric disorders.

Approximately 80% of TBIs are classified as MTBIs, defined as a brief loss of consciousness, a Glasgow Coma Scale score of ≥13, and a posttraumatic amnesia of ≤24 hours (Iverson 2006; Williams et al. 2010). In many clinical settings, the terms *mild traumatic brain injury* (or MTBI) and *concussion* are used interchangeably. The postconcussive syndrome is a set of symptoms that follows MTBI and produces disturbances in three domains: cognitive-intellectual (including attention and memory), affect (including depression, irritability, and lability) and physical well-being (including dizziness, fatigue, and headache). Approximately 80% of MTBI patients can expect to have full resolution of postconcussive symptoms within 6 months, and for most patients full resolution will occur within 2 weeks of the injury (McCrea et al. 2009). There is some evidence that cognitive-intellectual and physical symptoms may resolve before the affective symptoms.

Despite this generally good prognosis, up to 15% of patients with MTBI may have persistent symptoms (Williams et al. 2010). Risk factors for a poorer prognosis include preexisting psychiatric or neurological disorders, older age at the time of injury, female sex, and having a specific finding on a CT or MRI scan. Patients with an abnormality on neuroimaging are sometimes classified as having a "complicated" MTBI and may have worse cognitive-intellectual outcomes (Iverson 2006). As more sophisticated imaging techniques have been used, higher rates of brain lesions have been identified. In one series using both MRI and SPECT, nearly 80% of MTBI patients had identifiable lesions, most notably hypoperfusion on SPECT scanning. Six-month follow-up of patients with hypoperfusion demonstrated brain atrophy, suggesting the possibility of secondary ischemic brain damage. Interestingly, in this study there was only a weak correlation between neuroimaging findings and neurocognitive outcomes (Hoffman et al. 2001).

Depression after TBI is common, although incidence rates have varied widely. These widely varying rates may be due to difficulties determining whether symptoms should be ascribed to depression or are primarily related to the TBI, as well as to differences in rates of depression relative to TBI severity. For example, the most frequent symptoms following MTBI include fatigue, irritability, frustration, and poor concentration (Kreutzer et al. 2001), symptoms that overlap significantly with those of depression. A recent study by Bombardier et al. (2010) reported that the incidence of depression in the first year after TBI in a mixed group of patients with mild-to-severe injuries was approximately 50%, with most episodes having onset within the first 3 months after the TBI. Risk of depression in this mixed-severity TBI population was associated with a previous history of TBI, younger age, and lifetime history of alcohol dependence. Depression in the first year was also associated with greater problems with physical mobility, usual activities, pain/discomfort, and role functioning 12 months after the TBI (Bombardier et al. 2010). In a recent study of MTBI patients, depression was present in about 20% of patients (Rao et al. 2010).

The reason that the course of recovery from TBI is often complicated by depression is not yet well understood. Structural brain damage is but one of multiple factors that may be involved in the depression of individuals who have sustained a mechanical blow to the head. Psychosocial factors may be equally or more important. One report suggests a more direct effect of the injury itself, and left frontal lobe TBIs have been associated with post-TBI depression (Jorge et al. 2004). It is also important to note that MTBIs may initially cause white matter changes that localize to left hemisphere tracts as well as the corpus callosum. These changes may not be identified using standard imaging techniques, but they can be identified using diffusion tensor imaging (Mayer et al. 2010). Moreover, functional MRI studies have demonstrated that patients with MTBI have changes in activation and allocation of working memory processing circuits despite performing as well as healthy control subjects (McAllister et al. 2006). Although these imaging techniques are currently not indicated for routine use in the care of MTBI patients, in the near future it may be possible to link these discrete brain changes to the emotional and cognitive-intellectual symptoms experienced by patients with MTBI.

There is a paucity of literature on the treatment of post-TBI depression. A recent systematic review (Fann et al. 2009) found only one Class I study (evidence classified using American Academy of Neurology criteria), with 52 patients randomized to either sertraline or placebo. In this study, 59% of the sertraline group were responders (50% decrease in Hamilton Rating Scale for Depression score), whereas only 32% of the placebo group were responders (Ashman et al. 2009).

In a Class II study lasting only 4 weeks, 30 patients were randomly assigned to receive either sertraline or methylphenidate. Both interventions showed greater improvement in Hamilton Rating Scale for Depression scores compared with placebo. Patients receiving methylphenidate (but not sertraline) had additional improvements in cognition, alertness, and postconcussive symptoms (Fann et al. 2009). The systematic review (Fann et al. 2009) suggested that treatment begin with a low dose of an SSRI (sertraline or citalopram), with slow upward titration and close monitoring. No recommendations about psychotherapy or rehabilitation interventions could be made because of the poor quality of the trials.

Clinicians must take a careful history regarding TBI when seeing new patients with depression. For patients with a TBI, clinicians should develop a comprehensive formulation and treatment plan that takes into account all potential biological, psychological, and social issues. The organic workup in patients with TBI includes neuroimaging and preferably an MRI scan, which is much superior to a CT scan in identifying white matter disease and microhemorrhages. Taking a psychologically informed developmental history of events preceding the TBI is essential.

This patient's treatment included a pharmacological approach but also addressed long-standing vulnerabilities in her self-esteem from an early abusive environment. Patients with TBIs often have a sense of dependence on others and loss of control and self-esteem, which may activate latent psychological vulnerabilities that can be addressed in a supportive psychotherapy. In the social arena, there is inevitably family distress that can be mitigated through education of the patient and family members. This patient's family called her "crazy" when she was hearing the chewing sounds, before it was discovered that hyperacusis was the cause and that wearing earplugs helped. Engagement in work rehabilitation may allow the individual to resume former social roles. For some, joining a TBI support group and helping others with the condition is a meaningful intervention.

This patient had a postconcussive syndrome and depression after MTBI accompanied by significant decline in psychosocial functioning and distress in her family. She responded to a comprehensive intervention that included pharmacotherapy, psychotherapy, family therapy, and psychosocial rehabilitation.

Key Clinical Points

- Traumatic brain injuries are among the most frequent of neuropsychiatric disorders, and approximately 80% of TBIs are classified as mild TBIs.
- The cognitive-intellectual, emotional, and physical symptoms of

MTBI usually resolve within 2 weeks of injury.

- Complicated MTBIs may have persistent symptoms that can have devastating effects on psychosocial function.
- Depression after TBI is common and can add to functional impairment.
- Selective serotonin reuptake inhibitors are indicated for the treatment of depression following TBI.
- A comprehensive evaluation and biopsychosocial formulation are necessary to develop an individualized care plan that addresses workup, pharmacological and psychological treatments, and social and functional rehabilitation. A team of clinicians may be needed to fully implement the treatment plan.

Further Readings

McCrea M, Iverson GL, Hammeke TA, et al: An integrated review of recovery after mild traumatic brain injury (MTBI): implications for clinical management. Clin Neuropsychol 23:1368–1390, 2009

Williams WH, Potter S, Ryland H: Mild traumatic brain injury and postconcussion syndrome: a neuropsychological perspective. J Neurol Neurosurg Psychiatry 81:1116–1122, 2010

References

Ashman TA, Cantor JB, Katon WJ: A randomized controlled trial of sertraline for the treatment of depression in persons with traumatic brain injury. Arch Phys Med Rehabil 90:733–740, 2009

Bombardier CH, Fann JR, Temkin NR, et al: Rates of major depressive disorder and clinical outcomes following traumatic brain injury. JAMA 303:1938–1945, 2010

Fann JR, Hart T, Schomer KG: Treatment for depression after traumatic brain injury: a systematic review. J Neurotrauma 26:2383–2402, 2009

Hoffman PA, Stapert SZ, van Kroonenburgh MJPG, et al: MR imaging, single-photon emission CT, and neurocognitive performance after mild traumatic brain injury. AJNR Am J Neuroradiol 22:441–449, 2001

Iverson GL: Complicated vs uncomplicated mild traumatic brain injury: acute neuropsychological outcome. Brain Inj 20:13–14, 2006

Jorge RE, Robinson RG, Moser D, et al: Major depression following traumatic brain injury. Arch Gen Psychiatry 61:42–50, 2004

Kreutzer JS, Seel RT, Gourley E: The prevalence and symptom rates of depression after traumatic brain injury: a comprehensive examination. Brain Inj 15:563–576, 2001

Mayer AR, Ling J, Mannell MV, et al: A prospective diffusion tensor imaging study in mild traumatic brain injury. Neurology 74:643–650, 2010

McAllister TW, Flashman LA, McDonald BC, et al: Mechanisms of working memory dysfunction after mild and moderate TBI: evidence from functional MRI and neurogenetics. J Neurotrauma 23:1450–1467, 2006

Rao V, Bertrand M, Rosenberg P, et al: Predictors of new-onset depression after mild traumatic brain injury. J Neuropsychiatry Clin Neurosci 22:100–104, 2010

Tuberous Sclerosis Mistaken for Attention-Deficit/Hyperactivity Disorder

Pieter Joost van Wattum, M.D., M.A., D.F.A.A.C.A.P.

A 10-year-old boy was referred by his school to a child psychiatrist for assessment of possible attention-deficit/hyperactivity disorder (ADHD). In the classroom he was absentminded, needed regular prompts to pay attention, and was unable to finish his work on time. His grades were consequently poor. However, he was able to do his homework with minimal assistance and always received good grades for this. There was no evidence of hyperactive or impulsive behaviors. Although somewhat withdrawn, he was well liked by his peers. He was only recently enrolled in his current school, and due to frequent previous moves, sometimes more than once a year, there was no record of his academic performance, a history of special education services, or intelligence testing. His adoptive mother reported that she had not noticed inattention problems at home. However, several months prior to his visit to the psychiatrist's office, she had noticed that he had an occasional abnormal gait with instability while walking. In addition, she had noticed that he had difficulty following a two- or three-step command, particularly regarding self-care or minor chores in the home. She had not observed mood, anxiety, or psychotic symptoms, and his sleep pattern was age appropriate. She reported that a visit with the pediatrician for evaluation of his skin condition was pending.

Upon examination in the office, he appeared as a well-groomed, friendly, somewhat shy boy, looking his stated age. His eye contact was limited but improved as the interview progressed. Obvious light patches, some several inches long, were scattered on the skin of his face and bare arms. His mother stated that these had been present for a few months but with possible recent improvement. He was cooperative with the examination but, when addressed, seemed to have difficulty concentrating on the questions and there was a slight delay in his responses. He was soft-spoken, and his speech was mildly slurred. His affect was somewhat blunted. His mood was reported to be good, and he denied recent mood changes. His thought process was slow but coherent, logical, and goal directed. He denied suicidal or homicidal ideation, as well as delusions. There were no psychotic symptoms observed or reported. He was alert and oriented, following the conversation and confirming the facts stated by his mother or correcting them politely. He was able to recall three objects immediately and two objects after 3 minutes, the third with cues. He was able to follow a three-step command: taking a piece of paper, folding it, and handing it to the examiner. His insight and judgment were age appropriate.

A neurological examination revealed that he had motor difficulty. He could not stand on one leg and had difficulty placing one foot in front of the other when trying to walk a straight line. Strength in his left arm was slightly less than in his right arm. His tongue deviated to the right when protruded. The rest of the examination was unremarkable, including an absent Romberg sign.

Review of systems indicated that he did not have a previous psychiatric history. His medical history was unremarkable until recently. There was no history of seizures or head trauma. He had no drug allergies and was not taking any medication. His developmental history was significant for prematurity, but the extent was unclear due to his birth mother's absence from his life. No information was available about possible exposure to drugs in utero or developmental delays. He had been held back in school once. It was unclear whether this was simply related to his frequent moves and subsequent inability to adjust to different school curricula and catch up with his work. Although currently enrolled in the fourth-grade regular education class, he was overall functioning on a third-grade level. He excelled in spelling, was reading at a second-grade level, and had difficulty with mathematics. There were no behavioral concerns. He would quietly participate when engaged. His peer interactions were reported to be limited and mostly initiated by his classmates. There was no known history of obsessions, compulsions, preoccupations, or perceptual abnormalities. His biological family had a reported psychiatric history that included ADHD, substance dependence, and anxiety disorder.

His differential diagnosis included ADHD, predominantly inattentive type; reading disorder; mathematics disorder; pervasive developmental disorder; mild mental retardation; and cognitive disorder due to a general medical condition such as tuberous sclerosis. Vanderbilt rating scales (Wolraich et al. 2003) filled out by his adoptive mother and two of his teachers to assess for the presence of ADHD symptoms in school or at home revealed minor concentration problems but did not support a diagnosis of ADHD. Intelligence testing with the Wechsler Intelligence Scale for Children—Fourth Edition was performed and revealed the following scores: Verbal Comprehension Index, 83; Perceptual Reasoning Index, 75; Processing Speed Index, 60; Working Memory Index, 69; and Full Scale IQ, 72. These scores placed him in the borderline range of intellectual functioning.

A pediatrician-performed physical examination revealed a small tumor on the right side of his tongue; hypomelanotic macules on the skin of his face, upper body, and arms; and two raised, rough patches on his lower back. No other abnormalities were found. He was referred to the ear, nose, and throat specialist for assessment of the tumor on his tongue. An MRI scan of the head and neck revealed several cortical and subcortical lesions in the right temporal lobe. A neurological reassessment confirmed his previous gait ataxia. No other abnormalities were found. Genetic testing revealed a mutation on chromosome 9 of *TSC1*, confirming the diagnosis of tuberous sclerosis.

In the months following his evaluation and workup, his school implemented an individual education plan (IEP). He was placed in a smaller classroom and received special education services to remediate his reading and mathematics. He made significant gains in his reading skills within weeks of initiation of the IEP, indicating that his reading delay was due to the disruption from his frequent moves prior to placement in his current school rather than due to cognitive-intellectual compromise from tuberous sclerosis.

Discussion

Tuberous sclerosis, or tuberous sclerosis complex (TSC), is a rare multisystem autosomal dominant disorder characterized by benign tumors (hamartomas) in the brain, heart, kidneys, skin, and eyes as well as pulmonary lymphangioleiomyomatosis (pulmonary cyst formation). Comorbid neuropsychiatric disorders such as epilepsy, intellectual disability, behavioral dysregulation, and sleep disorders are common. Up to 50% of children with TSC meet criteria for autism or a pervasive developmental disorder, and ADHD is present in about half of children diagnosed with TSC. Learning disorders are also common in TSC patients with otherwise normal intelligence (Au et al. 2007; D'Agati et al. 2009; Jansen et al. 2008).

TSC can present at any age and affects all races and both sexes equally. TSC occurs in up to 60,000 individuals in the United States and 1–2 million worldwide, with an estimated prevalence of 1 in 6,000 newborns. Many patients have minimal symptoms and no neurological disease. The diagnosis is based on clinical findings (Yohay and Denckla 2008).

Epilepsy (often intractable), cognitive-intellectual delay, or autism is usually the first clue to the presence of TSC (Bolton 2004; Crino 2010). Other first signs include hypomelanotic macules, or "ash leaf spots," and a cardiac rhabdomyoma. In addition to the ash leaf spots, a variety of skin abnormalities may be present and can assist in the diagnosis. These abnormalities include facial angiofibromas (adenoma sebaceum), forehead plaques, shagreen patches (leathery skin found on the lower back), and ungual or subungual fibromas on the nails of fingers and toes.

Confirmation of the diagnosis is based on the demonstration of tubers in the brain through neuroimaging (CT or MRI); tubers in the kidneys, liver, or heart through ultrasound or CT; or typical retinal lesions through an eye examination. Infantile spasms (seizures) in infants may confirm a diagnosis in very young children, but many children are not diagnosed until later in life, coming to the attention of physicians because of angiofibromas, ash leaf spots, or seizures. The tubers in the brain are mostly responsible for the neurological manifestations of TSC; however, other neuropathological changes may also contribute, and the number of tubers has been shown to be correlated with the severity of symptoms (Crino 2010). Minor changes in the subcortical white matter and subcortical structures, such as the thalamus and cerebellum, may contribute to neuropsychological manifestations of TSC, including autism (Boer et al. 2008; Ridler et al. 2001).

TSC was first known as Bourneville's disease, named after a nineteenth-century French physician who, because of tubers' resemblance to potatoes, named the disorder *sclérose tubéreuse*. Initially considered a lifelong, potentially crippling disease, it is now considered a genetic disorder with a high spontaneous mutation rate, and less than a third of patients with TSC have the classic constellation of symptoms: seizures, mental retardation, and adenoma sebaceum (Crino et al. 2006). Genetic mutations on *TSC1* and *TSC2* are responsible for TSC, and mutation on only one gene is needed for expression of the disorder (Tsai and Sahin 2011). *TSC1*, located on chromosome 9q34, produces the TSC1 protein hamartin; *TSC2*, located on chromosome 16p33.3, produces the TSC2 protein tuberin. Together these proteins regulate the mTORC1 protein complex, forming a key cellular pathway for protein synthesis and cell size regulation (Tsai and Sahin 2011). Rheb, a small GTPase, is inhibited by the combined action of *TSC1* and *TSC2*, thus inhibiting protein synthesis.

Inactivation of either *TSC1* or *TSC2* leads to Rheb and mTORC1 overactivation and a subsequent increase in protein translation.

There is no cure for TSC. However, vigabatrin is approved for use in infantile spasms, and in 2010 the U.S. Food and Drug Administration approved the use of everolimus for the treatment of subependymal giant cell astrocytomas in patients who are not candidates for surgical removal. Parent training and education, behavior modification, and psychotropic medications may be helpful with behavior problems, and children with special needs may benefit from occupational therapy and special education services.

The prognosis of TSC depends on the severity of symptoms and is therefore highly variable. Patients with mild symptoms usually have a normal life expectancy. However, all TSC patients are at risk for life-threatening conditions related to the brain tumors, kidney lesions, or lung lesions, including lymphangioleiomyomatosis, a tumor-like disorder leading to lung destruction. Therefore, lifelong monitoring by physicians experienced with TSC is recommended.

Key Clinical Points

- Tuberous sclerosis complex is a rare multisystem genetic disorder that may present to a psychiatrist first, with symptoms of autism, cognitive-intellectual delays, learning disorders, or attention-deficit/hyperactivity disorder.
- The marked symptom variability and absence of visible dermatological or prominent neurological signs may lead to underrecognition of TSC.
- The diagnosis of TSC is based on clinical criteria and can be confirmed with computed tomography or magnetic resonance imaging and the finding of genetic mutations on *TSC1* and *TSC2*.
- Psychiatric treatment of TSC is symptomatic and may include psychotherapy, psychotropic medications, and school services, including special education and speech and language therapy.
- The prognosis of TSC is symptom dependent and highly variable, and lifelong monitoring of patients is recommended.

Further Readings

Roach ES, Gomez MR, Northrup H: Tuberous sclerosis complex consensus conference: revised clinical diagnostic criteria. J Child Neurol 13:624–628, 1998

Yohay KH, Denckla MB: Neurofibromatosis type 1 and tuberous sclerosis complex, in Child and Adolescent Neurology for Psychiatrists, 2nd Edition. Edited by Walker AM, Kaufman DM, Pfeffer CR, et al. Philadelphia, PA, Lippincott Williams & Wilkins, 2008, pp 212–221

References

Au KS, Williams AT, Roach ES, et al: Genotype/phenotype correlation in 325 individuals referred for a diagnosis of tuberous sclerosis complex in the United States. Genet Med 9:88–100, 2007

Boer K, Jansen F, Nellis M, et al: Inflammatory processes in cortical tubers and subependymal giant cell tumors of tuberous sclerosis complex. Epilepsy Res 78:7–21, 2008

Bolton PF: Neuroepileptic correlates of autistic symptomatology in tuberous sclerosis. Ment Retard Dev Disabil Res Rev 10:126–131, 2004

Crino PB: The pathophysiology of tuberous sclerosis complex. Epilepsia 51:27–29, 2010

Crino PB, Nathanson KL, Henske EP: The tuberous sclerosis complex. N Engl J Med 355:1345–1356, 2006

D'Agati E, Moavero R, Cerminara C, et al: Attention-deficit hyperactivity disorder (ADHD) and tuberous sclerosis complex. J Child Neurol 24:1282–1287, 2009

Jansen FE, Vincken KL, Algra A, et al: Cognitive impairment in tuberous sclerosis complex is a multifactorial condition. Neurology 70:916–923, 2008

Ridler K, Bullmore ET, De Vries PJ, et al: Widespread anatomical abnormalities of grey and white matter structure in tuberous sclerosis. Psychol Med 31:1437–1446, 2001

Tsai P, Sahin M: Mechanism of neurocognitive dysfunction and therapeutic considerations in tuberous sclerosis complex. Curr Opin Neurol 24:103–113, 2011

Wolraich ML, Lambert W, Doffing MA, et al: Psychometric properties of the Vanderbilt ADHD parent diagnostic rating scale in a referred population. J Pediatr Psychol 28:559–567, 2003

Yohay KH, Denckla MB: Neurofibromatosis type 1 and tuberous sclerosis complex, in Child and Adolescent Neurology for Psychiatrists, 2nd Edition. Edited by Walker AM, Kaufman DM, Pfeffer CR, et al. Philadelphia, PA, Lippincott, Williams & Wilkins, 2008, pp 212–221

FOCAL NEUROBEHAVIORAL SYNDROMES

Focal Neurobehavioral Syndromes

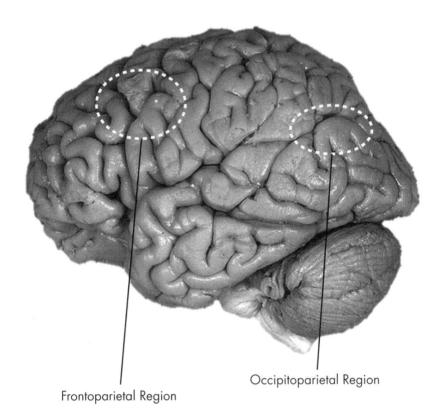

Frontoparietal Region

Occipitoparietal Region

INTRODUCTION

Focal neurobehavioral syndromes provide insight into the sequential and hierarchical organization of brain functions. Higher-order functions depend on intact lower-order functioning. Each higher-order function arises by mobilizing a distributed neural network but with a focal epicenter. This organization allows localization of injury in function-compromised individuals. Such capacities are innate and precede experience. Attention and space are examples of these inborn higher-order computational abilities.

Balint Syndrome

Trevor A. Hurwitz, M.B.Ch.B., M.R.C.P. (U.K.), F.R.C.P.C.

A 52-year-old man was visiting Asia on business when he experienced a sudden onset of vertigo, inverted vision, headaches, and palpitations. Most of his symptoms resolved over 2 days, but he had persistent and worsening visual symptoms. He found that he was only able to look at one object at a time. He was admitted to a local hospital, where he was investigated with magnetic resonance imaging (MRI) and lumbar puncture. His MRI scan showed new strokes. The lumbar puncture revealed normal findings. He was advised to return home, which he did the next day; upon arrival at the airport he went directly to the hospital.

His chief complaint at this time was persistent bilateral "blurry" vision. He did not, however, feel that his visual difficulties were a major problem. He had other symptoms, which included generalized throbbing headache, unsteady gait, vertigo with movement, and left-sided tinnitus. He reported intact dexterity, strength, sensation, and sphincter function. He had never had a seizure. His previous medical history was significant for a cholecystectomy, hypertension with known left ventricular hypertrophy, and stable pulmonary sarcoidosis, which was being managed by observation. He did not smoke, drink, or use any street drugs. He was taking aspirin, amlodipine, and ramipril. He worked as a cook and in construction but was negotiating a new business venture, hence his trip to Asia.

On examination his blood pressure was 171/104 mm Hg and pulse was 74 beats/minute, sinus rhythm. The findings of his general examination were normal. On neurological examination he was alert and oriented to person, place, and date. Verbal output was fluent, with intact comprehension, repetition, and naming. Writing and reading were poor because of his visuomotor difficulties. His visual fields were full on confrontation, and he was able to count fingers in all four quadrants of each field. Subsequent more careful assessment of vision confirmed a normal visual acuity (20/20 bilaterally). He was very slow because of difficulty finding the letters on the Snellen chart. Goldmann perimetry confirmed full visual fields. Despite these preserved visual abilities, he was not able to reach and locate objects under visual guidance (optic ataxia), nor could he voluntarily look at and find or track a moving finger with his eyes (ocular apraxia). He was still able to guide himself to his room door without bumping into objects.

He could not perceive his visual field as a whole. Thus, when looking at compound letters (large global letters made up of small local letters), he was able to identify the small Bs but not a larger A made up of the smaller Bs (Figure 11–1). Using the Cookie Theft picture from the Boston Diagnostic Aphasia Examination, he was only able to see some elements of this scene. These elements were experienced as isolated images with no object-object or object-action integration. When looking at the woman in the Cookie Theft picture who was holding and washing a plate, he could see a woman and "somebody holding a plate" but did not identify the two images as one and the same.

The findings from the rest of his cranial nerve examination were normal, including intact and full extraocular movements. Examination of his motor system revealed a right-arm drift but with normal power; bulk and tone were normal. Sensory examination and coordination were normal.

His MRI scan showed infarcts in the bilateral occipitoparietal regions but also smaller hypertension-linked old lacunar infarcts in the right caudate, right lentiform nucleus, and right corona radiata (Figures 11–2, 11–3, and 11–4). The MRI scan also demonstrated a small chronic left cerebellar infarct. The occipitoparietal infarcts demonstrated gyral enhancement but no restricted diffusion. This pattern indicated a subacute timeline of 1 week or longer. His intracranial circulation was abnormal on computed tomography angiogram. He had very small vertebral arteries and a very small and slightly irregular basilar artery. The pattern of anatomy suggested that most of the arterial supply of his brain was coming from his anterior circulation. His cardiac workup demonstrated a normal transthoracic echo. His cardiac Holter monitor findings were normal other than a shortened PR interval. The cause of his strokes was not identified. He was discharged to undergo rehabilitation and further cardiac investigations. A transesophageal echocardiogram showed moderate shunting from right to left across a patent foramen ovale (PFO).

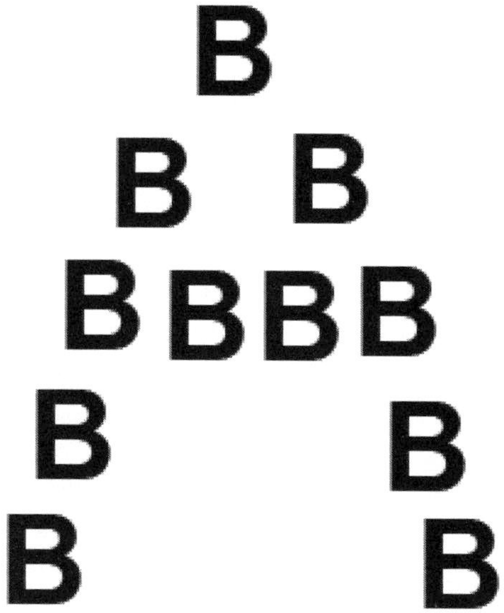

FIGURE 11–1. Compound letter (large global *A* made up of smaller *B*s).

He was seen 3 months after his initial strokes. He was left with a disabling neurobehavioral syndrome linked to his occipitoparietal infarcts, of which he was only minimally aware. From his perspective his chief ongoing problem was a problem with his sight, which he continued to describe as "blurry vision." His blurry vision had kept him confined at home.

On direct inquiry he acknowledged a problem with memory but was not aware of any difficulties in his other cognitive-intellectual capacities. He had occasional mild left-temple headaches. In all other respects he had no neurological complaints.

The full magnitude of his difficulties was clarified by his wife. She was not able to leave him unattended because he was overwhelmed by visual complexity. Within their small home he could find his way to various rooms, but he would not be able to find his way back home if he left the house. When the refrigerator was full he was not able to locate milk or orange juice even though he could see that the containers were in the refrigerator. Similarly, he could not locate a pair of socks among a collection of his socks. He struggled to open the refrigerator because it did not have an identifiable handle. When in a store he was often unable to locate a particular item on the shelves in front of him. He still was able to pick out his own clothes and dress himself.

On elementary neurological examination he was alert and fully oriented. Visual fields were full to confrontation. Optic disks were flat. Visual acu-

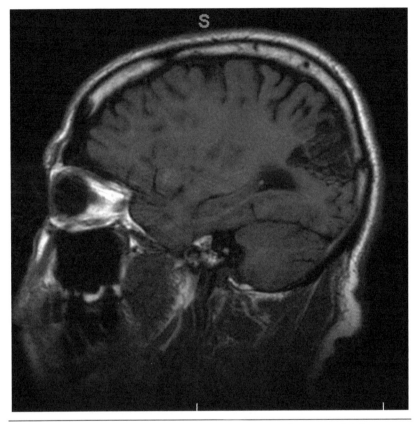

FIGURE 11–2. Magnetic resonance image: right sagittal T1 image, demonstrating occipitoparietal infarct.

ity was 20/20 without aids. Extraocular movements were full. He was now able to reach and locate objects under visual guidance and could voluntarily locate and track a moving finger with his eyes. The remainder of the cranial nerve examination was unremarkable.

Examination of the motor system revealed no drift. Fine motor movements and rapid alternating movements were normal bilaterally. Power, bulk, and tone were normal.

Reflexes were grade 2+ bilaterally, with bilaterally downgoing toes. Sensory examination, coordination, station, and gait were normal. The Romberg sign was absent.

On mental status and neurobehavioral examination his attention was impaired, with a digit span of 5 forward and 3 backward. Recent verbal memory was impaired. He recalled 1/3 words following distraction, increasing to

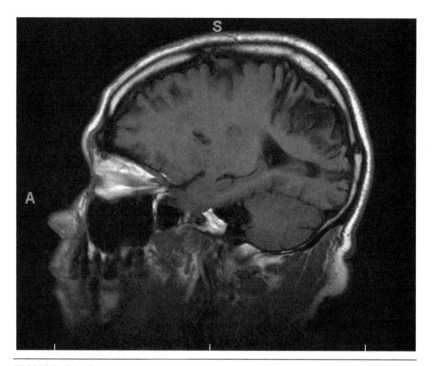

FIGURE 11–3.　Magnetic resonance image: left sagittal T1 image demonstrating occipitoparietal infarct.

2/3 with forced choice. He could not perform the three-shapes part of the Three Words–Three Shapes memory test because he was unable to copy the three figures. He was able to double numbers up to 32. Semantic memory was impaired. On the animal fluency test he was only able to name 8 animals in 1 minute (below the cutoff score of 15). He had no left-right disorientation and no finger agnosia. His verbal output was fluent, with intact comprehension and naming. Unlike in the first week after his initial stroke, he was able to read simple sentences but was slow. He still had severe agraphia. He was able to correctly identify the shape of the three-dimensional cross, calling it a plus sign, but he could not copy it as a result of his difficulty processing spatial objects. He could not copy the intersecting pentagons.

He remained unable to perceive his visual field as a whole. In a compound figure he was able to identify small *A*s but not a larger *B* made up of the smaller *A*s. He was able to correctly identify the shape of a clock, the short and long hands, and the numbers 12, 3, 6, and 9. Despite this intact capacity he could not correctly identify the time represented by three separate clocks (Figure 11–5).

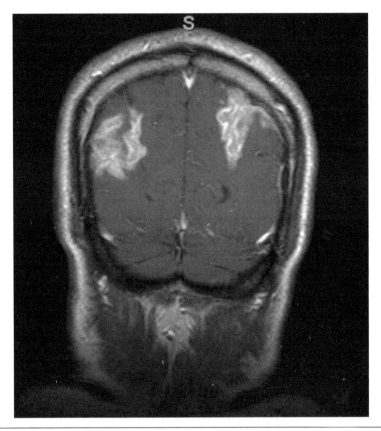

FIGURE 11–4. Magnetic resonance image: coronal T2 image demonstrating bilateral occipitoparietal infarcts.

All these difficulties could be attributed to simultanagnosia, the inability to capture, integrate, and bind the constituent elements of his perceptual scenes into meaningful wholes. On deeper analysis the failure of meaningful vision appeared to be due to a loss of a spatial reference grid onto which elements of his perceptual scene could be first mapped and then made available as a coherent object in external space. The problem went beyond visual information and involved his access to and grasp of three-dimensional space itself. The loss of this spatial map was demonstrated using a 2×1 grid labeled with the numbers 1 and 2, the letter *A*, and two different shapes. He was able to correctly name all individual components, but he could not identify which shape lay in the 1A or 1B position (Figure 11–6). He found more complex grids overwhelming. He was able to correctly name the shape and color of printed objects, but he

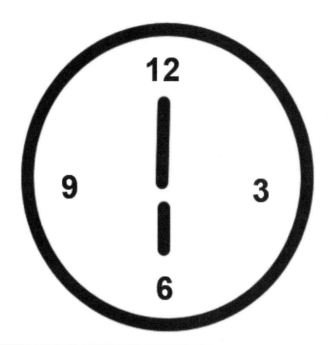

FIGURE 11–5. Clock example. The patient was unable to correctly identify the time indicated on the clock.

was unable to identify correctly the stacked order of these objects when superimposed on each other (Figure 11–7). He could identify arrows pointing left and right but not up or down. These spatial difficulties were all based on an external, object-centered reference frame.

To confirm that his difficulties also lay in the loss of an internal representation of a three-dimensional spatial map (topographic memory), he was asked to use himself as the center of spatial orientation (an egocentric reference frame). With respect to himself when told that he should imagine that he was facing north, he could not reliably identify the locations of the other three cardinal directions. When asked to imagine that he was a clock with his arms representing the hands of the clock, he could not reliably indicate positions of the hands for given times such as 6:00 or 9:15 (Figure 11–8).

One month later, he developed light-headedness followed by slurred speech, word-finding difficulties, and right-arm weakness 30 minutes after completing pulmonary function testing. On examination he had mild dysphasia with a mild right-arm drift, mild weakness in the finger abductors and extensors of the right hand, and mild weakness of the right-hip flexors.

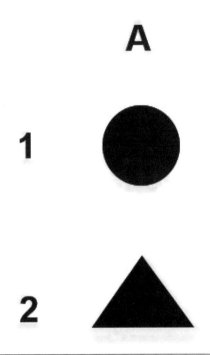

FIGURE 11–6.   Object-centered reference frame: 2×1 grid.

Computed tomography confirmed a new subcortical left middle cerebral artery (MCA) territory stroke. This stroke and possibly also his prior strokes were felt to have arisen from paradoxical emboli passing through his known PFO. The Valsalva maneuver, as part of pulmonary function testing, temporarily increases right atrial pressure, increasing the right-to-left shunt and the risk of paradoxical embolization. He underwent a leg ultrasound, which failed to identify any deep vein thrombosis as a source of emboli. There was also no evidence of a pulmonary arteriovenous fistula. His PFO was surgically closed, clopidogrel was added to aspirin in his medication regimen, and his hypertension management was optimized.

Discussion

Balint syndrome is named after the Hungarian physician Rezsö Bálint and consists of the triad of optic ataxia (an impairment of target pointing using visual guidance), ocular apraxia (the inability to voluntarily direct gaze to a particular location in space), and simultanagnosia (the inability to perceive the visual field as a whole; part recognition is retained but the

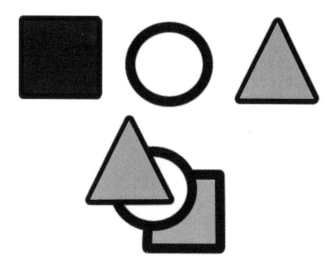

FIGURE 11–7. Object-centered reference frame: stacked objects.

FIGURE 11–8. Ego-centered reference frame: arms used to represent the times 3:45 or 9:15.

ability to integrate, bind, and unify the constituent elements of a perceptual scene into meaningful entities is impaired) (Rafal 1997). When severe the patient behaves like a blind person, does not blink to visual threat, and may bump into objects. The patient often locks onto a visual object and is not able to see anything else. Objects may vanish from or pop into view as fixation shifts. Given the location of the bilateral lesions and the causative pathologies, Balint syndrome is often not found in pure form and may occur together with visual field deficits, agnosia, prosopagnosia, alexia, and other cognitive-intellectual difficulties. Indeed, this patient had problems with calculation, reading, and writing, suggesting a partial Gerstmann syndrome (dyscalculia, alexia, agraphia, left-right disorientation, and finger agnosia).

Balint syndrome is due to occipitoparietal injury. Bilateral lesions are present and are most often due to watershed infarction between the middle and posterior cerebral artery territories secondary to global cerebral hypoperfusion. Other causes include bilateral penetrating missile injuries, strokes, butterfly glioma, multiple metastases, and degenerative disorders such as Alzheimer's disease.

Balint syndrome is not due to constriction of the visual fields, which are usually normal, nor to spatial neglect. Patients can detect movement and have intact depth perception and color vision. At a superficial level the patient appears to be able to see only a small fraction of the visual scene—seemingly a constriction of visual attention to a single object (Rafal 1997). However, the fundamental problem appears to be caused by the disruption of the three-dimensional spatial reference grid (an inadequate spatial representation) to which visual attention can be applied (Friedman-Hill et al. 1995). Spatial disorientation is thus the cardinal and common underlying feature of this syndrome; it accounts for compromise in both object- and ego-centered spatial frames of reference and unifies simultanagnosia, ocular apraxia, and the optic ataxia by a common mechanism:

- Simultanagnosia is caused by the inability to map elements of a visual scene onto a compromised spatial grid to allow the correct binding of these visual elements into recognizable coherent entities.
- Ocular apraxia and optic ataxia are caused by an inability to accurately direct eyes and hands, respectively, because of a damaged three-dimensional spatial reference grid that maps the coordinates of external space.

Loss of this central template for the representation of space also accounts for the failure of ego-centered spatial frames of reference, as reflected in the failure of topographic memory.

Balint's neurobehavioral syndrome provides a striking window into the construction of the mind. The lived world is experienced as objects and actions that take place in space, unfold in time, and obey causal laws. Incoming data received through the senses must be actively processed by neural templates into meaningful cognitive experiences. These templates are innate and precede experience. Space is one such preset format that specifies how incoming sensory information is encoded as a location in a three-dimensional grid, thus allowing the binding and integration of the constituent elements into meaningful wholes to capture the emergent properties that relate to the distribution of spread-out but interacting data points. Recent animal models support this Kantian view that spatial representation includes an innate component prior to experience (Palmer and Lynch 2010). Balint syndrome is the living human model of spatial disorientation caused by disruption of the three-dimensional spatial reference grid. Without this template located in the occipitoparietal regions, the individual, despite intact senses, is "lost in space."

Key Clinical Points

- Balint syndrome is the triad of simultanagnosia, optic ataxia, and optic apraxia.
- The syndrome is caused by bilateral injury to the occipitoparietal regions.
- Spatial disorientation is the cardinal feature of this syndrome and is caused by the disruption of the three-dimensional spatial reference grid to which visual attention can be applied.
- Despite intact senses, the patient is "lost in space."

Further Readings

Rizzo M, Vecera SP: Psychoanatomical substrates of Bálint's syndrome. J Neurol Neurosurg Psychiatry 72:162–178, 2002
Robertson LC: Binding, spatial attention and perceptual awareness. Nat Rev Neurosci 4:93–102, 2003

References

Friedman-Hill SR, Robertson LC, Treisman A: Parietal contributions to visual feature binding: evidence from a patient with bilateral lesions. Science 269:853–855, 1995
Moreaud O: Balint syndrome. Arch Neurol 60:1329–1331, 2003
Palmer L, Lynch G: Neuroscience: a Kantian view of space. Science 328:1487–1488, 2010
Rafal RD: Balint syndrome, in Behavioral Neurology and Neuropsychology. Edited by Feinberg TE, Farah MJ. New York, McGraw-Hill, 1997, pp 337–356

Left Hemispatial Neglect[1]

Robert Stowe, M.D., F.R.C.P.C.

A 63-year-old right-handed man was transferred to a neuropsychiatric unit for an assessment because of irritability, dysphoria, agitation, and aggression.

One year earlier, he had developed acute left-sided numbness and confusion while driving and had driven his car into a stranger's front yard. The police who attended the scene found him to be confused, and he was hospitalized. He was diagnosed with a stroke but recovered within a week and returned to his job upholstering furniture.

Two months later, he became unresponsive while watching television. He recalled his wife slapping him in the face, trying to arouse him. Although his entire left side was numb, he failed to recognize that anything was seriously wrong at the time. He was again hospitalized for about a week for a presumed ischemic event and recovered rapidly.

About a month thereafter, another stroke ensued when he suddenly became confused and complained of feeling "as though someone had knocked me out." This time, left-sided numbness was accompanied by left upper-extremity weakness and persisting urinary incontinence. He had retained awareness of the urge to void but lacked voluntary control. He was hospitalized and heparinized, but his condition progressed to a dense left hemiparesis. Carotid Doppler studies showed total occlusion of the left carotid artery with good collateral flow. He was started on ticlopidine and underwent 2 months of inpatient rehabilitation.

Following the third stroke, his wife left him, and he was discharged to a nursing facility. After brief rehospitalization and transfer to a different facility, and a visit from a former female lover, he became depressed. Two weeks prior to neuropsychiatric admission, he became paranoid and delusional, and he swore at and pushed other residents with his wheelchair. Haloperidol was

[1]The author wishes to acknowledge the contribution of Dr. Joseph Pierri, who examined the patient with the author, to the data collection used to write the case history. Neuropsychological testing was performed by Carol Schramke, Ph.D.

instituted, without improvement; it was discontinued, and sertraline was started. Other medications on admission included digoxin, oxybutynin, aspirin, isosorbide dinitrate, and lactulose as needed for constipation.

When he was assessed several weeks thereafter, dysphoria and irritability had markedly improved, and there were no further aggressive incidents.

There was no history suggestive of a seizure disorder. Past medical history included long-standing hypertension and non-insulin-dependent diabetes mellitus; and coronary artery disease with two remote myocardial infarctions, triple-vessel coronary artery bypass grafts, and stable angina relieved by nitroglycerin. Holter monitoring showed supraventricular tachyarrhythmias. A thallium stress test showed an ejection fraction of 55% and anterior wall akinesia. Transurethral prostatic resection for benign prostatic hypertrophy had been performed 6 months, and cervical fusion 8 years, prior to presentation. Chronic mild hearing loss was attributed to noise exposure.

One year prior to presentation he quit smoking cigarettes; before that time he had smoked a pack a day for 20 years. There was no other history of substance abuse.

Family history included death of his father at age 55 of a myocardial infarction and unexplained sudden death of a brother at age 35. Another brother had insulin-dependent diabetes. His mother died of tuberculosis at age 52.

He had obtained a GED and worked as a tool and die maker for 35 years. He moved to a different state 6 years prior to presentation to marry for the third time, starting his own reupholstering business with his new wife. He loved to fish, boat, and hunt.

Mental status examination revealed him to be alert and spatially oriented, but disoriented to date, month, and year. There was persistent rightward head and eye deviation. Hygiene and grooming were adequate. He was mildly abulic in conversation, but he put forth good effort on neurocognitive testing. Mood was described as "normal, with occasional bitterness and sadness," attributed to the breakup of his marriage. His Geriatric Depression Scale score was 13/30 (mild depression). Baseline affect appeared euthymic, but range was reduced because of aprosodia. Thought processes were generally logical, coherent, and goal directed. Egocentricity and deficits in temporal ordering of events were, however, evident during history taking. Thought content was unremarkable. Perceptual abnormalities and suicidal and homicidal ideations were denied. Insight into behavioral and personality changes and hemispatial neglect was poor, and judgment was impaired based on history.

Neurocognitive examination revealed a digit span of 4 forward and 4 backward and a pointing span of 5 forward and 4 backward. A random letter cancellation test took almost 5 minutes and demonstrated severe left neglect (Figure 11–9). There was minimal improvement on a structured version. Spontaneous speech was fluent and grammatical, without paraphasias or word-finding difficulty. He had mild aprosodia and dysarthria. Performance was normal on screening tests of naming, comprehension, repetition, and reading. Fluency was unimpaired (12/15/12 words on the Controlled Oral Word Association Test ["FAS test"—name as many words in 1 minute for each of the letters F, A, and S], and 15 on animal naming). Writing was extremely micrographic and was initiated in the middle of the page. Left-right orientation was intact. Buccofacial praxis was normal. He demonstrated extensional errors on limb praxis testing. He could not make change from $10 accurately, but he could perform two-digit subtractions with pencil and paper. Comprehension and expression of affective prosody were extremely impaired; repetition was slightly less so. He omitted the number 12 on clock drawing, and there was failure to close the external configuration of drawings (see Figure 11–10). There was a depressed learning curve and poor uncued retrieval on a 10-item story, improving after cues. On the Three Words–Three Shapes memory test, copying was very disorganized and showed mild left neglect. On incidental recall, he produced one shape but no words. After five study periods, this improved to two words and parts of three shapes, decreasing to one word and parts of two shapes after 5, 15, and 30 minutes. He recognized two words and three shapes, endorsing a synonym for the missing word. Recall of recent news items was somewhat better. Interpretation of similarities was abstract, but he was concrete on unfamiliar proverbs. Graphomotor sequences were very impaired (Figure 11–11).

General neurological examination revealed intact visual acuity, pupillary responses, and extraocular movements. Visual fields showed extinction on the left to double simultaneous stimulation. There was left upper motor neuron facial weakness. Hearing was decreased to finger rubbing bilaterally. He had intermittent left-sided auditory extinction to double simultaneous finger snaps. Pharyngeal reflexes were intact, but the uvula deviated to the right. Speech was dysarthric, and there was weakness of tongue protrusion to the left. A dense flaccid left upper- and lower-extremity paresis was unimproved by positioning left-sided extremities in right hemispace. He had left hyperreflexia and a left extensor plantar response. Light touch sensation appeared absent on the left, with subjectively decreased but grossly intact pinprick perception. Vibration sense was decreased in the left upper extremities and absent in the lower extremities; proprioception was absent in both. Cerebellar testing was normal on the right. He was mobile only by wheelchair.

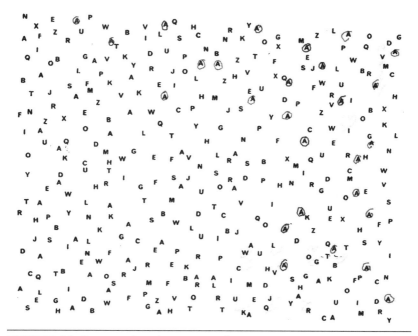

FIGURE 11–9.   Random letter cancellation test showing rightward exploratory bias.

He was asked to circle all the *A*s while keeping the page squarely in front of him. Targets are symmetrically arranged in quadrants (15 targets in each), but this is not apparent to subjects because distractor letters are randomly distributed. He used a typical left-to-right, top-down scanning strategy, detecting 22/30 targets on the right but only 5/30 on the left. Note the progressive rightward shift of target detection, with detection of only the rightmost targets by the end.

Investigations revealed markedly elevated blood sugars in the 300–400 mg/dL (16–22 mmol/L) range, and mildly elevated triglycerides.

The results of imaging studies were not available at the time of assessment. Localization strongly suggested a large right MCA infarction (see "Discussion" section).

On neuropsychological testing (age-scaled Wechsler Adult Intelligence Scale—Revised) he obtained normal scores on Information, Comprehension, and Similarities, but Picture Completion was 7, Digit Span 6, and Block Design 2. He correctly named 55/60 line drawings from the Boston Naming Test, plus 2 more after phonemic cues. Hemispatial neglect was again evident in drawings of a flower, a house, and a clock. The California Verbal Learning Test demonstrated significant trial-to-trial variability and a relatively flat learning curve, with very impaired uncued retrieval but mildly impaired cued retrieval (12/12 hits, but 2 false positives). Wechsler

A

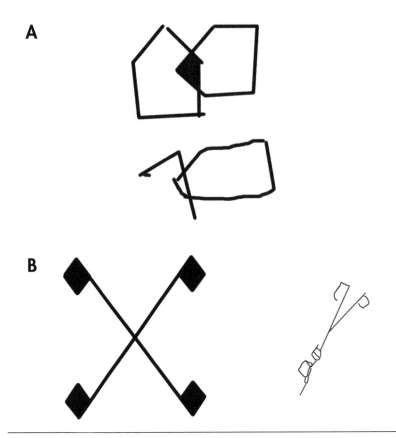

B

FIGURE 11–10.   Left neglect and constructional dyspraxia.
(A) His copying (bottom) of intersecting pentagons demonstrates left neglect and failure to close the external configuration of the leftmost pentagon. (B) His copying (right) of the Wechsler Memory Scale design demonstrates distortion and micrographia.

Memory Scale scores were at the 34th and 11th percentiles on Logical Memory I (immediate) and II (delayed) recall, respectively, with much better recognition memory (7/9 on both subtests), contrasting with the 1st percentile on both Visual Reproduction I and II, with only 20% accuracy on recognition. On the Wisconsin Card Sorting Test, he achieved no sorts, perseverative responding/errors were high, and there was one loss of set.

Oxybutynin was discontinued because anticholinergic side effects could have been worsening his neurocognitive capacities. His behavior stabilized and his depression remitted on sertraline, and he was discharged soon thereafter to the same nursing facility. Six months later he was admitted to a general psychiatric unit after making sexual advances

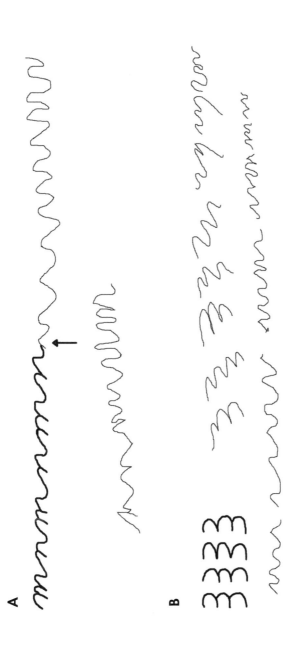

FIGURE 11–11. Impaired reproduction of graphomotor sequences (A) and Luria loops (B). (A) He was asked to "copy and continue" alternating *m*s and *n*s. Note the initial "frontal pull" to the stimulus—that is, his attempt to continue it (at arrow) rather than copying it below as instructed, and the disintegration of the sequence in his subsequent attempt. (B) When asked to "make a whole row of these designs, with the same number of loops" shown in the stimulus designs, he perseverated with attempts to produce *m*s and *n*s and then distorted and rotated the loops, likely reflecting perseverative carryover from the graphomotor sequence.

to an older female patient with dementia. Two months thereafter he had an acute myocardial infarction and died in the intensive care unit the same day.

Discussion

The history suggested at least three episodes of right hemisphere ischemia, the last resulting in a profound left hemiparesis, hemispatial neglect, dysarthria, and incontinence. (The second episode might have involved a complex partial seizure, given a period of apparent unresponsiveness; however, if this was the case it was likely secondary to an ischemic event, given his subsequent course.) Sudden onset in an MCA distribution suggested an embolic source, given a history of paroxysmal supraventricular tachyarrhythmias and left ventricular anterior wall hypokinesis. The absence of spasticity, and maximal deficit in the arm relative to the face and leg, argued for a cortical, rather than a capsular, hemiparesis. Loss of light touch and impaired vibration with diminished but present pain perception suggested suprathalamic involvement, implicating somatosensory cortex or thalamocortical radiations.

Neurocognitive examination was notable for constructional dyspraxia and hemispatial neglect, consistent with a large right MCA territory infarction. Involvement of all aspects of prosody (comprehension, repetition, and expression) implicated both frontal and parietal lobes and their interhemispheric white matter connections (Ross and Monnot 2008). Additional evidence of potential prefrontal cortical involvement in this case came in the form of impaired graphomotor sequences, impaired temporal orientation and temporal ordering of autobiographical events, impaired uncued retrieval of visual information, and poor set maintenance and shifting, abstract reasoning, and judgment (Royall et al. 2002). Impairment of verbal encoding and retrieval (given relative preservation of recognition memory) suggested the possibility of additional frontal-subcortical pathology in the left hemisphere, such as vascular leukoencephalopathy and/or basal ganglia lacunae, a superimposed "dementia syndrome of depression," and anticholinergic toxicity. The latter two possibilities were supported by neurocognitive and affective improvement after institution of sertraline and discontinuation of oxybutynin. Preservation of verbal fluency and upgaze argued against the development of hydrocephalus. Micrographia was likely attributable to recent treatment with haloperidol, in the absence of resting tremor and other features of Parkinson's disease or dementia with Lewy bodies.

Hemispatial neglect is a complex syndrome characterized by the failure to orient to, respond to, or explore the contralesional hemispace (Adair and

Barrett 2008). Motor neglect may be so severe that it is mistaken for hemiparesis; however, effort may improve if the neglected limbs are positioned in the nonneglected hemispace. The perceived locus of sensory stimuli on the neglected side may be displaced to the nonneglected side (allesthesia).

In some cases there is also "personal" neglect of the contralesional side of the body (e.g., failing to shave the left side of the face). Typically there is lack of awareness of deficits (*anosognosia*) in various forms, including the failure to recognize contralesional plegic limbs as paralyzed, or even failure to recognize paralyzed limbs as one's own (*hemiasomatognosia*). Anosognosia for neglect may be quite persistent, even after patients become aware of other deficits (Carota et al. 2002). Patients may acknowledge their paralysis but appear indifferent to it, a phenomenon termed *anosodiaphoria*.

While deficits in cancellation tasks and line bisection, extinction, and constructional dyspraxia are seen more commonly with parietal than frontal involvement, there is substantial overlap in the phenomenology of neglect created by damage to the right frontal eye fields (FEFs), posterior parietal cortex, and cingulate gyrus, the areas most commonly implicated in neglect (Leibovitch et al. 1998). Damage to right temporal neocortex, thalamus, striatum, and especially white matter bundles connecting the occipitoparietal junction region with frontal areas can also produce elements of the neglect syndrome. This anatomical heterogeneity led to the first distributed neuroanatomical network models of neurocognitive capacities (Mesulam 1981; Watson et al. 1981), so elegantly validated by today's functional imaging experiments.

In nonhuman primates and other mammals, neglect occurs contralateral to the damaged hemisphere, regardless of laterality. However, the vast majority of human cases are left-sided. In simple terms, while the left hemisphere orients to and attributes motivational salience to events primarily in right hemispace, development of language in the left hemisphere forced the development of bilateral attentional/exploratory capacities in the right hemisphere of humans. Thus when the left hemisphere is damaged, the expected neglect in right hemispace does not occur, because it is masked by the *ipsilateral* attentive capacity of the right hemisphere, but when the right is damaged instead, contralateral neglect emerges (Mesulam 2000).

The neglect syndrome observed in this patient included several components. *Representational neglect* was manifested by multimodal left-sided extinction to double simultaneous stimulation in the face of preserved perception of unilateral stimuli, and by omission of left-sided elements in drawings (Figure 11–10A). These findings likely represent involvement of the posterior parietal cortex, a critical gateway integrating cross-modal and sensorimotor spatially relevant information streams with frontally predominant motor output channels related to orienting, reaching, grasping, and exploration of the environment (Mesulam 2000). Extinction reflects the role of these areas in *disengaging* attentional focus from the current location, to permit a spatial shift of attention to a new target (Lundervold et al. 2002).

Motor-exploratory neglect was evident in ipsilesional motor bias (head and eye deviation to the right) and on cancellation tests (Figure 11–9). The head and eye deviation to the right implicates the right FEF and/or its connections; the FEF in each hemisphere, which moves the head and eyes contralaterally, being tonically active. Damage to one side results in ipsilesional deviation, because the contralateral FEF is unopposed.

Finally, *anosognosia* was evidenced by his vague and nonlocalizing description ("I felt as though someone had knocked me out") at the time of his final catastrophic stroke, and by persisting relative lack of awareness of left-sided deficits, while *anosodiaphoria* was reflected in the absence of appropriate concern during his previous strokes. His characterization of his recent mood as "normal, with occasional bitterness and sadness" in the face of a psychotic-depressive illness suggests a relative *anosognosia for mood* (or perhaps alexithymia) that contributes to underdiagnosis of poststroke depression in patients following right hemisphere damage (Schramke et al. 1998). Psychotic depression, manifested by dysphoria, delusions, irritability, and aggressive outbursts, developed about 8 months after his major stroke, within the 1-year time window containing most poststroke depressions. This event was overdetermined, with both biological and psychosocial factors (e.g., his wife's decision to file for divorce, and a recent visit from a former girlfriend) being plausible triggers. These symptoms were refractory to haloperidol (albeit a brief trial) but responded rapidly to low-dose sertraline.

Key Clinical Points

- Examination of a patient with a possible right hemisphere lesion should include evaluation of prosody, the spatial distribution of attention (e.g., testing for extinction, cancellation tests, line bisection, reading), visuoperceptual and visuoconstructive functions, and visual memory.

- Diagnosis of depression after right hemisphere stroke can be complicated by aprosodia, anosodiaphoria, and alexithymia.

- Depression following right hemisphere damage may present primarily with irritability, aggression, and delusions.

- Hemispatial neglect is a multifaceted syndrome characterized most prominently by the failure to orient to, respond to, or explore the contralesional hemispace.

- Hemispatial neglect in humans is most often left-sided and results most often from right frontoparietal damage. It is often accompanied by anosognosia and anosodiaphoria.

Further Readings

Adair JC, Barrett AM: Spatial neglect—clinical and neuroscience review: a wealth of information on the poverty of spatial attention. Ann N Y Acad Sci 1142:21–43, 2008

Barrett AM, Buxbaum LJ, Coslett HB, et al: Cognitive rehabilitation interventions for neglect and related disorders: moving from bench to bedside in stroke patients. J Cogn Neurosci 18:1223–1236, 2006

Mesulam M-M: Attentional networks, confusional states, and neglect syndromes, in Principles of Behavioral and Cognitive Neurology, 2nd Edition. Edited by Mesulam M-M. New York, Oxford University Press, 2000, pp 174–256

References

Adair JC, Barrett AM: Spatial neglect—clinical and neuroscience review: a wealth of information on the poverty of spatial attention. Ann N Y Acad Sci 1142:21–43, 2008

Carota A, Staub F, Bogousslavsky J: Emotions, behaviours and mood changes in stroke. Curr Opin Neurol 15:57–69, 2002

Leibovitch FS, Black SE, Caldwell CB, et al: Brain-behavior correlations in hemispatial neglect using CT and SPECT: the Sunnybrook Stroke Study. Neurology 50:901–908, 1998

Lundervold AJ, Lundervold A, Hugdahl K: A multivariate classification study of attentional orienting in patients with right hemisphere lesions. Neuropsychiatry Neuropsychol Behav Neurol 15:232–246, 2002

Mesulam M-M: A cortical network for directed attention and unilateral neglect. Ann Neurol 10:309–325, 1981

Mesulam M-M: Attentional networks, confusional states, and neglect syndromes, in Principles of Behavioral and Cognitive Neurology, 2nd Edition. Edited by Mesulam M-M. New York, Oxford University Press, 2000, pp 174–256

Ross ED, Monnot M: Neurology of affective prosody and its functional-anatomic organization in right hemisphere. Brain Lang 104:51–74, 2008

Royall DR, Lauterbach EC, Cummings JL, et al: Executive control function: a review of its promise and challenges for clinical research. J Neuropsychiatry Clin Neurosci 14:377–405, 2002

Schramke CJ, Stowe RM, Ratcliff G, et al: Poststroke depression and anxiety: different assessment methods result in variations in incidence and severity estimates. J Clin Exp Neuropsychol 20:723–737, 1998

Watson RT, Valenstein E, Heilman KM: Thalamic neglect: possible role of the medial thalamus and nucleus reticularis in behavior. Arch Neurol 38:501–506, 1981

Index

*Page numbers printed in **boldface** type refer to tables or figures.*